Nursing Delegation and Management of Patient Care

Nursing Delegation and Management of Patient Care

KATHLEEN MOTACKI, MSN, RN, BC
Clinical Associate Professor of Nursing
Saint Peter's College School of Nursing
Jersey City, New Jersey

KATHLEEN BURKE, PhD, RN
Assistant Dean in Charge of Nursing Programs
Professor of Nursing
Ramapo College of New Jersey
Mahwah, New Jersey

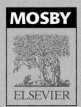

MOSBY
ELSEVIER

MOSBY
ELSEVIER

3251 Riverport Lane
St. Louis, Missouri 63043

Nursing Delegation and Management of Patient Care   ISBN: 978-0-323-05306-8

Notice

Neither the Publisher nor the Authors assume any responsibility for any loss or injury and/or damage to persons or property arising out of or related to any use of the material contained in this book. It is the responsibility of the treating practitioner, relying on independent expertise and knowledge of the patient, to determine the best treatment and method of application for the patient.

The Publisher

ISBN: 978-0-323-05306-8

Senior Editor: Yvonne Alexopoulos
Senior Developmental Editor: Danielle M. Frazier
Publishing Services Manager: Deborah L. Vogel
Project Manager: Pat Costigan
Design Direction: Kimberly Denando

Printed in Canada
Last digit is the print number: 9 8 7 6 5 4 3 2 1

*I dedicate this book to my loving family: my husband Robert, my son Robert,
my lovely daughter Lisa, my baby John, and to my in-laws, Edward and
Irene Motacki, Uncle Ted Tatarek, and brother-in-law Brian Motacki.
Thank you for your support in my nursing endeavors and philanthropy work.
Thank you and I love you.*
Kathleen Motacki

*For all of the marvelous nurses I have worked with over the years …
and to Elaine, Peggy, Jody, Kathleen, Cristina, Asha, and Ulysses at Ramapo.*
Kathleen Burke

About the Authors

Kathleen Motacki, MSN, RN, BC

Associate Clinical Professor at Saint Peter's College School of Nursing, Jersey City, New Jersey, has more than 33 years of experience in nursing, 7 years as a Professor of Nursing, and currently teaches traditional 4-year nursing courses at the Jesuit College of New Jersey. Her areas of clinical and classroom expertise include: pediatric nursing, nursing leadership and management, community health, Lifespan, and Prep for Success programs. She has taught pediatric NCLEX® review sessions. She is a referral liaison at Children's Specialized Hospital, New Brunswick, New Jersey. She holds board certification in pediatric nursing from the American Nurses Credentialing Center (ANCC). She was on the ANCC examination-standard-setting committee for the new pediatric credentialing examination. She was the lead investigator for the American Nurses Association School of Nursing Curriculum Study on Safe Patient Handling and Movement. She received the 2008 National Occupational Research Agenda (NORA) Partnering Award for the American Nurses Association Safe Patient Handling and Movement Training Program for her role in the Schools of Nursing research project. She is past president of the Epsilon Rho Chapter Sigma Theta Tau International Nursing Honor Society and is presently the Vice-President for Saint Peter's College for Mu Theta Chapter-At-Large, Sigma Theta Tau International Nursing Honor Society. Professor Motacki obtained her BSN and MSN in transcultural nursing administration from Kean University, Union, New Jersey. She has published several articles in nursing journals, her latest a continuing nursing education series for contact hours, "Safe Patient Handling in Pediatrics" in the *Journal of Pediatric Nursing*. She has published several books including *The Illustrated Guide to Safe Patient Handling and Movement*, Springer Publishing; *Silent Medical Errors,* Publish America; *Life is Ridiculous*, Dorrance Publishing; and *My Friends*, Dorrance Publishing. She has presented at conferences on Safe Patient Handling and Movement in New Jersey, Florida, Rhode Island, at The Sigma Theta Tau International Nursing Honor Society Biennium in Indianapolis, and the Annual Safe Patient Handling and Movement Conference. She was the keynote speaker at the Founders Day Dinner for the New Jersey Consortium of Chapters at Rutgers University. She is a nurse philanthropist and her volunteer efforts include: Our Lady of Fatima Rehabilitation Hospital in Liberia, Africa; Children's Specialized Hospital, New Brunswick, New Jersey; Children's Miracle Network; The International Wheelchair and Amputee Athletic Games; Lupus Foundation; Holy Spirit Church; Sigma Theta Tau International Nursing Honor Society; and American Cancer Society for Breast Cancer Research. Professor Motacki is married to a dialysis health care administrator and has three children: Robert, a Master's Prepared Special Education Teacher; Lisa, who is attending the school counseling Graduate Program at Caldwell College; and John, who attends New Jersey City University.

Kathleen Burke, RN, PhD

Professor of Nursing, and Assistant Dean in Charge of Nursing at Ramapo College of New Jersey, she has more than 36 years of experience in nursing and has served in a wide variety of positions over the years. As an educator, she has taught at the diploma, associate, baccalaureate, masters, and doctoral levels. She has been a Senior Vice President of a local community based hospital, and later served as an Assistant Dean at the University of Medicine and Dentistry of New Jersey (UMDNJ). Since 2007, she has led the Nursing Programs at Ramapo College of New Jersey. Her clinical and academic expertise includes nursing informatics, leadership, performance improvement and program evaluation. She also serves as a nurse research consultant to two local Magnet Hospitals. As a consultant to the Centers of Excellence program of the National League for Nursing (NLN), she works with nursing programs to further develop their innovative programs. Dr. Burke also assisted with the development of the Certified Nurse Educator exam of the NLN. She also serves as a Senior Examiner to the Malcolm Baldrige National Quality Program as well as being a site examiner for the National League for Nursing Accrediting Commission. In her role as the leader of the Nursing Programs at Ramapo, she has been instrumental in working with the faculty to develop both local and international partnerships of benefit to the student population. Local partnerships include the partnering with local magnet hospitals to combine both academic and clinical expertise, resulting in positive outcomes for both the clinical and academic partners. On an international level, she has worked with faculty to develop a partnership with the University of Sierra Leone faculty of nursing to further model the globalization of nursing.

She received a BS from Rutgers University College of Nursing, and MA and PhD from New York University, Division of Nursing. She presents frequently on innovations in nursing education, technology in the curriculum, performance excellence and the partnering of academic and clinical institutions. She holds membership in Sigma Theta Tau, Phi Delta Kappa, and Omicron Delta Kappa. She has been inducted into the Stuart Cook Master Educators' Guild at UMDNJ and has received numerous Who's Who citations. She has also received numerous grants in support of the Nursing Programs at Ramapo.

Contributors

EVIDENCE-BASED PRACTICE BOXES

Amy Mitchell, RN, MSN
Nurse Manager, MICU
Hackensack University Medical Center
Hackensack, New Jersey

Judy Urgo, RN, MSN
Staff Nurse
Hackensack University Medical Center
Hackensack, New Jersey

CLINICAL CORNER BOXES

Denise Addison, RN, MSN
Manager Nursing Education
Hackensack University Medical Center
Hackensack, New Jersey

Mary Jo Assi, MS, RN, APRN, BC, AHN-BC
Director, Advanced Practice Nursing
The Valley Hospital
Ridgewood, New Jersey

Joan Brennan, DNP, RN
Vice President Quality and Performance Excellence
AtlantiCare
Egg Harbor Township, New Jersey

Edna Cadmus, PhD, RN, CNAA, BC
Senior Vice President, Patient Care Services
Englewood Hospital and Medical Center
Englewood, New Jersey

Joan Shinkus Clark, MSN, RN, NEA-BC, CENP
SVP & Texas Health Chief Nurse Executive
Texas Health Resources
Arlington, Texas

Joy Espejo, RN, BSN, CCRN
ICU Staff Nurse
St. Joseph's Regional Medical Center
Paterson, New Jersey

Patricia D. Fonder, MSN, RN BC, CCRN
Patient Care Manager
Englewood Hospital and Medical Center
Englewood, New Jersey

Mary Frey, RN
Nurse Manager, Palliative Care and Admissions
Chair, Mountainside Hospital Ethics Committee
Mountainside Hospital
Montclair, New Jersey

Mary Ann Hozak, MSN, RN, CCRN
Magnet Program Manager
St. Joseph's Regional Medical Center
Paterson, New Jersey

Catherine Hughes, RN, BSN, CCRN
Co-Chairperson
Recruitment and Retention Committee of
the Professional Nurse Practice Council
St. Joseph's Hospital and Medical Center
Paterson, New Jersey

Beverly S. Karas-Irwin, MS, MSN, RN, APN-C, HN-BC
Director, Clinical Partnerships & Nursing Programs
The Valley Hospital
Ridgewood, New Jersey

Bonnie Michaels, RN, MA, NEA-BC, FACHE
Vice President, CNO
The Mountainside Hospital
Montclair, New Jersey

Denise L. Occhiuzzo, MS, RNC
Administrative Director of Nursing
Clinical Education and Nursing Practice
Magnet Program Director
Hackensack University Medical Center
Hackensack, New Jersey

Jane O'Rourke, DNP, RN, NEA-BC, CENP
Chief Nurse Executive
Bergen Regional Medical Center
Paramus, New Jersey

Joan Orseck, RN
Director of Nurse Recruitment
Hackensack University Medical Center
Hackensack, New Jersey

Rosemarie D. Rosales, BSN, MPA, RN, CCRN
Director, Nursing Education and Infection Control
East Orange General Hospital
East Orange, New Jersey

Gina Sallustio, RN, BSN
Staff Nurse
Hackensack University Medical Center
Hackensack, New Jersey

Karen M. Stanley, MS, PMHCNS-BC
Psychiatric Consultation Liaison Nurse
Medical University of South Carolina
Charleston, South Carolina

Julie Sturbaum, RN, BSN, RNFA, CIC
Program Manager, Infection Prevention and Control
St. Luke's Hospital
Cedar Rapids, Iowa

Elvira Usinowicz, RN, MS, CCRN, CCNS, APN-C
Chairperson, Nursing Research Council
The Valley Hospital
Ridgewood, New Jersey

Reviewers

Carole A. Baxter, MSN, EdD, RN
Dean, RN Program
St. Joseph's Hospital School of Nursing
Philadelphia, Pennsylvania

Kathleen Becker, RN, BSN, MEd, MSN
Associate Professor of Nursing
St. Louis Community College—Forest Park
St. Louis, Missouri

Katherine H. Dimmock, JD, EdD, MSN, RN
Dean, Professor of Nursing
Columbia College of Nursing
Milwaukee, Wisconsin

Susan Draine, MSN, CNS, CCRN, MBA
Chair, Department of Nursing
Associate Professor of Nursing
Olivet Nazarene University
Bourbonnais, Illinois

Joyce Foresman-Capuzzi, RN, BSN, CEN, CPN, CTRN, CCRN, EMT-P
Clinical Nurse Educator
Emergency Department
The Lankenau Hospital
Wynnewood, Pennsylvania

Shirley Garrick, PhD, MSN, BSN
Professor of Nursing
Texas A&M University
Texarkana, Texas

Judith Ann Gentry, APRN, MSN, OCN
Assistant Professor of Clinical Nursing
LSUHSC School of Nursing
New Orleans, Louisiana

Gloria Green-Ridley, MSN
Associate Professor
Department of Nursing and Allied Health
University of the District of Columbia
Washington, DC

Sharron Guillett, PhD, RN
Associate Professor and Chair of BSN Program
School of Health Professions
Marymount University
Arlington, Virginia

Arlene Haddon, RN, BN, MN, MSM
Instructor
College of Nursing
Valdosta State University
Valdosta, Georgia

Josephine Kahler, EdD, RN, CS
Dean and Professor of Nursing
College of Health and Behavioral Sciences
Texas A&M University—Texarkana
Texarkana, Texas

Patricia A. Keresztes, PhD, RN, CCRN
Assistant Professor of Nursing
Saint Mary's College
Notre Dame, Indiana
Staff Nurse
Cardiovascular Intensive Care Unit
Memorial Hospital
South Bend, Indiana

Marilyn Lee, RN, PhD
Associate Professor
University of North Alabama
Florence, Alabama

Susan H. Lynch, MSN, RN
RN BSN Coordinator
School of Nursing
UNC Charlotte
Charlotte, North Carolina

Dimitra Loukissa, PhD, RN
Associate Professor
North Park University
Chicago, Illinois

Dorothea McDowell, PhD, RN
Professor and Associate Chair
Department of Nursing
Salisbury University
Salisbury, Maryland

Susan Meyer, RN, MSN
Chair of the Nursing Department
Mount St. Mary's College
Los Angeles, California

Kereen Mullenbach, RN, PhD
Assisstant Professor
School of Nursing
Radford University
Radford, Virginia

Jack Rydell, RN, MS
Assistant Professor
Nursing Department
Concordia College
Moorhead, Minnesota

Teresa Saxton, MSN, RN
Instructional Assistant Professor
Mennonite College of Nursing
Illinois State University
Normal, Illinois

Susan Turner, RN, MSN, FNP
Professor of Nursing
Gavilan College
Gilroy, California

Karen Ward, PhD, RN, COI
Professor and Associate Director for Online Programs
Middle Tennessee State University
Murfreesboro, Tennessee

Cheryl Webb, PhD, RN, CS
Assistant Professor
Community College of Beaver County
Monaca, Pennsylvania

Debra Webster, EdD, MSN, RNBC
Nursing Instructor
Salisbury University
Salisbury, Maryland

Preface to the Instructor

Nursing Delegation and Management of Patient Care is designed to assist nursing students and novice nurses to begin to develop an understanding of the myriad of issues facing them as managers of care and the potential nursing leaders of tomorrow. This is only a beginning; the concepts of management and leadership are changing daily. Health care is moving at an unprecedented speed, and it is imperative that we all attempt to keep up. What is the important lesson here is that as nurses, we need to keep current, questioning, and focused on what is "best" for our patients and practice.

There is massive information, both in the scholarly and commercial literature, that focuses on what makes a good manager or leader. It is important that nurses keep in touch with this literature, but they need to be able to differentiate between what is "best evidence" and what is best-selling fiction. As you move into practice, your professional organizations, your health care library/librarian, and your own engagement in the profession will be your best allies. Keep in touch with the current literature and strive to continually improve the care that you deliver to patients and families. Remember: continuous improvement is continuous!

This book is divided into 5 sections, each dealing with a concept of leadership and management. American Organization of Nurse Executives (AONE) (2005) delineated five areas of competency for the nurse manager. These areas are: communication and relationship building, knowledge of the health care environment, leadership, professionalism, and business skills. The emphasis on particular competencies will be different depending on the position in the organization. There are skills necessary for managing the business of health care. These would include:

- Financial Management
- Human Resource Management
- Performance Improvement
- Foundational Thinking Skills
- Technology
- Strategic Management
- Clinical Practice Management

Other competencies are necessary for the art of managing health care. This is leading the people of health care. These competencies would include:

- Human Resource Skills
- Relationship Management and Influencing Behaviors
- Diversity
- Shared Decision Making

And lastly, there are competencies for creating the leader in yourself:

- Personal and Professional Accountability
- Career Planning
- Personal Journey Disciplines
- Optimizing the Leader Within

FEATURES

The text is organized according to these competencies of nurse leaders and managers. Each chapter includes a Clinical Corner box written by a nurse leader that shares a current practice that is utilized in practice. Additionally, there is an evidence-based discussion from a current piece of literature that reviews current research and/or best practice. It is our hope that the reader gleans some ideas from these sections to spark their own practice. Each chapter concludes with some NCLEX®-exam style question that may prove helpful in reviewing the content.

ANCILLARIES

Evolve Resources for Nursing Delegation and Management of Patient Care, first edition is available at http://evolve.elsevier.com/Motacki/delegation/ to enhance student instruction. This online resource is organized by chapter and includes the following:

For instructors:
- Case Studies
- Test Bank Questions
- PowerPoint Slides

For students:
- NCLEX®-exam style practice questions with answers and rationales

Preface for the Students

Nursing Delegation and Management of Patient Care is designed to assist you as you prepare to become the nursing leaders of tomorrow. To help you make the most of your learning experience, here are the key features that you will find in this text:

CHAPTER 12

Monitoring Outcomes and Use of Data for Improvement

Objectives begin each chapter and explain what you should accomplish upon completion of each chapter.

Key terms with definitions are placed at the beginning of each chapter for quick reference.

Summaries review key points covered in the chapter.

Clinical Corner boxes discuss topics related to practice process improvements made by nurses.

Evidence-Based Practice boxes review current research and/or best practice.

Each chapter ends with NCLEX®-exam style review questions.

Acknowledgments

Thank you to Dr. Kathleen Burke who agreed to take on this project with me. Her knowledge and expertise has made this book an excellent and exceptional resource for senior-level students and new graduate nurses. Her lead on the clinical corners and the evidence-based practice boxes make this book unique. Thank you to the contributors and reviewers for their expertise and input. Thank you to senior acquisitions editor Yvonne Alexopoulos, senior developmental editor Danielle Frazier, editorial assistant Heather Rippetoe, and project manager Pat Costigan for their unending patience with this project. Finally, thank you to my daughter Lisa for assisting me with permissions and references.

Kathleen Motacki

Thank you to Kathleen Motacki for asking me to assist her in this project. Also to Jean Kenworthy of Elsevier who suggested my name to Kathleen. Thank you to the contributors and reviewers for their expertise and input. Thank you to senior acquisitions editor Yvonne Alexopoulos, senior developmental editor Danielle Frazier, editorial assistant Heather Rippetoe, and project manager Pat Costigan for their unending patience with this project. I would also like to thank my many colleagues who assisted with the evidence-based practice boxes and clinical corners. Their names are listed under contributors.

Kathleen Burke

Contents

Patient Care Management

This section of the text deals with issues of importance in the management of patient care and will assist you to gain competence in the frontline management of patient care. While you have had experience in dealing with the care planning and delivery for one or more individual patients, the experience of managing the care delivered by other members of the health care team is the culmination of your initial nursing education. Patient care management is the process of planning, organizing, leading, and improving all of the activities centered on the delivery of care to a group of patients.

You will not be expected to manage an entire patient unit on graduation but will be in charge of the delivery of care to a group of patients. As you mature in your professional role, you may be asked to take a management role within your institution. You first need to become comfortable with the practice of management of patient care for a group of patients, and then move toward unit management of care. Numerous processes and governance structures will assist you to achieve positive patient outcomes.

The process of patient care management includes skills such as delegation, patient assignment, coordination, collaboration, communication, and outcome monitoring. This process occurs in an interdisciplinary work environment, and skill in working in such environments is necessary. The American Organization of Nurse Executives (AONE) (2006) delineated five areas of competency for the nurse manager: communication and relationship building, knowledge of the health care environment, leadership, professionalism, and business skills. The emphasis on particular competencies will differ depending on the position in the organization. There are skills necessary for managing the business of health care:

- Financial management
- Human resource management
- Performance improvement
- Foundational thinking skills
- Technology
- Strategic management
- Clinical practice management

Other competencies are necessary for the art of managing health care—this is leading the people of health care. These competencies include the following:

- Human resource skills
- Relationship management and influencing behaviors
- Diversity
- Shared decision making

And, last, there are competencies for creating the leader in yourself:
- Personal and professional accountability
- Career planning
- Personal journey disciplines
- Optimizing the leader within

This section will deal with the knowledge and skills necessary to assist you in achievement of some of the competencies of the management of patient care—managing the business of health care.

CHAPTER 1

Patient Care Management

Chapter Objectives

1. Differentiate between leadership and management.
2. Identify the management structures of patient care.
3. Describe the various modes of patient care delivery systems.
4. Discuss the pros and cons of each of the delivery systems.
5. Determine the responsibility of the nurse in the various care delivery systems.
6. Identify outcome measures of patient care management.
7. Relate a clinical scenario to each of the delivery models.

Definitions

Leadership Ability to influence people to work toward the meeting of stated goals

Management Act of planning, organizing, staffing, directing, and controlling for the present

Total patient care Model of care in which nurse assumes full accountability for care of a group of patients

Case management Model of care in which nurse integrates delivery of clinical services in combination with financial services

Primary nursing Model of care in which one nurse assumes accountability for care delivered by other personnel in a 24-hour time period

Team nursing Model of care in which a group of staff members led by a nurse provides care

Functional nursing Model of care in which nursing work is allocated according to specific tasks and skills

LEADERSHIP VERSUS MANAGEMENT

Just because someone is in a leadership position, it does not automatically follow that this person is a leader. Some people have false assumptions about leaders and leadership. Many people believe that the position and title are the same as true leadership. Having the title of chief nurse does not necessarily mean that the person in that position is a leader, while being a staff nurse does not mean that person is not a leader. New nurse managers often make the mistake of believing that along with the new title comes the mantle of leadership. Leadership takes a tremendous amount of effort, time, and energy. *Leadership* can be defined as the

3

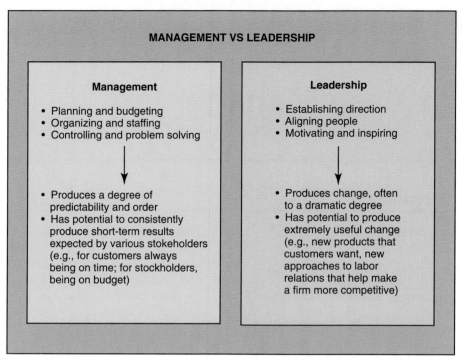

Figure 1-1 • Management versus leadership. Data from Kotter, J. (1996). *Leading change.* Boston, MA: Harvard Business School.

use of individual traits and personal power to influence and guide strategy development. Leaders need to "do the right thing," be future oriented, be visionary, focus on purposes, and empower others to set and achieve organizational goals. *Management* is the act of planning, organizing, staffing, directing, and controlling for the present. Management can be taught, whereas leadership is usually a reflection of personal experience.

As shown in Figure 1-1, leaders show the way, while managers labor to produce the day-to-day outcomes. Leaders focus on effectiveness, and managers deal with efficiencies.

COMPARISON OF LEADERSHIP AND MANAGEMENT

A further review of leadership and management focuses on the major themes of each role (Table 1-1). The nurse, as manager, works collaboratively to achieve the desired outcomes of quality care, fiscal responsibility, and customer satisfaction by coordinating the care of individuals, families, groups, or populations through

Table 1-1	COMPARISON OF LEADERSHIP AND MANAGEMENT		
	Leadership	**Management**
Motto	Do the right thing	Do things right
Challenge	Change	Continuity
Focus	Purposes	Structures and procedures
Time frame	Future	Present
Methods	Strategy	Schedule
Questions	Why?	Who, what, when, where, how?
Outcomes	Journeys	Destinations
Human	Potential	Performance

Bennis, W., & Nanus, B. (1997). *Leaders: the strategies for taking charge.* New York: Harper and Row.

the effective use of technology, resources, information, and systems. Some health care agencies will differentiate between the level of academic preparation of the nurse and the expected competency of the manager (Table 1-2).

Table 1-2	COMPETENCIES OF ADN AND BSN NURSES	

Skill	ADN	BSN
Management of care	Coordinates, organizes, prioritizes and modifies care provided for the individual, family or group. Assigns and delegates care appropriately.	Coordinates, organizes, prioritizes and modifies care provided for the individual, family, group or population. Assigns and delegates care appropriately. Develops, implements, and evaluates population-based health care programs.
Management and leadership concepts	Applies management and leadership concepts. Uses effective communication and conflict management skills in promoting a positive milieu.	Analyzes the management process and leadership concepts for implementation. Uses and coaches others to use effective communication and conflict management skills in creating a positive milieu.
Professional development	Contributes to the professional development of health care providers.	Promotes and evaluates professional development of health care providers.
Nursing care delivery systems	Participates in implementing and evaluating traditional and alternative nursing care delivery systems.	Develops and evaluates traditional and alternative nursing care delivery systems.
Management goals	Identifies and participates in influencing management goals.	Demonstrates a beginning leadership role in establishing and influencing management goals.
Standards of care	Participates in evaluation and development of standards of nursing care.	Develops and evaluates standards of nursing care.
Change	Demonstrates flexibility and effectively influences the change process.	Evaluates the need for change and demonstrates flexibility in promoting planned change.

ADN, Associate degree in nursing; *BSN,* Bachelor of Science in Nursing.
Copyright 2000, by the Colorado Council on Nursing Education.

THEORIES OF LEADERSHIP

There are numerous theories of leadership. How the leader approaches leadership is often very dependent on his or her personal experiences. Leadership also relies on the organizational structure and culture of the health care facility. Two leadership theories prevalent within health care today are transactional leadership and transformational leadership. In *transactional leadership,* there is an exchange between the leader and the employee. The needs of the employees are identified, and the leader provides rewards to meet those needs in exchange for performance. This type of leadership usually takes place in a hierarchal organization. A hierarchal organization is one where decision making occurs at the top of the structure and is communicated to the employees. *Transformational leadership* is more consultative and collaborative. Kouzes and Posner

(2002) identify five basic practices in transformational leadership:

1. Challenging the process, questioning the ways that things have always been done, and creatively thinking of new ways of doing things
2. Motivating and inspiring shared vision or bringing everyone together, moving toward the shared goal
3. Empowering others to act
4. Modeling the change
5. Praising the employee for the work done

One form of governance often used by transformational leaders is *shared governance.* This is a democratic, dynamic process resulting from shared decision making and accountability (Porter-O'Grady, 2001). In shared governance, there is the creation of organizational structures that allow nursing staff autonomy to govern their practice (Batson, 2004).

LEADERSHIP STRUCTURE IN HEALTH CARE

Health care institutions are usually organized according to lines of authority, power, and communication. Structures are defined as centralized or decentralized depending on the degree to which the organization has spread its lines of authority.

ORGANIZATIONAL STRUCTURES

An organizational chart is a visual means for determining the level of centralization or decentralization. A flat organizational structure signifies the removal of hierarchal layers, demonstrating that the authority for action occurs at the point of service (Figure 1-2).

FUNCTIONAL STRUCTURES

Functional structures arrange services and departments according to their function (Figure 1-3). Departments providing similar functions would all report to a common manager or vice president. This type of structure supports professional expertise but can result in the "silo" effect, where departments become separate silos with little interaction.

PRODUCT LINE STRUCTURES

In product line structures, the functions necessary to produce a specific service are brought together into an integrated unit under the control of a single manager (Figure 1-4). For example, the orthopedic service line at a hospital would include all personnel providing services to the orthopedic service population. This might include the orthopedic ambulatory care service, the orthopedic operating rooms, the orthopedic trauma center of the emergency department, and the orthopedic rehabilitation center. Benefits of this model include coordination of all services within the specialty and a similarity of focus. A limitation would be increased expense due to duplication of services.

MATRIX STRUCTURES

Matrix structures combine both function and service line in an integrated service structure (Figure 1-5). In

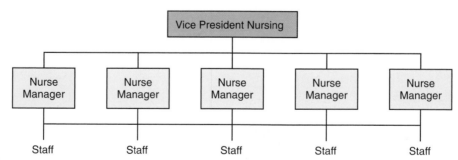

Figure 1-2 ● Organizational structure. (From Yoder-Wise, P. S. [2007]. *Leading and managing in nursing,* ed. 4. St. Louis: Mosby.)

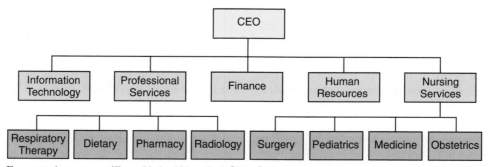

Figure 1-3 ● Functional structure. (From Yoder-Wise, P. S. [2007]. *Leading and managing in nursing,* ed. 4. St. Louis: Mosby.)

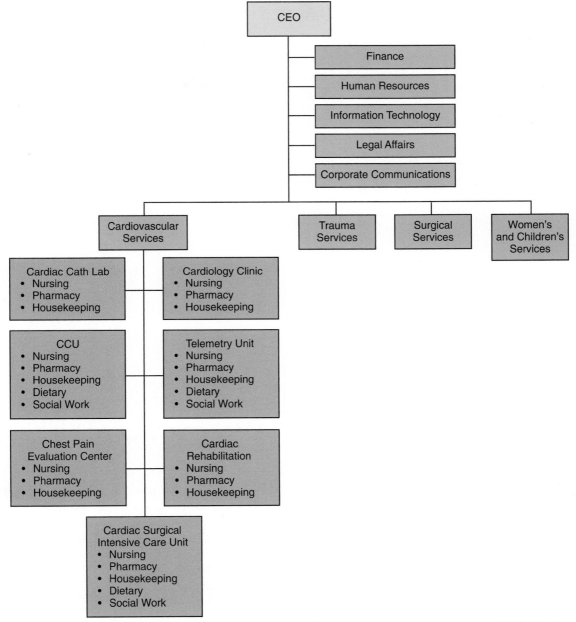

Figure 1-4 • Product line structure. (From Yoder-Wise, P. S. [2007]. *Leading and managing in nursing,* ed. 4. St. Louis: Mosby.)

a matrix organization, the manager of a unit responsible for a service reports both to a functional manager (vice president for nursing) and a service manager (directors of the services: cardiovascular services, trauma services, surgical services, or women's and children's services). Such a structure requires a collaborative relationship between the service line and func-

tional manager. The nurse is responsible to the nurse manager and vice president of nursing for nursing care and to the program director when working within the matrix.

In the organizational structure, the nursing department is usually listed on the senior leadership level. The chief nursing officer (senior vice president of patient

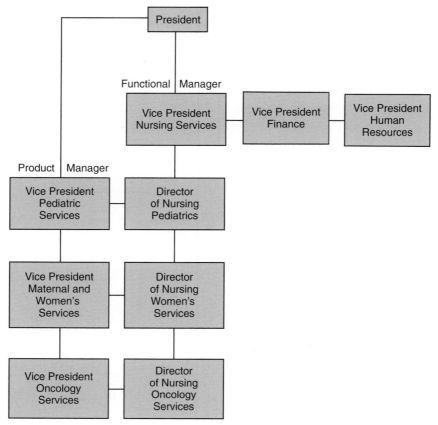

Figure 1-5 • Matrix structure. (From Yoder-Wise, P. S. [2007]. *Leading and managing in nursing*, ed. 4. St. Louis: Mosby.)

care, vice president of nursing, etc.) is the highest-level reporting nursing officer in an organization.

As a new staff nurse, you will report to a unit-based manager. Yes, you will be ultimately responsible to the vice president of nursing (chief nursing officer) but, during the workday, you may report to a shift charge nurse. This charge nurse (patient care manager) will have the overall responsibility for the patient care delivered during the work shift. There are many delivery systems, and the titles and responsibilities of the nurse and nurse manager vary according to the delivery system.

MAJOR TYPES OF CARE DELIVERY SYSTEMS

A patient care delivery model is the method used to deliver care to patients. There are multiple care delivery models, and the choice of a model within an organiza-

tion is dependent on many factors: financial, staffing capabilities, patient population, and organizational mission and philosophy. The fundamental element of any patient care delivery system (Manthey, 1990) is a combination of the following:
- Clinical decision making
- Work allocation
- Communication
- Management
- Coordination
- Accountability

The following are the models associated with hospital practice:
- Total patient care
- Functional nursing
- Team nursing
  - Modular nursing
- Primary nursing
- Case management

TOTAL PATIENT CARE

Total patient care is the oldest method of providing care to a patient. It is sometimes called case method (not to be confused with case management). It was the primary care delivery model until the 1930s, and it had a resurgence in the 1990s. In this model, one nurse assumes accountability for the complete care of a group of patients. It has been described as a type of primary nursing (Reverby, 1987), but in total patient care the accountability for coordination of care does not extend beyond the assigned shift. This is the type of care seen in private duty nursing and some intensive care units and was the model of care used by Florence Nightingale.

Advantages of total patient care:
- Quality of care—all care is delivered by a registered nurse
- Continuity of care for a given shift
- High patient satisfaction
- Decreases communication time between staff
- Reduces the need for supervision
- Allows one person to perform more than one task

Disadvantages of total patient care:
- May not be cost effective because of the number of registered nurses needed to provide care
- Some nurses dislike this model because they believe that some of the patient care activities could be done by others with less skill

An example of a patient care assignment using the total patient care model is shown in Table 1-3.

FUNCTIONAL NURSING

Functional nursing is a model in which work is allocated according to specific tasks and technical skills. This model was popular from the late 1800s to the end of World War II. In this model, the "charge nurse" identifies the tasks/work that need to be completed during the shift. These tasks/work are then divided and assigned to personnel. In this model, there would be a "medication nurse," a "dressing nurse," etc. This model of care delivery is oriented to the accomplishment of tasks. It is efficient in times of staff shortages, and you will see patient care units reverting to this delivery mode in times of staff shortage, such as "snow emergencies" when the number of staff is limited. Some institutions with a large variation in the classification

Table 1-3	PATIENT CARE ASSIGNMENT USING THE TOTAL CARE MODEL
Hester B., RN, MSN	Patient Care Manager 4 West
Joseph Z., RN, BSN	Full patient care, documentation, orders, admissions, discharges—rooms 410-414
Maria C., RN	Full patient care, documentation, orders, admissions, discharges—rooms 415-417
Joy T., RN, BSN	Full patient care, documentation, orders, admissions, discharges—rooms 418-420
Michael Y., RN	Full patient care, documentation, orders, admissions, discharges—rooms 421 and 422
Clarisa T., RN	Full patient care, documentation, orders, admissions, discharges—rooms 423-425

of staff (registered nurses, licensed practical nurses, nurse aides, and technicians) to care for patients may also use functional nursing.

Advantages of functional nursing are:
- A large number of tasks can be completed in a shift
- Ability to mix staff classifications
- Efficient financially
- Staff members can be trained to master one task

Disadvantages of functional nursing are:
- Charge nurse may be only one with total view of patient
- Decreased patient satisfaction
- Decreased nurse satisfaction
- Fragmented communication
- Unit coordination becomes responsibility of charge nurse
- Fragmented accountability

An example of a patient care assignment using the functional nursing method is shown in Table 1-4. In this assignment, everyone is accountable for a portion of care. A challenge is that all aspects of patient care need to be communicated to the next shift, and the charge nurse must make sure that all pertinent information is known by her and that she is then able to communicate it to the next shift. This can lead to fragmented patient knowledge and a lack of holistic care.

Table 1-4	PATIENT CARE ASSIGNMENT USING THE FUNCTIONAL NURSING METHOD
Unit 4 West Telemetry—30 patients	
Mary L., RN, BSN, charge nurse	All orders, rounds, report
Bob W., telemetry technician	All monitors, rhythm strips Q 4, and chart
Lisa N., RN	Medications rooms 401-415, oversee nurse aide Tom R. rooms 401-415, charting for rooms 401-415, admissions/discharges rooms 401-415
Tom R., nurse aide	Hygienic care rooms 401-415, feeding, line cart restock

Table 1-5	PATIENT CARE ASSIGNMENT USING THE TEAM NURSING MODEL
Mary B., RN, BSN	Charge nurse Oversight of patients Rooms 410-422
Team A	
Betty K., RN	Team leader, Team A Rooms 410-416 Documentation, orders admissions/discharges, charting for PCA. Restocks cardiac arrest cart
Maria B., RN	Rooms 410-412 patient care Medications Team A
Sara N., LPN	Rooms 413-416 Blood sugars, rooms 414, 416
Edith, W., PCA	Hygienic care, rooms 410, 412, 414, 415 Assists patients, rooms 411, 413, 416 Vital signs 8a and 12n
Team B	
Tom A., RN	Team leader, Team B Rooms 417-422 Documentation, orders admissions/discharges, charting for PCA
Marci S., RN	Rooms 418, 420 patient care
Michael T., PCA	Rooms 417, 422 hygienic care Vital signs 8a and 12n, Team B Blood sugars rooms 417, 422

TEAM NURSING

Team nursing is a delivery approach that uses a group of staff members led by a nurse to provide care. The team is composed of health care workers with a diversity of skills, education, licensure, and ability who work collaboratively to provide care to a group of patients. The registered nurse is the team leader, and she supervises and evaluates team members delivering care. The team leader can provide care to a patient with complex care needs but usually does not provide hands-on care. Strong communication skills are essential. This model supports group work and productivity.

Advantages of team nursing are:
- Facilitation and oversight of novice nurses
- Smaller group of patients allows for higher quality of care than with functional nursing
- Team leader has knowledge of patient needs and can provide coordination of care
- Fixed teams relate to higher-quality patient care

Disadvantages of team nursing are:
- Increased time to communicate within the team
- Expensive due to the increased number of staff needed
- Increased time needed to supervise, coordinate, and delegate
- Can lead to omissions in care

- Most educated staff relegated to role of supervision, not direct delivery of care

An example of a patient care assignment using the team nursing model is shown in Table 1-5. In this assignment, care is delivered by a group of staff, all of whom report back to the team leader. It is the team leader who has the decision-making responsibility for the care delivered to the group of patients.

Modular Nursing

A variation of team nursing is modular nursing (Anderson and Hughes, 1993). Modular nursing is based on the physical layout of the unit. Some hospital units were designed to house a number of smaller patient "pods" and as such are structurally divided into smaller patient care areas or substations. Nurses are stationed near the patients. The essential components of modular nursing are as follows:

- A module consists of a group of staff members and a group of patients.
- Patients are grouped by spatial or floor plan clustering.
- Nurse/patient assignment is standardized by cluster.

Advantages of this model center on the physical layout of the assignment and the ease of working in such an environment. Disadvantages center on the need to have consistent numbers of staff members in such a physical environment.

PRIMARY NURSING

Primary nursing is a one-to-one approach to patient care. Each patient is assigned a specific nurse, who assumes 24-hour responsibility for the delivery, implementation, evaluation, and coordination of care for the duration of the hospital stay. The primary nurse works in conjunction with nurses (associate nurses) on the other shifts to coordinate all care for the patient and family. The primary nurse is responsible for the development and evaluation of the plan of care for the patient. Decision making is decentralized and takes place at the patient's bedside. This is a flexible model and can include a variety of skill mixes. It does not mean that only registered nurses care for patients. The primary nurse plans, coordinates, and evaluates the plan of care, but the care can be delegated to appropriate staff members depending on the severity of the patient condition.

Advantages of primary nursing are:
- Improved quality and continuity of care
- Simplified communication
- Increased nurse satisfaction in nurses prepared for the role
- Patients perceive care to be more personalized

Disadvantages of primary nursing are:
- Increased number of hours of care per day requires greater number of registered nurses
- Overall patient satisfaction results are inconclusive
- Can be difficult to implement if patient has multiple unit transfers

An example of a patient care assignment using the primary nursing model is shown in Table 1-6.

CASE MANAGEMENT

Case management is a model that mixes both process and care delivery. In hospital nursing, it focuses on the

Table 1-6	PATIENT CARE ASSIGNMENT USING THE PRIMARY NURSING MODEL
Hester A., RN, MSN	Patient Care Manager 4 West
Joseph T., RN, BSN (primary nurse) 7-3 Jody N. (associate nurse) 3-11 Evelyn B. (associate nurse) 11-7	Full patient care, documentation, orders, admissions, discharges —rooms 410-414
Maria C., RN 7-3 Cathy C., RN, BSN (primary nurse) 3-11 Evelyn L. (associate nurse) 11-7	Full patient care, documentation, orders, admissions, discharges —rooms 415-417
Joy T., RN, BSN (primary nurse) 7-3 Peter U., RN (associate nurse) 3-11 Barbara S., RN (associate nurse) 11-7	Full patient care, documentation, orders, admissions, discharges —rooms 418-420
Michael T., RN, BSN (primary nurse) 7-3 Peter B., RN (associate nurse) 3-11 Barbara S., RN (associate nurse) 11-7	Full patient care, documentation, orders, admissions, discharges —rooms 421 and 422
Clarisa I., RN 7-3 Diane O. (associate nurse) 3-11 Erline P., RN, BSN (primary nurse) 11-7	Full patient care, documentation, orders, admissions, discharges —rooms 422-425

achievement of patient outcomes within an effective and appropriate time frame. It is focused on the entire illness episode and can cross all units in which the patient receives care. It is associated with the use of care pathways/order sets/care maps/protocols/clinical practice guidelines, which are written plans that identify critical and predictable events that must occur throughout a hospitalization. The assigned case manager works with the assigned nursing staff to coordinate patient

Table 1-7   OVERVIEW OF MAJOR TYPES OF NURSING CARE DELIVERY MODELS

Model	Focus	Clinical Decision Making	Work Allocation	Time Span
Total patient care	Total patient care	Nurse at bedside, charge nurse makes some decisions	Assigning patients	One shift
Functional	Tasks	Charge nurses make most decisions	Assigning tasks	One shift
Team	Group task	Team leader makes most decisions	Assigning tasks	One shift
Primary	Total patient care	Nurse at bedside	Assigning patients	24 Hours/7 days a week

Model	Communication	Documentation	Outcomes	Quality
Total patient care	Hierarchical—charge nurse gives and receives report	Unknown	May lack continuity of care between caregivers	High—all care delivered by RN
Functional	Hierarchical—charge nurse gives and receives report	Tasks	Fragmented care	Omissions and errors can occur
Team	Hierarchical—charge nurse to charge nurse, or charge nurse to team leaders, or team leaders to team members	Tasks and care plan	Fragmented care	Omissions and errors can occur
Primary	Lateral—caregiver to caregiver	Individualized plan	Continuity of care	Process oriented

From Tiedman, M., & Lookinland, S. (2004). Traditional models of care delivery: what have we learned? *Journal of Nursing Administration, 34*(6), 291-297.

progress through the pathway. The Case Management Society of America defines *case management* as "a collaborative process of assessment, planning, facilitation and advocacy for options and services to meet an individual's health needs through communication and available resources to promote cost-effective outcomes" (CMSA, 2002).

Case managers are often population based, so that one case manager may work with all surgical patients within a hospital, although some institutions do use unit-based case managers. The case manager is assigned to the patient on admission and follows the patient for the entire hospital stay and performs all post hospital care coordination. Not all case managers are nurses.

Advantages of case management are that it:
- Provides a professional practice model for nurses
- Is cost effective

Disadvantages of case management are that it:
- May lead to fragmented communication
- Needs to be integrated into the care delivery model

- May lead to nurses caring for patients to become more skills focused if the case manager makes all the decisions

Table 1-7 provides an overview of the major types of nursing care delivery models.

SUMMARY

New nurse managers often make the mistake that along with the new title comes the mantle of leadership. Leadership takes a tremendous amount of effort, time, and energy. *Leadership* can be defined as the use of individual traits and personal power to influence and guide strategy development. Leaders need to "do the right thing"; they are future oriented and visionary, focus on purposes, empower others to set and achieve organizational goals. *Management* is the act of planning, organizing, staffing, directing, and controlling for the present. Management can be taught, while leadership is usually a reflection of personal experience.

The manner in which patient care is delivered to patients and families is reflective of the nursing philosophy of the organization. Each model of patient care delivery has advantages and disadvantages for both the patient and the nurse. The role of the nurse in each type of model differs according to the delivery system. It is important to acknowledge your role and responsibilities in the model being used in your institution.

New models of patient care are being developed and used across the United States. Some of the newer models combine aspects of the models already in existence. As research and evidence concerning the successes and challenges of the new models evolve, care delivery will change.

 CLINICAL CORNER

The Twelve Bed Hospital Model
Joan Shinkus Clark

At Baptist Hospital of Miami, Florida, a care delivery model has been evolving since 2000 as a hybrid of many of the popular models of delivery, taking some of the best elements of each of the traditional models and combining them in a model that helps the hospital address some of the most perplexing issues faced in the current environment. The model is based on clinical leadership provided by a nursing role called a patient care facilitator (PCF). The PCF role was originally conceptualized by nurses in direct care positions, as an approach to ensuring that nurses on the unit have the leadership needed to deal with all of the complexity that characterizes the hospital environment today.

One of the most significant changes in the staffing of inpatient units over the years has been 12-hour shifts and flexible scheduling. Along with the changes, continuity of care from a particular nurse has markedly diminished, leaving patients to meet new faces on practically every new shift. With the advent of hospitalists, many hospitals have also accommodated their scheduling around the nursing model, which has further fragmented the continuity of caregivers. With lengths of stays dramatically shortened and comorbidities on the rise, patient complexity has also increased. The unfortunate reality is that despite all the differences, patient expectations for nursing care have not changed! Nurses at Baptist recognized the need to change the model to promote improved continuity through identifying one person whom patients admitted to their unit could call "their nurse."

In early 2000, nurses on a busy 52-bed cardiovascular unit were asked to provide input on the ideal staffing pattern, as well as to make recommendations on whether some of the support functions (housekeeping, dietary, phlebotomy, etc.), decentralized during the reengineering efforts in the 1990s, should be recentralized. What emerged in the discussion was the need for a consistent nursing figure for staff, physicians, patients, and families to act as a point person. It was preferred that this individual be an expert nurse and that the patient caseload be kept to around 12 (no more

that 16) patients. The nursing director for the cardiovascular nursing encouraged the staff to write a job description that described this role; some of the experts complied, and the nursing director received the approval of the chief nursing officer (CNO) to pilot the first PCF on a 12-bed section of the unit in late 2000.

Results of the pilot were so encouraging in the initial phases that discussions immediately began around extending the number of PCFs to cover the other beds on the unit, which slowly occurred in the early part of 2001, one section of the unit at a time. Patients, physicians, and other supportive caregivers voiced such a resounding approval of the concept that the momentum carried to other departments within the hospital. The medical-surgical nursing director soon submitted a proposal to the CNO to further the pilot to two additional medical-surgical units, each at 48 beds, but to add all four PCFs on each unit simultaneously. The CNO received the CEO's approval to move forward with the phase 2 pilot and the CNO appointed a project manager from among the original staff nurses involved in authoring the original job description to ensure continuity with the original concept.

As the PCF role was piloted on these units, the total concept as a *model* came together. Broken down into small manageable segments led by a PCF, what was a large urban hospital, growing quickly away from *acting small* (a concept passionately promoted by the CEO as a vision for staff at Baptist Hospital), now was able to reproduce some of that personal touch of yesteryears. It was out of this concept that the idea of naming the model a "Twelve Bed Hospital" emerged. With the Twelve Bed Hospital, care delivery revolves around the patient, and because the caseload is held at about 12 to 16 patients, the PCF can follow every patient in the Twelve Bed Hospital, acting as an advocate, a liaison, and a support for the patient as well as significant others. In past experiences, similar roles at Baptist had much broader assignments, necessitating a prioritization of patients who were most complex or had acute problems. The PCF has the responsibility to know all the patients in the Twelve Bed Hospital and act much like a traffic controller for all parties involved in care.

Continued

The PCF also coordinates the patient needs related to a safe and effective plan for discharge and work with care managers to ensure that arrangements are made to enhance continuity in the posthospital setting.

Staff assigned to work with a PCF within a consistent geographic area of the patient care center are scheduled consistently within each Twelve Bed Hospital. This promotes a team approach to care delivery, one that enhances overall efficiency as staff work together on a consistent basis. The positions designated for PCFs are an addition to the staffing pattern on each nursing unit, and although they do not factor into the direct care component relative to staffing, they provide care as needed, especially during emergencies or to assist novice staff in their care.

The Twelve Bed Hospital model is in many ways the best aspect of a number of traditional delivery models. It is *primary nursing* because one nurse (PCF) oversees the care while the patient is admitted to that 12-bed area. It is *team nursing* because the same staff works together consistently and the PCF acts a team leader, assisting the team to adjust flexibly to the demands of each particular Twelve Bed Hospital. The model is also *modular*, in that it is confined to specific geographic regions of a patient care center. And the PCF acts as the primary *nursing case manager*, in the coordination of the discharge plan. With the help of the other team members, such as social workers' utilization review, or care managers focused on reimbursement for care, improved communication and efficiencies can result in improved length of stay and coordination. The PCF is accountable for their patients' care day and night. They carry beepers, allowing staff, patients, and families to have constant accessibility.

During a nursing retreat in fall 2002, the CNO presented a report to nursing leadership and others, including the CEO, on the early results of the newly named Twelve Bed Hospital on three nursing units. The idea of the model as a hospitalwide model emerged as the CNO presented, and spontaneous discussion from managers of the emergency department and critical care addressed applicability of the role within their specialties. As a result of this presentation and the reaction of the other specialty leaders, the CEO approached the

CNO about moving the model quickly to other areas of the hospital. An implementation plan was developed that spanned an additional 2 budget years, accommodating about 45 total positions (less offsets) when fully deployed. The return on investment for the cost of the model was the ability to focus a group of 45 people on achieving key clinical and operational organization objectives.

The CNO and other nursing leaders orchestrated the roll-out plan for the Twelve Bed Hospital beginning in 2003, and the model was fully implemented by late 2004. Nursing units that were exceptions to housewide implementation were inpatient rehabilitation, the interventional nursing areas, postacute care unit/surgery, radiation oncology, and diagnostic areas that employ nurses.

Perhaps one of the most compelling issues for this model as it has been replicated in other settings or has evolved around the development of the clinical nurse leader (CNL) role in more recent times is building the business case for the model. The CEO's and CNO's vision for the model is its alignment to key organizational goals. Key performance improvements around length of stay, patient throughput (11 AM discharge), core measure top decile performance, and 90th percentile satisfaction among patients, physicians, and staff are tracked to document the business case. In addition, an even more compelling case is made around patient safety metrics, in looking at improvements in nurse outcomes, avoidance of adverse patient outcomes, and improved continuity of communication between the patient, family, and the health care team.

As the model has evolved over the past few years, an increasing number of the PCFs have pursued master's preparation in nursing, either as CNLs, nurse practitioners, or specialists. With the transition of the role to expert generalists and advanced practice roles, additional benefits have been realized around improved coordination with hospitalists in patient care planning, application of complex adaptive theory and microsystems thinking, and concepts of transforming care at the bedside. The result is a landscape that is dramatically different and has forever changed the patient care experience at Baptist Hospital.

EVIDENCE-BASED PRACTICE

"How Well Do You Know Your Patients?"

Potter, P. & Mueller, J. R. (2007): Nursing Management 38*(2),* *40–48.*

Experts warn that when nurses work in situations where it is impossible to sufficiently "know" patients, nursing is reduced to a technology and loses its ground as a practice. In this environment, nurses are also unable to see changing relevance, recognize early warnings, or protect patients from threats to their well-being. This undermines the foundation for safe and astute nursing care. The concept of "knowing the patient" refers to the therapeutic decision making that enables registered nurses (RNs) to individualize patient care. "Knowing the patient" has been explored through qualitative research to reveal two components: a nurse's understanding of a patient and the selection of individualized interventions. It has also been found through research that the working relationships between RNs and patient care technicians (PCTs) are critical to the delivery of care. It is known that nurse understaffing is a major public health issue that affects patient outcomes and nurse retention. Nurse administrators need to ask themselves whether their staffing levels, work environment, and delivery of care design promote nurses' ability to know their patients.

One acute care Midwestern medical center envisioned developing and instituting a new delivery of care model. The goals were to improve the ability of RNs and PCTs to better know patients, to create a more professional care environment, and to improve the quality of patient care. The model included the following:

- A 1:1 RN/PCT assignment was implemented.
- RNs and PCTs conducted patient rounds together. This increased the RN's time at the bedside and improved the socialization of PCTs to the RN role.
- During rounds, the goals for the day were determined and communicated via a board in the patient's room to the patient, family, and other members of the health care team.
- Change-of-shift reports now included the PCTs.
- A clinical nurse specialist was added to the staff to act as a mentor to the care model.

Each RN was assigned to a single PCT during a shift of care. However, if staffing did not allow for each RN to have a PCT, RNs without PCTs were given a lighter assignment.

There was extensive education provided to the staff before implementation. This included a 4-hour in-service for PCTs and RNs. A video titled "Knowing the Patient" was viewed, and conflict management, assessment skills, and end-of-shift reporting were stressed. Team-building classes were provided, and each session covered the elements of good teamwork as well as barriers to avoid when working as a team. Measurement tools were created for both patient and provider; they were used 3 months before implementation and then monthly or quarterly.

The model was successful as long as the 1:1 RN/PCT assignments could be maintained. Staff perceived better working relationships and an improvement in being able to know who to go to for information. RNs reported a better sense of understanding their patients' needs and anticipating priorities for the day. PCTs were better able to prioritize and complete care activities. Staff satisfaction increased and stress levels decreased.

This care delivery model gives nurses a means to form important relational connections with patients as well as other caregivers so that more effective priority setting and decision making can occur.

NCLEX® EXAM QUESTIONS

1. In a team nursing delivery model, the nurse would have the following assignment:
   1. total care for a select group of patients
   2. responsibility for a particular function, such as medications
   3. an oversight role for care delivered by self and staff
   4. a combination role integrating financial and insurance decisions

2. The type of patient care in which the nurse caring for the patient makes most decisions is:
   1. functional
   2. team
   3. case management
   4. total patient care

3. The most flexible model of patient care, which can include a variety of skill mixes, is:
   1. team
   2. functional
   3. case management
   4. primary

4. The fundamental elements of any patient care delivery system combine clinical decision making with:
   1. leadership style
   2. work allocation
   3. nursing productivity
   4. patient acuity

5. A decentralized leadership structure would be one that allows decision making:
   1. at senior levels
   2. by the board of trustees
   3. at point of care
   4. by all involved

6. You are a nurse working in a primary care model. You are presently working during a snowstorm. Your staff has been cut in half. You need to change the manner in which you assign patient care. One method of care delivery that might assist is:
   1. case management
   2. team nursing
   3. modular nursing
   4. functional nursing

7. The difference between management and leadership is that leadership:
   1. organizes and assigns staff
   2. plans and budgets
   3. motivates and inspires
   4. controls and problem solves

8. In a leadership role, a chief nurse executive would:
   1. manage day-to-day operations
   2. create a long-term vision of patient care
   3. work to increase patient satisfaction
   4. supervise the work of all patient care

9. Which of the following roles is the charge nurse applying when assigning unlicensed assistive personnel to tasks such as vital signs, measuring intake and output, and bathing on the unit?
   1. Accountability
   2. Responsibility
   3. Delegation
   4. Prioritization

10. The nurse manager is planning a meeting with the staff members on group process. Which of the following functional roles should be discussed?
    1. Each group needs an individual with responsibility to coordinate and maintain records.
    2. An effective team needs a spokesperson.
    3. The group needs to have equal roles with no leader.
    4. The team rallies around group leader.

Answers: 1. 3   2. 4   3. 4   4. 2   5. 3   6. 4   7. 3   8. 2   9. 3   10. 1

REFERENCES

American Organization of Nurse Executives. (2006). *AONE competencies for nurse managers and nurse executives*. Chicago: Author.

American Organization of Nurse Executives. (February 2005). *AONE nurse executive competencies: nurse leader*. Chicago: Author.

Anderson, C., & Hughes, E. (1993). Implementing modular nursing in a long term facility. *Journal of Nursing Administration, 23*(6), 23-35.

Batson, V. (2004). Shared governance in an integrated health care system. *AORN Online, 80*(3), 493-514.

Bennis, W., & Nanus, B. (1985, 1997). *Leaders: the strategies for taking charge*. New York: Harper and Row.

Case Management Society of America (CMSA). (2002). *Standards of practice for case management* (2nd ed.). Little Rock, AK: Author.

Gardner, K. (1991). A summary of findings of five year comparison study of primary and team nursing. *Nursing Research, 40*(2), 113-117.

Kotter, J. (1990). A Force for Change: How Leadership differs from management. In J. Kotter (Ed.), (1996) *Leading Change*. Boston. MA: Harvard Business School.

Kouzes & Posner (2002). *The Leadership Challenge*. San Francisco, CA: Jossey Bass.

Manthey, M. (1990). Definitions and basic elements of a patient care delivery system with an emphasis on primary nursing. In G. Meyer, M. Madden, & E. Lawrence (Eds.). *Patient care delivery models* (pp. 201-211). Rockville, MD: Aspen.

O'Connor, S. E. (1994). A re-organization that improves patient care: an evaluation of team nursing in acute clinical setting. *Professional Nurse, 9*, 808-811.

O'Connor, B., Bennett, M., Crawford, S., & Korfiatis, V. (2006). The trials and tribulations of team nursing. *Collegian, 13*(3), 11-17.

Porter-O'Grady, T. (2001). Is shared governance still relevant? *Journal of Nursing Administration, 31*, 468-473.

Reverby, S. (1987). *Ordered to care: the dilemma of American nursing 1850-1945*. Cambridge: Cambridge University Press.

Sherman, R. (1990). Team nursing revisited. *Journal of Nursing Administration, 20*(11), 43-46.

Tiedman, M., & Lookinland, S. (2004). Traditional models of care delivery: what have we learned? *Journal of Nursing Administration, 34*(6), 291-297.

Yoder-Wise, P. S. (2007). *Leading and managing in nursing* (4th ed.). St. Louis: Mosby.

CHAPTER 2

Communication in the Work Environment

Chapter Objectives

1. Identify the principles of good communication.
2. Discuss the importance of good communication in the management of care.
3. Identify various means of communication used in health care.
4. Review the components of a change-of-shift report.
5. Discuss SBAR communication and its use in health care.
6. Identify principles of communication when dealing with patients/families and staff members.
7. Review communication principles when dealing with conflict resolution.

Definitions

Communication Process by which information is shared between and among individuals

Computerized physician order entry Process by which clinician orders are entered through electronic information systems

SBAR Template for communication among professionals that includes communication about Situation, Background, Assessment, and Recommendation

Change-of-shift report Process by which patient information is shared by nurses who have taken care of the patient for the previous shift and are reporting to the incoming caregivers

COMMUNICATION

Communication forms the basic principle when managing and coordinating care. Much of what nurses do needs to be communicated to the patient, family, and fellow staff members. Professional communication sets the tone of our management style and often the tone of the unit in which we work. Communication and the lack of a consistent process for communication of patient condition have been cited as variables in the number of medical errors that occur in hospitals. A recommendation of the Institute of Medicine calls for hospitals to "develop a working culture in which communication flows freely" (1999, p. 180).

Sullivan and Decker (1992) note five principles of effective communication:

- Giving information is not the same as communication, which requires interaction, understanding, and response. For example, if a nurse asks a staff member to do something but the staff member does not understand, information has been given but communication has not occurred.

- The sender of the communication is responsible for clarity. Nurses as well as nurse managers must make sure that their communication is clear—it is not the job of the receiver of the message "to translate." If the receiver of the message has to translate the message, the possibility of error increases. For example, if you expect the unlicensed nursing personnel to report back to you immediately if a patient's temperature increases, you need to specifically say just that.
- Use simple, exact language. The sender of the message needs to use words that are easily understood by the receiver of the communication. The words need to be precise and unambiguous. A word about e-mail communication—"I" message language is inappropriate...professional e-mail needs to avoid the use of all slang and shortcuts.
- Communication encourages feedback. Although feedback is not always positive, it is essential for making sure that the receiver understands the message. It is not enough to ask, "Did you understand?" because the answer may be an automatic "yes" because the receiver expects that is what you want to hear. Feedback can be verbal ("I do not understand what you said") or nonverbal (rolling of eyes when asked to do a task).
- Sender must have credibility. A credible sender is perceived as trustworthy and reliable. Receivers who think the sender is not reliable may ignore the message.
- Use direct communication channels when possible. Direct communication (person to person, face to face, or in writing) is best because there is less chance of the message being distorted as it passes through senders. Face-to-face communication is preferred as it allows the sender to get immediate feedback about the message.

E-mail

In the new technological age, much of the interdepartmental and staff-to-staff communication involves electronic mail, or e-mail. Communication using such technology should follow the principles just stated but also needs to follow the basic principles of *e-mail netiquette*. Tschabitscher (2009) offers 10 rules for e-mail netiquette, which have been adapted as follows:

1. **Use e-mail the way you want everybody to use it:** Do not use it to send nonprofessional concerns.
2. **Take another look before you send the message:** Proofread your comments for appropriateness and confidentiality.
3. **Quote original messages properly in replies:** Make your e-mail replies easy to read by quoting in a useful manner.
4. **Avoid irony, sarcasm, and emotional tones in e-mail:** Keep the message objective.
5. **Clean up e-mails before forwarding them:** Forwarding e-mails is a great way of keeping track of a concern but make sure that the original idea is not lost.
6. **Send plain text e-mails**: Avoid fancy formatting of e-mails. Cutesy pictures are for personal, not professional, communication.
7. **Writing in all caps is shouting:** Caps are also difficult to read.
8. **Ask before you send large attachments:** Large attachments may clog e-mail systems.
9. **The use of "smileys" raises an alarm:** Avoid the use of emoticons, IM language, and Internet slang.
10. **Avoid "me, too" messages:** Content needs to be specific and complete.

(Adapted from *Top 26 Most Important Rules of Email Etiquette.* Copyright 2009 by Heinz Tschabitscher, http://email.about.com/od/emailnetiquette/tp/core_netiquette.htm. Used with permission.)

COMMUNICATION WITH PATIENTS AND STAFF

Nurses and nurse leaders also communicate with families and staff. Difficult situations often involve patients and staff and disagreements or complaints about the delivery of or assignments of care. According to Sullivan and Decker (1992), nurse leaders need to keep the following in mind when dealing with patient or staff issues:

- Patients and their families are customers and should be communicated to with honesty and respect. Even if the communication involves dealing with a complaint, the customer needs to receive prompt and tactful assistance. The same philosophy is appropriate for an employee—he or she is a stakeholder in the work environment and also requires honesty and respect in communication.

- Nurses need to find a balance between avoiding medical jargon that is too complex and using terms that are too simple and condescending. Paying attention to both verbal and nonverbal feedback will help nurse managers negotiate this challenge.
- Provide angry or upset customers or staff members a private, neutral place for communicating their concerns.
- When possible, if customers or stakeholders are not native speakers and/or are not fluent in English, try to provide interpreter service. For patients, professional interpreters (including those for American Sign Language) should be used. Unless it is an emergency, do not use family members, as the practice is a potential violation of patient privacy. Family members may also have an agenda that will bias their communication with the patient. Each hospital has specific regulations about patient translation and privacy regulations. When communicating to fellow employees with limited language skills, make sure that the message is clear and understood.
- Learn about cultural issues to be able to recognize communication issues with both patients and staff members that are culturally based. Culturally competent responses to patients and fellow staff greatly enhance communication.

There are many modes of communication in the health care organization. One mode is used to *communicate with* the patient and family. Much of the nursing curricula have been spend on the theories and principles of professional and therapeutic communication. The Joint Commission (2007) also has some very specific regulations dealing with patient/family communication and the necessity of open and honest communication. It is crucial that patients and families understand the communication that is directed toward them. Cultural competence in communication is a vital skill of every nurse.

Another mode of communication deals with communication *about the patient*. Hospitals are institutions that are operational on a 24-hours/7-days-a-week basis and therefore require communication processes that are sound and reliable with which to communicate vital patient information. The communication processes also need to follow Health Insurance Portability and Accountability Act (HIPAA) guidelines (see Chapter 7). Processes that are used in the communication of patient care include transcription of orders, change-of-shift report, and SBAR (**S**ituation, **B**ackground, **A**ssessment, **R**ecommendation) reporting.

COMMUNICATION ABOUT THE PATIENT—TRANSCRIPTION OF ORDERS

The creation of physicians' and nursing orders in patient care forms the basis of the therapeutic regimen for the patient. This was often divided into two processes: the transcription of the physician's orders and the creation of the nursing care plan. Both of these documents need to be communicated effectively to all members of the health care team. Historically, the nurse has been responsible and accountable for the transcription process. This accountability was and remains documented by the nurse "signing off" the order as it is transcribed. With the increasing use of computerized physician order entry (CPOE), the role of the nurse in the transcription process is changing (Box 2-1). The order is transmitted directly by the physician or

---

Box 2-1   IMPACT OF COMPUTERIZED PHYSICIAN ORDER ENTRY

Handwritten orders have become a thing of the past for patients and their caregivers in the John Dempsey Hospital (UConn Health Center, Farmington, CT) intensive care and cardiac step-down units, where an electronic system for entering physicians' orders was recently adopted. The system, introduced on a pilot basis on one of the surgical floors last spring, is designed to improve patient safety and reduce medical errors.

"The electronic physician order entry system not only eliminates handwriting and transcription errors, it provides many online alerts and warnings for clinical caregivers, and distributes orders as they are written directly and immediately to ancillary units," says Roberta Luby, assistant vice president for information technology strategic projects, who supervised the rollout. "The process is much safer and more streamlined."

When a physician orders a medication for a patient with the new electronic system, the order goes to the pharmacy with no manual intervention.

Goodenough, K. (2007). Electronic system for physician orders improves patient safety. *UConn Advance*, April 23, 2007.

practitioner to the specific patient department and is automatically placed on the order sheets. A new order alert is highlighted on the computer system when a new order is entered. These orders are then integrated with the existing therapeutic regimen that is part of the computerized record. The electronic medical record is further discussed in Chapter 11.

In agencies where there is no CPOE, it will be important to follow the policy for transcription of orders. Each institution has specific guidelines dealing with the transcription of orders and one must be familiar with institution's guidelines. A sample policy for the transcription of orders is shown in Figure 2-1.

The communication of these orders to all caregivers is the responsibility of the nurse. The order needs to be communicated directly to others as it was entered. The manner in which these orders are communicated varies, but many institutions use a nursing care plan, medication/therapeutic orders, and nursing flow sheet to communicate the plan of care. These plans are also communicated via the change-of-shift report.

COMMUNICATION ABOUT THE PATIENT—CHANGES IN CONDITION

Nurses are also expected to communicate *changes in patient conditions* to the team caring for the patient. This communication may be made to the physician to receive a new set of medical orders or to members of the health care team to update them on a patient's condition or to a rapid response team. SBAR is a communication mechanism useful for framing any conversation, especially those requiring a rapid response from a clinician (Institute for Healthcare Improvement, 2007). Figure 2-2 shows a template for an SBAR report to a physician, which can be used in a number of situations requiring communication about a patient's condition.

The following guidelines need to be followed:
1. Before calling the physician, follow these steps:
   * Have I seen and assessed the patient myself before calling?
   * Has the situation been discussed with the nursing coordinator?
   * Review the chart for the appropriate physician to call.
   * Know the admitting diagnosis and date of admission.
   * Have I read the most recent physician's progress notes and notes from the nurse who worked the shift before me?

* Have available the following when speaking with the physician:
   * Patient's chart
   * List of current medications, allergies, intravenous fluids, and labs
   * Most recent vital signs
   * Reporting lab results: provide the date and time test was done and results of previous tests for comparison
   * Code status
2. When calling the physician, follow the SBAR process:
   (S) Situation: What is the situation you are calling about?
   * Identify self, unit, patient, and room number.
   * Briefly state the problem, what is it, when it happened or started, and the severity.
   (B) Background: Pertinent background information related to the situation could include the following:
   * Admitting diagnosis and date of admission
   * List of current medications, allergies, intravenous fluids, and labs
   * Most recent vital signs
   * Lab results: provide the date and time test was done and results of previous tests for comparison
   * Other clinical information
   * Code status
   (A) Assessment: What is the nurse's assessment of the situation?
   (R) Recommendation: What is the nurse's recommendation, or what does he or she want?
   Examples:
   * Notification that patient has been admitted
   * Patient needs to be seen now
   * Order change
3. Document the change in the patient's condition and physician notification.

COMMUNICATION ABOUT THE PATIENT—CHANGE OF SHIFT

Change-of-shift reports vary across institutions. The purposes of the report are to exchange information that is necessary for future patient care and to discuss the present status of the patient. These reports occur during the overlapping time between shifts. They occur in a variety of ways, with the most common being (1) change-of-shift meetings where the outgoing and

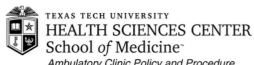

TEXAS TECH UNIVERSITY
HEALTH SCIENCES CENTER
School *of* Medicine™
Ambulatory Clinic Policy and Procedure

Title: **ORDERS, RECEIVING AND NOTING**	Policy Number: **3.04**
Regulation Reference: **JCAHO: PC.4.10, NPSG #2**	Effective Date: **12/2007**

Policy Statement:

It is the policy of TTUHSC SOM Clinics to accurately transcribe orders and to implement the orders correctly and efficiently. Orders transcription may be done by a RN or LVN.

Scope and Distribution:

This policy applies and will be distributed to all TTUHSC School of Medicine Clinics, also known as Texas Tech Physicians.

Procedure:

1. Who May Give or Write Orders

   Only licensed providers (attending physician, consultant, fellow, resident, physician assistant or nurse practitioner) may give or write orders. Orders written by medical students will not be honored by the nursing staff or ancillary personnel unless validated/countersigned by a licensed physician.

2. Verbal and Telephone Orders

   Verbal orders, except telephone orders, will be accepted in emergencies or when it is not practical for the physician to write the order. Orders must be given to an RN or LVN.

   - The RN or LVN should record the order directly onto a clinic progress note, labeled "T.O" or "V.O."
   - The RN or LVN should **read back** what has been written to the ordering physician, validating the accuracy of the order.

   The verbal order and documentation should include:

   - Date and time received
   - Patient name, age, weight (when appropriate)
   - Drug name
   - Dosage form
   - Exact strength or concentration
   - Dose frequency and route
   - Purpose indication (as appropriate)

3. Registered Nurse or Licensed Vocational Nurse

   a. Reviews orders and identifies those needing immediate attention
   b. Documents final validation or orders by signing first initial, last name, title, date, and time (as appropriate to clinic documentation).
   c. The order should be signed by the physician or practitioner as soon as possible.

Approval Authority:

This policy shall be recommended for approval by the Joint SOM Policy Committee to the Regional Deans with final signatory authority by both Deans, School of Medicine, Lubbock and El Paso.

Responsibility and Revisions:

It is the responsibility of the Joint SOM Policy Committee to review and initiate necessary revisions based on collaboration and input by and through Quality Improvement/Performance Improvement and Risk Management. Administrative and technical management of this policy, including web site maintenance, will be the responsibility of the Lubbock Office of Performance Improvement.

Policy Number: 3.04	Original Approval Date: 4/2002
Version Number: 3	Effective Date: 12/2007
Signatory approval on file by: Steven L. Berk, MD Dean, School of Medicine Jose Manuel De La Rosa, M.D. Founding Dean, School of Medicine, El Paso	

Figure 2-1 • Sample policy for transcription of orders. Texas Tech University Health Sciences Center. (2007). Orders, receiving and noting. Policy No. 3.04. Retrieved November 30, 2007, from www.ttuhsc.edu/som/clinic/policies/ACPolicy3.04.pdf.

S	**Situation**
	I am calling about <u><patient name and location></u>
	The patient's code status is <u><code status></u>
	The problem I am calling about is_____
	    I am afraid the patient is going to arrest
	
	I have just assessed the patient personally:
	
	Vital signs are: Blood pressure_____/_____Pulse_____ Respiration_____Temperature_____
	
	I am concerned about the:
	    Blood pressure because it is over 200 or less than 100 or 30 mmHg below usual
	    Pulse because it is over 140 or less than 50
	    Respiration because it is less than 5 or over 40
	    Temperature because it is less than 96 or over 104

B	**Background**
	The patient's mental status is:
	    Alert and oriented to person place and time
	    Confused and cooperative or non-cooperative
	    Agitated or combative
	    Lethargic but conversant and able to swallow
	    Comatose, eyes closed, not responding to stimulation
	The skin is:
	    Warm and dry
	    Pale
	    Mottled
	    Diaphoretic
	    Extremities are cold
	    Extremities are warm
	The patient is not or is on oxygen
	    The patient has been on _____ (l/min) or (percent) oxygen for _____ minutes (hours)

A	**Assessment**
	    This is what I think the problem is: <u><say what you think is the problem></u>
	    The problem seems to be Cardiac infection neurologic respiratory
	    I am not sure what the problem is, but the patient is deteriorating
	    The patient seems to be unstable and may get worse, we need to do something

R	**Recommendation**
	I suggest or request that you <u><say what you would like to see done></u>
	    Transfer the patient to critical care
	    Come to see the patient at this time
	    Talk to the patient or family about code status
	    Ask the on-call family practice resident to see the patient now
	    Ask for a consultant to see the patient now
	Are any tests needed:
	    Do you need any tests like CXR ABG EKG CBC or BMP?
	    Others?
	If a change in treatment is ordered then ask:
	    How often do you want vital signs?
	    How long do you expect this problem will last?
	    If the patient does not get better, when would you want us to call again?

Figure 2-2 • SBAR report to physician about a critical situation. Institute for Healthcare Improvement (2007). *SBAR technique for communication: a situational briefing model.* Retrieved March 30, 2009, from http://www.ihi.org/IHI/Topics/ PatientSafety/SafetyGeneral/Tools/SBARTechniqueforCommunicationASituationalBriefingModel.htm.

the incoming nurses meet face to face for a review of the pertinent information; (2) tape-recorded reports in which the outgoing nurse "reports" all pertinent information to the incoming nurse; and (3) "walking" reports where the incoming and the outgoing nurses "walk" to the patient room and report the pertinent information while observing the patient.

There are advantages and disadvantages to each form of change-of-shift report. The face-to-face meetings and walking reports allow for questions to be exchanged between the nurses. The walking report also has the added advantages of both nurses assessing the patient's situation and of patient participation. Both of these face-to-face reports, however, can be costly if they are not completed in a timely manner. The taped report can be a more efficient way to impart the necessary information, but there is little opportunity for questioning and sharing of information, which may be important to the plan of care.

Regardless of the type of change-of-shift report, there are some pointers that may assist the incoming nurse.
1. Report vital information—allergies, code status, diagnosis, critical laboratory values, and family and medical team information.
2. Review current status and therapeutics of the patient—This may be done in a systems approach (head to toe) or using an organization-specific report document.
3. Discuss upcoming plans—This is important so the incoming nurse can prepare for events, such as a patient who is going for an examination and needs to be NPO.
4. Review discharge plan as appropriate.
5. Discuss any other information pertinent to the patient's care—This may include family responses to care and results of multidisciplinary team meetings.

The report is a vital link in the communication of patient status and needs. It is a crucial time to communicate accurate information about the patient status and the plan of care. One of the most frequent errors in shift report is the omission of critically important safety information. A change-of-shift report may be given orally in person, by audiotape recording, or during walking-planning rounds at the patient's bedside. Many hospitals are moving toward the use of walking reports (in the patient room) at the end of shifts. This type of change-of-shift reporting allows the incoming nurse to assess the patient situation and to ask ques-

tions of the outgoing nurse based on the assessment. It also allows the patient to participate and to confirm what the outgoing nurse is communicating.

There are several options for organizing the information that one passes on to the next shift. Some hospitals have templates for the report that are used by all staff members. SBAR is used in some institutions. Some institutions organize the report according to body systems—the report is presented based on the patient's body systems. Some organize the report on a "head-to-toe" assessment. Some report by exception—focusing solely on variances or patient problems. No matter what style of report is used, it should be done professionally using the guidelines given in Table 2-1.

CONFLICT RESOLUTION

Conflict resolution among staff members or patients and families is a challenging part of the profession. The resolution process includes using the principles of negotiation, which can result in one group winning or both groups winning. In situations where the outcome is a win/win result for both sides, collaboration and negotiation are required.

In dealing with conflict resolution, the following communication principles apply (adapted from Jones, 2007, p. 214):
- Identify who is involved in or who is the source of the conflict.
- Identify interests and clarify issues.
- Build mutual trust.
- Separate the individuals from the conflict.
- Stay in the present; avoid dwelling in the past.
- Avoid placing blame.
- Remain focused on the identified issues.
- Discover options.
- Develop outcomes.
- Come to a consensus.

Remember that, as a nurse, you will communicate information about patients to staff and to families so that all team members can make appropriate decisions about patient care. It is important that all forms of communication are timely, accurate, and relevant.

ORGANIZATION-WIDE COMMUNICATION

The last type of communication is organization-wide communication. Organization-wide communication

Table 2-1	COMPARISON OF DO'S AND DON'TS OF CHANGE-OF-SHIFT REPORT
Do's	**Don'ts**
Provide only essential background information about the client (name, age, sex, physician's diagnosis, medical history, allergies).	Don't review all routine care procedures or tasks (e.g., bathing scheduled changes).
Identify the client's nursing diagnosis or health care problems and their related causes.	Don't review all biographical information already available in written form.
Describe objective measurements or observations about client's condition and response to health problem; emphasize recent changes.	Don't use critical comments about a client's behavior, such as, "Mrs. Willis is so demanding."
Share significant information about family members as it relates to client's problems.	Don't make assumptions about relationships between family members.
Continuously review ongoing discharge plan (e.g., need for resources, client's level of preparation to go home).	Don't engage in idle gossip.
Relay to staff significant changes in the way therapies are given (e.g., different position for pain relief, new medication).	Don't describe the basic steps of a procedure.
Describe instructions given in teaching plans and the client's response.	Don't explain detailed content unless staff members ask for clarification.
Evaluate results of nursing or medical care measures (e.g., effect of back rub or analgesic administration).	Don't simply describe results as "good" or "poor." Be specific.
Be clear about priorities to which oncoming shift must attend.	Don't force oncoming staff to guess what to do first.

Adapted from Potter, P. A., & Perry, A. G. (2008). *Fundamentals of nursing*, ed. 7. St. Louis, MO: Mosby.

occurs in many formats. Formal communication about changes in practice, policy, and other important institution-wide activities often occurs formally through newsletters, intranet communication, formal education, or other methods of structured communication. Such formal communication usually is governed by the organizational culture and is defined by a specific flow. That is, the communication is directed to the specific individuals and groups that need the communication. A change is nursing policy is communicated from the nursing practice council to the care unit and then to the individual nurses. This top-to-bottom communication often follows defined distribution channels. Formal communication also occurs from the bottom up. Health care organizations have methods of collecting information from point-of-care workers that is delivered up the chain of command. It is important for all employees to know the chain of command. Employees are expected to respect the chain of command. For example, if a staff nurse has a concern, she is to communicate it to the person who is next in the chain of command, her immediate supervisor. The supervisor then brings the communication up the chain of command. The chain of command follows the organizational structure of the organization. Some of this formal information may take the form of data collection through the use of employee surveys, customer complaints, budget requests, or strategic planning information. This information is further discussed in Chapters 12 and 14.

Informal communication also occurs in all institutions. Informal communication occurs in many situations, but it often occurs with individuals who are not part of the organizational hierarchy. Nurses often talk during breaks about patient conditions, suggestions for plans of care, and policies and procedures. The content may be perceived as formal, but the actual communication is occurring in a nonstructured setting. Another type of informal communication is the "grapevine." Communication that occurs via the grapevine occurs outside of the traditional formal structures. A challenge with grapevine communication is that it is often altered as it moves across the grapevine. Another concern about informal communication is its lack of defined lines of communication. Information communicated via an informal network may not reach all parties.

Therefore, it is vital that information about the patient, staff policies and rules, and any information that is necessary for practice be communicated via a formal structure so that receipt of the information can be validated.

SUMMARY

Good communication is essential to the operations of all patient care activities. Communication occurs among staff and patients and families, from staff to staff, and among departments. Professional communication forms the basis for the delivery of patient care from shift to shift and from staff member to staff member. The communication needs to be timely, efficient, correct, and respectful, and it needs to be delivered to all in need of the information and understood by those who receive it.

CLINICAL CORNER

SBAR as a Communication Tool

Beverly S. Karas-Irwin

The communication of patient handoffs—end-of-shift report, which transfers information to the next provider of care—can cause problems. It is a challenge to provide pertinent, accurate information in this age of multiple patient diagnoses, with a multitude of over-the-counter and prescription medications, multiple practitioners, and advanced technology, without omission of crucial information that would be potentially harmful to the patient's safety.

One of the 2009 Joint Commission Patient Safety Goals is to improve the effectiveness of communication among caregivers in managing the handoff of communication. To comply with this expectation, a standard communication tool needs to be adopted by organizations so that all involved in patient care are speaking and listening in the same framework.

In December 2006, the Patient Care Services Department of the Valley Hospital in Ridgewood, New Jersey, embarked on an initiative to set a department goal to implement a standardized communication tool. SBAR (situation, background, assessment, and recommendation) was adopted. This communication tool is a structured framework that ensures all parties have the same mental model. The tool was first developed in the armed forces to try to standardize communication and has since been adapted for use in various other industries. Many health care organizations have adopted the tool to improve end-of-shift report and patient handoffs.

SBAR allows all parties to have a common expectation—to focus on the problem, not the people. It takes the emotional component out of the exchange.

An overview of SBAR:

Situation: stating the problem

Background: brief statement or statements related to the problem

Assessment: judgment, what was identified

Recommendation: what you want done/what needs to be the outcome

To have staff incorporate this into their daily practice, leadership must first incorporate this tool into their daily practice and role model. SBAR was incorporated into the computerized documentation screens and procedural checklist, and a standard template was developed for end-of-shift report. SBAR was incorporated into rounds and was used to relay information and change of practice in emails. During daily rounds, managers need to observe peer-to-peer reports and recognize staff for the use of SBAR. As one becomes more comfortable, one will not only speak in SBAR but also listen in SBAR! The staff should receive assistance in framing information as they struggle to become comfortable with the SBAR format.

The benefits of SBAR are improved communication, both written and oral. SBAR provides a clear, accurate feedback of information between caregivers. There is a reduction in the omission of information during handoffs. Staff should always be encouraged to recommend solutions when they identify a problem area; this empowers staff and increases staff satisfaction, enhancing the workplace environment and reducing stress.

Shift Report Redesign: A Midwest Medical Center Uses Server-Based Telephone Technology to Streamline Shift Reporting.

Brown, E. Victor Health Management Technology, August 1, 2007. Brown, E. Victor. (2007, August 1). Shift report redesign: a midwest medical center uses server-based phone technology to streamline shift reporting. The Free Library. (2007). Retrieved April 28, 2009 from http://www.thefreelibrary.com/Shift report redesign: a midwest medical center uses server-based...-a0167345215

Provena Saint Joseph Medical Center (PSJMC) in Joliet, Illinois, is an acute care hospital with more than 24,000 admissions yearly. CNO Kathy Mikos and other managers decided to solve the dilemma of lengthy shift handoff reporting. According to Mikos, PSJMC has large nursing units consisting of 53 to 55 beds. The reporting system that has been used was verbal and was a lengthy process that was often noisy and chaotic. Mikos became committed to finding a way to standardize and streamline this process.

PSJMC decided to work with The White Stone Group (TWSG) on integrating a voice technology system into shift handoff reporting. They used a process improvement model that allowed them to evaluate the process and then make rapid changes if needed, reevaluate, and continue to make those process improvements quickly.

After multiple revisions, the system was installed and integrated into the telephone technology rather than a stand-alone recorder. Prompts were built in that nurses thought would provide the necessary consistency, such as code status. Nurses were given PIN numbers to access the system and a 10-minute individual training session. Landlines and the institution's wireless patient-to-caregiver telephone system could be used. Education was further reinforced with the distribution of individual reference cards.

Improvements and refinements could be made almost daily due to the collaborative effort between staff and TWSG. This proved to be great for staff morale and "buy in." There could be immediate action on their feedback. The nurse preparing to end a shift could complete patient reports anytime that was convenient. Night shift nurses could also do this before things got too hectic around 6 AM. When the day shift comes onto the unit, they can retrieve the report while the nighttime nurse is still taking care of the patients. There is time allotted for the oncoming nurse to ask questions and interact with the off-going nurses. After a nurse gives report, she can go back into the system if a patient's status changes and create an addendum to the report. Case managers will soon be able to facilitate the discharge process by leaving pertinent information for the registered nurses in their reports. Furthermore, the unit manager's messages for the entire unit can now be broadcast to every nurse at the beginning of his or her shift. In addition, a preceptor or mentor of a new nurse can review the quality of her reports, critique them, and provide constructive feedback.

PSJMC is approaching their 2-year anniversary with the system they have named OptVox. They report having reduced the time of the handoff process from 60 to 90 minutes for a nurse with a five- or six-patient assignment to just 15 minutes. They are currently introducing the SBAR reporting methodology into the already successful process. The SBAR prompts require the nurse to describe the patient's medical situation and background information, which is followed by recent assessment and recommendation. They are now focusing on expanding the system to allow for multidisciplinary access. This will provide other members of the health care team the opportunity to contribute pertinent information through the OptVox system. The hope is that in the near future, family members will be given a PIN number to access a *Family Link* that will assist them in remaining connected and updated on the patient's progress.

According to Mikos, PSJMC has been able to show a yearly savings of nearly $120,000 from reducing overtime related to shift reporting. This alone has easily paid for the system in 1 year.

NCLEX® EXAM QUESTIONS

1. The communication process is essential to the leader or manager role and to the client's care. Effective communication is crucial. As a nurse, you understand that messages are:
   1. native and foreign
   2. verbal and nonverbal
   3. coded and encoded
   4. clear and unclear

2. Nurse leaders need to keep all of the following in mind when dealing with patient or staff issues *except:*
   1. Patients and their families are customers and should be communicated to with honesty and respect.
   2. Nurses should always use medical jargon in explanations.
   3. Provide angry or upset customers or staff members a private, neutral place for communicating their concerns.
   4. When possible, if customers or stakeholders are not native speakers and/or not fluent in English, try to provide interpreter service.

3. The electronic physician order entry system:
   1. prevents all medication errors
   2. provides many online alerts and warnings for clinical caregivers
   3. poses problems when the system is done
   4. is not the most acceptable type of physician's orders

4. SBAR stands for:
   1. **S**ituation, **B**ackground, **A**ssessment, **R**ecommendation
   2. **S**ituation, **B**ackground, **A**ssessment, **R**eaction
   3. **S**ituation, **B**ackground, **A**ssessment, **R**eply
   4. **S**ituation, **B**ackground, **A**ction, **R**ecommendation

5. When calling the physician and following the SBAR process, which of the following items is included under the Situation criteria?
   1. Identify the patient's ethnicity and religious affiliation.
   2. Briefly state the problem, what is it, when it happened or started, and its severity.

3. Inform the physician regarding the patient's roommates.
   4. Describe patient's mental status.

6. Regarding the SBAR process, pertinent Background information related to the situation includes:
   1. socioeconomic status of the family
   2. list of current medications, allergies, intravenous fluids, and laboratory results
   3. patient's dietary needs before hospitalization
   4. family history of disease

7. One of the most frequent errors in a change-of-shift report is the omission of:
   1. critically important safety information
   2. site of the intravenous line
   3. diagnosis of the patient
   4. last dose of pain medication

8. A change-of-shift report may be given:
   1. orally in person, by audiotape recording, or during walking-planning rounds at the patient's bedside
   2. orally in person only
   3. orally in person or by audiotape recording only
   4. during walking-planning rounds at the patient's bedside only

9. Which of the following is on the list of "do's" regarding the change-of-shift report?
   1. Provide essential background information about the patient.
   2. Identify the patient's discharge plans.
   3. Share significant information about family friends.
   4. Discuss every routine order for the patient.

10. Which of the following is on the list of "don'ts" regarding the change-of-shift report?
    1. Share significant information about family members.
    2. Relay to staff significant changes in the way therapies are given.
    3. Continuously review ongoing discharge plan.
    4. Review all routine care procedures.

Answers: 1. 2   2. 2   3. 2   4. 1   5. 2   6. 2   7. 1   8. 1   9. 1   10. 4

REFERENCES

Goodenough, K. (2007). Electronic system for physician orders improves patient safety. *UConn Advance*, April 23, 2007.

Institute for Healthcare Improvement. (2007). *SBAR technique for communication: a situational briefing model.* Retrieved March 30, 2009, from http://www.ihi.org/IHI/Topics/PatientSafety/SafetyGeneral/Tools/SBARTechniqueforCommunicationASituationalBriefingModel.htm.

Institute of Medicine. (1999). *To err is human.* Washington, DC: Author.

Jones, R. (2007). *Nursing leadership and management.* Philadelphia, PA: FA Davis.

Potter, P. A., & Perry, A. G. (2008). *Fundamentals of nursing*, ed. 7. St. Louis, MO: Mosby.

Sullivan, E., & Decker, P. (1992). *Effective management in nursing*, ed. 3. Redwood City, CA: Addison-Wesley Publishing.

Texas Tech University Health Sciences Center. (2007). Physician's orders, receiving and noting. Policy No. 3.04. Retrieved November 30, 2007, from www.ttuhsc.edu/som/clinic/policies/CPolicy3.04.pdf.

The Joint Commission. (2007). *Comprehensive Accreditation Manual: The Official handbook.* Update 2.

Tschabitscher, H. (2005). *Top ten most important rules of e-mail netiquette.* Retrieved June 16, 2008, from http://e-mail.about.com/cs/netiquettetips/tp/core_netiquette.htm.

CHAPTER 3

Delegation of Nursing Tasks

Chapter Objectives

1. Define *delegation.*
2. Identify the five rights of delegation.
3. Review the circumstances where delegation is appropriate.
4. Identify tasks appropriate for delegation.
5. Discuss the role of unlicensed personnel in the delivery of health care.
6. Identify the role of the nurse in the delegation of health care.
7. Review the legal ramifications of delegation of care.

Definitions

Accountability Acknowledgment and assumption of responsibility for actions, decisions, and policies within the scope of the role or employment position and encompassing the obligation to report, explain, and be answerable for resulting consequences

Delegation Transferring the authority to perform a selected nursing task in a selected situation to a competent individual

Assignment Delegation of work to a selected group of patient caregivers. The downward or lateral transfer of the responsibility of an activity from one individual to another while retaining accountability for the outcome

Supervision Active process of directing, guiding, and influencing the outcome of an individual's performance of an activity

Unlicensed assistive personnel Individuals who are not licensed by the state and are trained to assist nurses by performing patient care tasks as allowed by the organization. There are many job titles for such employees, such as nursing assistant (NA), patient care associate (PCA), and unlicensed assistive personnel (UAP)

Direct patient care activities Activities such as hygienic care, feeding patients, taking vital signs, and so on that are performed on the patient

Indirect patient care activities Routine activities of the patient unit that deal with the day-to-day functioning of the unit, such as restocking supplies

DELEGATION

Delegation is defined as the "transfer of responsibility for the performance of an activity from one individual to another while retaining accountability for the outcome. Example: the nurse, in delegating an activity to an unlicensed individual, transfers the responsibility for the performance of the activity but retains professional accountability for the overall care" (ANA, 1992). It is the entrusting of a selected nursing task to an individual who is qualified, competent, and able to perform such a task.

The majority of health care institutions have care delivery systems that include various levels of caregivers. The acuity of patients within hospitals has increased during the past 10 years, and many hospitals have moved from total patient care, primary care, and other care delivery systems that require an all–registered nurse staff. To meet the needs of the higher-acuity patients, nurses must delegate aspects of care to non–registered nurse team members. Delegation changes as the health care environment changes. Since the advent of the nursing shortage, unlicensed assistive personnel (UAP) have been used to help fill the workforce gaps. The role of these assistive personnel is defined by the institution that employs them and defines their practice. In addition to UAP, they are called **noncredentialed assistive personnel.** Individuals hired into these jobs are trained by the facility and by facility personnel and are evaluated by the facility. They may use a variety of titles, such as nursing assistant (NA), patient care associate (PCA), nursing technician, unit technician, and others (Carroll, 1998). They cannot practice nursing, and they must be directed, supervised, and evaluated by a registered nurse, who is ultimately responsible for all patient care (see Box 3-1 for the nurse's responsibility in delegation). One form of licensed personnel, the licensed practical nurse (LPN), is used by many facilities. The LPN works under the direction and supervision of the registered nurse. Licensed personnel work according to the state board regulations (see Chapter 7), but the job descriptions will vary from institution to institution. Sample job descriptions can be obtained at the websites listed in Table 3-1.

There are two types of nursing activities that may be delegated: direct patient care activities and indirect

Table 3-1	SAMPLE JOB DESCRIPTIONS

Director of Medical Surgical Services—http://www.hospitalsoup.com/public/jd-1-10.pdf

Licensed Practical Nurse—http://www.hr.duke.edu/jobs/descr_duhs/printer.php?ID=4086

Nursing Care Assistant I—http://www.hr.duke.edu/jobs/descr_duhs/printer.php?ID=4105

Nursing Care Assistant II—http://www.hr.duke.edu/jobs/descr_duhs/printer.php?ID=4106

RN Medical Surgical Unit—http://www.hospitalsoup.com/public/jd-1-111.pdf

Unit Services Coordinator—http://www.hr.duke.edu/jobs/descr_duhs/select.php?ID=4165

Unlicensed Assistive Personnel (Patient Care Technician)—http://www.hospitalsoup.com/public/aca-1-18.pdf

Box 3-1   NURSE'S RESPONSIBILITY IN DELEGATION

1. Prior to delegating a nursing task, the nurse shall determine the nursing care needs of the patient. The nurse shall retain responsibility and accountability for the nursing care of the patient, including nursing assessment, planning, evaluation, and nursing documentation.
2. Prior to the delegation of the nursing task to unlicensed assistive personnel, the nurse shall determine that the unlicensed person has been trained in the task and determined to be competent.

Criteria for Delegation

1. The delegated nursing task shall be a task that a reasonable and prudent nurse would find within the scope of sound nursing judgment and practice to delegate.
2. The delegated nursing task shall be a task that can be competently and safely performed by the unlicensed personnel without compromising the patient's safety.

3. The nursing task shall not require the unlicensed personnel to exercise independent nursing judgment or intervention.
4. The nurse shall be responsible for ensuring that the delegated task is performed in a competent manger by the unlicensed personnel.

Supervision

1. The nurse shall provide supervision of the delegated nursing task.
2. The degree of supervision required shall be determined by the nurse after an evaluation of the following factors:
   a. Stability and acuity of the patient's condition
   b. Training and competency of the unlicensed personnel
   c. Complexity of the nursing task being delegated
   d. Proximity and availability of the nurse to the unlicensed personnel when the nursing task is being performed

Adapted from State of Kentucky. (1999). Delegation of nursing tasks. KRS 311A.170, 314.011, 201 KAR 20:400. Retrieved July 2, 2007, from http://www.lrc.state.ky.us/kar/201/020/400.htm.

patient care activities. *Direct patient care activities* include activities such as assisting with feeding, grooming, hygienic care, taking vital signs, ambulation, electrocardiogram tracing, and measuring blood sugar levels. *Indirect patient care activities* are those activities that are routinely done to support the functioning of the patient care unit. Such activities include the restocking of supplies, the transport of patients, and clerical activities.

THE FIVE RIGHTS OF DELEGATION

The National Council of State Boards of Nursing (1997) has defined the Five Rights of Delegation, as follows:
1. Right task
2. Right circumstance
3. Right person
4. Right direction/communication
5. Right supervision

To assist you in reviewing these five rights, Box 3-2 will help you to determine if you are following these rights in your delegation (ANA and NCSBN, 2008).

RIGHT TASK

State boards of nursing relegate the nursing practice within each state. It is important for you to know the nurse practice act of the state in which you are practicing and to be aware of the delegation regulation within your state. In addition, most hospitals have policies that very carefully describe what nursing tasks can be delegated to whom. This is important, because you will see differing standards of delegation depending on the type of health care facility in which you practice. Many long-term care facilities assign LPNs as charge nurses, with registered nurses supervising that care. In ambulatory care settings, medical assistants play a major role in the delivery of care. Just because your institution uses patient care technicians to measure all vital signs and blood sugar levels and to make blood draws does not mean that all facilities can or do use such personnel. It is vital to know your institution's standard on delegation and the specific job descriptions and competencies of each level of personnel with whom you will be working. A sample hospital policy on delegation is shown in Figure 3-1. The scope of practice will vary from state to state, so this will vary across the country.

Box 3-2   THE FIVE RIGHTS OF DELEGATION

Right Task
- Has the nursing department established policies and standards consistent with the nurse practice act of the state and professional nursing standards?
- Are you aware of the specific polices and standards of your institution?
- Do you know to whom you can delegate what?
- Can this task be delegated to any staff, or only to certain staff?

Right Circumstance
- Are the setting and resources conducive to safe care?
- Do the job description and competency of the caregiver match the patient requirements?
- Do staff members understand how to do the task safely?
- Do staff members have the appropriate resources and equipments to carry out the task safety?
- Do staff members have the appropriate supervision to carry out the task safely?

Right Person
- Is the right person delegating the task, and is the right person being delegated to?

- Is the patient condition appropriate for the level of delegation?
- Does hospital policy and the nurse practice act of the state allow delegating this activity?
- Can you verify the knowledge and competency of the staff member to whom you are delegating a specific task?

Right Direction/Communication
- Have you clearly communicated the task? With directions, limits, and expected outcomes?
- Are the times for feedback specified in your assignment?
- Does the staff member understand what is to be done?
- Can the staff member ask questions as needed?

Right Supervision
- Will you be able to appropriately monitor and evaluate patient response to the delegated task?
- Will you be able to give feedback to the staff member if needed?

THE VALLEY HOSPITAL
Ridgewood, New Jersey

PATIENT CARE SERVICES (PCS) POLICY AND PROCEDURE

SUBJECT: Delegation – Nursing Tasks

POLICY:

1. In delegating selected nursing tasks to licensed practice nurses and other health care team members, the registered professional nurse shall be responsible for exercising that degree of judgment and knowledge reasonably expected to assure that a proper delegation has been made.

2. A registered professional nurse may not delegate the performance of a nursing task to persons who have not been adequately prepared by verifiable training and education and have not demonstrated the adequacy of their knowledge, skill and competency to perform the task being delegated.

3. A RN may not delegate non-PCA tasks to staff employed as PCA II or PCA I who are RNs from a foreign country or those enrolled in nursing school. In order to function/perform tasks that are approved under the scope of practice of a RN, staff must be licensed as a RN in New Jersey.

4. No task may be delegated which is within the scope of nursing practice and requires:
   a. The substantial knowledge and skill derived from completion of a nursing education program and the specialized skill, judgment and knowledge of a registered nurse; and
   b. An understanding of nursing principles necessary to recognize and manage complications which may result in harm to the health and safety of the patient.

WHO CAN PERFORM: RN

RESPONSIBILITY:

It is the responsibility of nursing leadership or management member, as appropriate to implement, maintain, evaluate, review and revise this policy.

APPROVED: Nurse Practice Education Council, January 10, 2003.

Beverly S. Karas-Irwin, RN
Chairperson, Nurse Practice Education Council

Linda C. Lewis, RN
Vice President, Paient Care Services

Figure 3-1 • Sample hospital policy on delegation. (With permission from Valley Hospital.)

Tasks which could be delegated based on patient condition and staff ability

TASK	PRACTICE ACT		REGULATORY		VALLEY POLICY	PRACTICE			
	RN	LPN	DOH	JCAHO		RN	LPN	PCA2	PCA1
Abdominal binders/breast binders, Apply					X	X	X	X	X
Advance Directive-determine intent					X	X			
Air casts to sprains/Strains, Apply						X	ED only		
Assess effects of teaching	X		X	X	X	X			
Assessment, Family	X		X	X	X	X			
Assessment, need fall protocol	X		X	X	X	X			
Assessment, Physical, patient	X		X	X	X	X			
Assessment, Psycho Social					X	X			
Assignments	X		X	X	X	X			
Bath, Sitz					X	X	X	X	X
Bed Making					X	X	X	X	X
Bili Lights					X	X	X		
Blood Transfusions					X	X			
Bowel Disimpaction					X	X	X		
Buddy tape to toes, Apply							ED only		
Call Lights					X	X	X	X	X
Care Plan – evaluate, update					X	X	X		
Care Plan – initiate	X		X	X	X	X			
Chest Pt.					X	X	X		
Chest Tube Drainage System:									
- Adjust amount of suction					X	X			
- Change drainage system					X	X			
- Maintain Water Seal					X	X	X		
- Measure/mark drainage					X	X	X		
Circumcision Care	X				X	X	X		
Code Cart Teach/Education, Check					X	X			
Cold/Heat, Apply					X	X	X	X	X
Communication					X	X	X	X	X
Cough/Deep Breath					X	X	X	X	X
Count Controlled Substances					X	X	X		
Crutch walking & crutch use, Demonstrate						X	ED only		
Douche					X	X	X		
Drains:									
- Biliary, measure output					X	X	X	X	
- Hemovac, empty/recharge					X	X	X		

Figure 3-1 • cont'd

RIGHT CIRCUMSTANCE

The right circumstance refers to the workplace. The circumstance is the context in which the delegation takes place. As stated earlier, an LPN will be performing different tasks under different circumstances. In a long-term facility, it is not unusual to have an LPN as "charge nurse" with a registered nurse covering multiple units for supervision. However, it would be unusual to have an LPN assigned as a "charge nurse" in an acute care facility with a high acuity of patients. There may be differences in extreme circumstances, such as disasters, but in such a situation, the right communication/direction needs to occur.

RIGHT PERSON

The requirement of the right person means that you must know the competency level, job description, individual level of skill, and education of the individual to whom you are delegating. Job descriptions will give you a broad view of what an individual is expected to do, but you must know the individual's capabilities, experience, attitude, and skills. A novice nurse will not have the competency that a nurse with 10 years of experience, a professional certification, and a clinical ladder position will have. It is also necessary to have knowledge of the individual strengths and weaknesses of each team member. A team member who just lost her mother to breast cancer may not be the best person to delegate to perform tasks for a patient with breast cancer.

THE RIGHT DIRECTION/ COMMUNICATION

The right direction/communication is required of the nurse as she delegates the task to a staff member. It is not enough to assign the task to a staff member; the staff member must know what is expected of him or her. "You will take Ms. Smith's temperature every hour starting at 8 AM, and report the temperature back to me immediately." If you tell the staff member to take the temperature every hour, he or she may not know when to start and may report a sudden increase in temperature to you because he or she has not been trained to determine when an independent nursing action is needed. Your directions must follow the 4Cs—be clear, concise, correct, and complete. A *clear* communication is one that is understood by the listener. If you say, "Can you get Mrs. Jones," what are you asking? For that patient to be transported back to the unit from a test? For the staff member to assume full care for Mrs. Jones? Or to answer Mrs. Jones's bell? Tell the staff member exactly what you want done. A *concise* communication is one in which the right amount of communication has been given. If you are asking a PCA to take a patient's temperature, he does not need to know the physiological response to an increased temperature. It confuses the communication and wastes time. Tell the associate what he needs to know. A *correct* communication is one that is accurate. You may have two patients named Edward Norton on your unit. It is not enough to tell the LPN to give Mr. Norton his pain medication. Which Mr. Norton are you referring to? Last, a *complete* communication leaves no questions on the part of the delegate. Do not assume that just because you asked a PCA to take a patient's temperature that she will know to report it to you.

Communication is a two-way activity, and it is important to create an environment where the staff member feels free to say that he is not comfortable doing a task because he has not done it for a long time.

RIGHT SUPERVISION

The nurse remains accountable for the total care delivered to the patients on the unit. The right supervision includes "the provision of guidance, direction, oversight, evaluation and follow up by the licensed nurse

for accomplishment of a nursing task delegated to nursing assistive personnel" (NCSBN, 2005). While you will not directly perform the tasks delegated, you will be responsible to determine the patient progress and outcomes of the care delivered, as well as evaluating and improving staff performance. This requires you to be able to communicate effectively to support team performance.

ACCEPTANCE OF DELEGATED ASSIGNMENT

In accepting a delegated assignment, the following decision-making algorithm is appropriate (State of New Jersey, 1999):

- Is the act consistent with your defined scope of practice?
- Is the activity authorized by a valid order and in accordance with established institutional/agency or provider protocols, policies, and procedures?
- Is the act supported by research data from nursing literature/or research from a health-related field? Has a national nursing organization issued a position statement on this practice? (See Chapter 4.)
- Do you possess the knowledge and clinical competence to perform the act safely?
- Is the act to be performed within acceptable "standards of care" that would be provided under similar circumstances by reasonable, prudent nurses with similar education and clinical skills?
- Are you prepared to assume accountability for the provision of safe care?

This model will assist you if you have a question about nursing practice or the delegation of work to you.

DELEGATION FACTORS

To recap, what to delegate will depend on a number of factors (adapted from Heidenthal & Marthaler, 2005):

- Your state's nurse practice act
- Hospital policies and procedures
- Job descriptions
- Staff competencies
- Clinical situation
- Professional standards
- Patient needs

What *can* be delegated?

- Noninvasive and nonsterile treatments such as emptying Foley catheters and providing hot/cold soaks
- Collection of and reporting data such as vital signs, height and weight, and capillary blood sugar results
- Hygienic care activities such as bathing and toileting, assistance with feeding, and assisting with ambulation
- Socialization activities

What *cannot* be delegated?

- Patient assessments (data collection is not assessment; assessments require interpretation)
- Planning and evaluation of nursing care
- Development of plan of care
- Health teaching and health counseling (unless it is reinforcement of previously taught material)

OBSTACLES TO DELEGATION

There are obstacles to delegation. They include some organizational issues, as well as personal issues, and include the following (Sullivan & Decker, 2001):

- Lack of training for nurses on how to delegate
- Personal qualities, such as poor communication or interpersonal skills
- Lack of resources
- Insecure delegator
- Unwilling delegate
- Nurse unwillingness to trust in others, or let go of tasks with personal importance

LEVELS OF CLINICAL EXPERIENCE

As a nurse grows professionally, the use of effective delegation has been related to levels of clinical experience (Benner & Benner, 1984, cited in Carroll, 2006):

The novice nurse has limited experience with tasks and needs rules to guide actions.

The advanced beginner has enough experience to recognize patterns in work but continues to need help in setting priorities; relies on rules and protocols.

The competent nurse has been practicing 2 to 3 years; can prioritize and cope with various contingencies; requires assistance working through various situations not yet experienced.

The proficient nurse has enough experience to see the "big picture" rather than a series of individual accidents/actions; decision making is more efficient and accurate; able to prioritize and plan even more challenging patient care.

The expert no longer relies on rules to understand a situation or to act appropriately; focuses quickly on viable solutions; able to lead a team efficiently; can organize others' work and supervise them effectively.

So, it is important to know the nurses with whom you are working on any given day, so that you can also use their level of expertise in the planning of your delegation.

PRIORITY SETTING

Proper delegation also requires priority setting. One of the most difficult challenges facing both the nurse and the nurse manager is the prioritization of care delivered to the patients on a unit. The priorities change rapidly and the nurse manager needs to be aware of the unit needs at all times. To manage your priorities and to control the activity of the workplace around you, Carrick et al. (2007) suggest the three "I"s:

1. Identify your priorities.
2. Interact differently with others.
3. Initiate action.

To *identify your priorities,* list your entire job-related responsibilities on a piece of paper. Then classify the top priorities, and create a "to-do" list that you can work from during the day. Remember, this list will change as the day progresses, but keep updating it and rank your priorities as they change. This list serves as a reference for the actions of the day.

To *interact differently with others,* Carrick et al. (2007) recommend the following four tactics to maintain control over your time, energy, and priorities:

- Identify a time when you can handle an issue— You cannot refuse a task or patient request, but you will be able to say when you will be available to do the task. Reassuring a person that you will complete the task and giving a timeline help to control requests and interruptions that compete for your time.
- Ask questions before taking on an assignment— Before you take on any assignment, you need to

understand the scope, the intended outcome, and the deadlines.

- Ask for help when you need it—Quickly do a reality check of your time, prioritize alternatives, and then meet with the person who can help you make the right decision or complete the assignment. When asking for help, be realistic about the expectation of the other person, and be open to alternative decision making.
- Use delegation to manage your responsibilities— You CANNOT do it all! When delegating, be sure to explain the scope, expectations, roles, responsibilities, and authority for the task. Always be available as a resource.

To *initiate action*, you need to set realistic goals. To set realistic goals, be SMART—the goals need to be **S**pecific, **M**easurable, **A**ttainable, **R**elevant, and **T**ime bound.

As a nurse manager, you have a responsibility to control time, set appropriate priorities, and act on the priorities. In setting priorities, you will always need to keep in mind the following question: "Of all of the important things that I need to do right now, which is the most important for the patient(s)?" Is it urgent? Or just important?

SUMMARY

Delegation is one of the most challenging activities of the new manager. There is more nursing care than nurses to provide that care. In addition, not all care needed for a patient requires a professional nurse. Nurses must work within an interdisciplinary team and work with individuals of varying capabilities and talents.

Delegation skills are developed by the new nurse over time. It involves an awareness of the total patient care needs for the patients assigned, as well as a thorough knowledge of the capabilities and competencies of staff members. Delegation is a process that results in safe and efficient patient care if it is used appropriately. It is a critical step in the delivery of nursing care.

CLINICAL CORNER

New Nurses' Experience with Delegation
Gina Sallustio

As a new nurse, there are many tasks that you must learn to carry out in a safe and efficient manner. These tasks include things taught in nursing school such as safe medication administration and physical assessment of a patient. However, there were tasks that you were taught in classes but usually did not have enough experience with, for example, delegation.

During my first year as a nurse, I worked on a pediatric hematology/oncology floor where I had been a student nurse extern and nursing assistant for a year before I graduated. Along with making the transition to my new role as a registered nurse, I had to learn how to delegate to others instead of being delegated to. Because of my previous position on the floor, learning this task sometimes seemed more challenging than learning other nursing skills. At times I thought it would be OK for me to do a simple task myself instead of delegating it to someone else who was qualified to do it. For example, when I assess my patient at the beginning of my shift, I would take their vital signs at the same time, regardless of the fact that we had a nursing assistant whose job was to do so. Having been in the position of the nursing assistant, I know how overwhelming it is when every room on the floor is occupied. So, with this in mind, I would repeatedly avoid delegating because I felt bad asking the nursing assistant to do another task.

My preceptor was the person who noticed that I was not delegating tasks, so we decided that this was something I had to work on. She taught me how to use my resources to complete simple tasks so that more time could be spent completing nursing tasks like administering medications and providing patient education. We would then discuss what kinds of tasks could be safely delegated and to whom they could be delegated. She would often remind me by saying, "Gina, can that be delegated?" And it didn't take long for me to answer, "Yes." I then began to understand that we were all there working as a patient care team, and we had to help each other so we can carry out our responsibilities. But she didn't fail to remind me that I was ultimately accountable for the task and for evaluating the care provided. If I had asked a nursing assistant to take a blood sugar level on a patient, I was responsible for evaluating the result and taking any action needed.

I learned that successful delegation also requires good communication between the nurse and the person

CLINICAL CORNER—cont'd

being delegated to. I have found that it is beneficial to delegates if they are given an explanation about the patient and their plan of care so they understand their responsibility. For example, a nursing assistant should understand why a patient's urine has to be dipped and tested for specific gravity with each void so that they are aware of how important their role is to the patient's care.

When I finished my orientation and I became more comfortable completing my own tasks, I felt more comfortable delegating as well. As a new nurse, it is very easy to become overwhelmed with all of the work that has to be completed. But by learning how to appropriately delegate, it can make things a little easier to handle and allow more time for the nursing tasks that cannot be delegated.

EVIDENCE-BASED PRACTICE

Delegation of Medication Administration

Dickens, G., Stubbs, J., & Haw C. (2008) Delegation of medication administration: an exploratory study. Nursing Standard, 22(22), 35–40.

Medication management in nursing homes and in psychiatric facilities caring for older adults can be described as grim and chaotic. This study done in England stated that the Commission for Social Care Inspection recommends that all care homes urgently review their medication management policies and practices due to findings that show an increase in medication errors.

This exploratory study was designed to look at whether it was feasible, prudent, and practical for the RN who prepares the medication to delegate the delivery of it to another RN or to a caregiver (both would be called runners). It was an observational study that only observed the runner when she/he was in sight of the RN who had prepared the medications. The results

showed that the medication errors made during the observational period all occurred during preparation or recording rather than final administration. The errors made by the runners had to do with unauthorized crushing of medication into foods.

Should runners be used in medication administration? It seems sensible to have the person who prepares the medications also administer them and sign the record as it reduces the number of transition points with the administration process. However, it will also inevitably increase the already considerable time taken to conduct a medication round. On these units older patients are often mobile, confused and nonconcordant. The authors believe it is sensible to use runners to ensure that medication is administered safely and effectively. They also found after reviewing the literature that the process will be more successful if the caregiver runners are given guidelines and education regarding medication administration.

NCLEX® EXAM QUESTIONS

1. You are taking care of a patient with an acute myocardial infarction. You want to assign a PCA to this patient. Which of the following tasks would be appropriate to delegate to the PCA?
   1. Teaching about low sodium diet
   2. Assisting with bathing
   3. Pain assessment
   4. Nothing
2. You are caring for a patient with anorexia nervosa. Which of the following tasks could be delegated to the licensed practical nurse?
   1. Initiation of daily weights

   2. Oral hygiene
   3. Intravenous push medications
   4. Diet teaching
3. Which of the following patients can be assigned to a PCA?
   1. A patient with sudden unexplained bleeding
   2. A patient with frequent breakthrough pain for the past 8 hours
   3. A patient scheduled for a chest radiograph this morning
   4. A patient with multiple allergic reactions to medication

Continued

4. You are the leader of a team that consists of a new registered nurse and a PCA. The following are your patients:
   - Mrs. C, a 58-year-old with unstable blood sugars who is scheduled for a pancreatic scan this morning
   - Mr. W, a 49-year-old with a history of chest pain admitted because of shortness of breath
   - Ms. K, a 22-year-old in sickle cell crisis, with multiple intravenous lines
   - Mr. F, an 83-year-old with a history of chronic leukemia admitted with an increased temperature and shortness of breath
   - Mrs. U, a 40-year-old 1 day postoperative for laparoscopic cholecystectomy

   Which patients should you assign to the new nurse? (Choose all who apply.)
   1. Mrs. C
   2. Mr. W
   3. Ms. K
   4. Mr. F
   5. Mrs. U

5. On completing her shift, the new nurse lets you know that she has not completed the medication documentation for her assigned patients. You would:
   1. question her why she has not completed her work
   2. assist her with the documentation so that you can both go home
   3. grant her overtime to complete the necessary documentation
   4. notify your nurse manager to include this on her evaluation

6. You are the charge nurse on the 11 PM to 7 AM shift. One of your tasks is to assign both direct patient care activities and indirect patient care activities to the staff. You are aware that one of the direct patient care activities is:
   1. restocking supplies
   2. transport patients
   3. clerical activities
   4. electrocardiogram tracing

7. Nurses can be placed into different levels of clinical experience. You are aware that the _____ has enough experience to recognize patterns in work but continues to need help in setting priorities; relies on rules and protocols.

   1. novice nurse
   2. advanced beginner
   3. competent nurse
   4. proficient nurse

8. Which of the following is a list of delegation factors?
   1. Your state's nurse practice act, hospital policies and procedures, job descriptions, patient needs, staff competencies, clinical situation, professional standards
   2. Your state's nurse practice act, hospital policies and procedures, job descriptions, patient needs, staff competencies, clinical situation
   3. Your state's nurse practice act, hospital policies and procedures, job descriptions, patient needs, staff competencies, professional standards
   4. Your state's nurse practice act, hospital policies and procedures, patient needs, staff competencies, clinical situation, professional standards

9. To manage your priorities and to control the activity of the workplace around you, Carrick et al. (2007) suggest the three "I"s; they are:
   1. identify your problems, interact differently with others, and initiate activities
   2. identify your problems, interact similarly with others, and initiate action
   3. identify your issues, interact differently with others, and initiate action
   4. identify your problems, interact differently with others, and initiate action

10. You are listening as your colleague, an RN, is giving out her assignments to her team, which consists of 2 LPNs and 2 nursing assistants. She is considered a *competent nurse* and has been practicing 2 years. You are aware that one of the tasks she is assigning to the nursing assistant should only be done by a licensed professional. What should you do?
    1. Bring the issue to the charge nurse who is at a meeting
    2. Discuss at the next staff meeting and say she was wrong
    3. Openly discuss that she is wrong and report her to nurse manager
    4. Discuss why the task is not appropriate for the non-licensed personnel

Answers: 1. 2   2. 2   3. 3   4. 1, 2, 4, 5   5. 1   6. 4   7. 2   8. 1   9. 4   10. 4

REFERENCES

American Nurses Association (ANA). (1992). Position statement: registered nurse education relating to the utilization of unlicensed assistive personnel. Retrieved July 2, 2007, from http://ana.org/readroom/position/uap/uaprned.htm.

American Nurses Association (ANA) and National Council of State Boards of Nursing (NCSBN). (2008). *Joint Statement of Delegation*. Retrieved June 20, 2008, from https://www.ncsbn.org/index.htm.

Benner, P., & Benner, R. (1984). *From novice to expert: excellence and power in clinical nursing practice.* Menlo Park, CA: Addison-Wesley Publishing.

Carrick, L., Carrick, L., & Yurkow, J. (2007). A nurse leader's guide to managing priorities. *American Nurse Today, July,* 40-41.

Carroll, P. (1998) Buyer beware? Using non-credentialed assistive personnel: clinical and management perspectives. *Subacute Care Today, 1*(5), 24-28.

Carroll, P. (2006). *Nursing leadership and management: a practical guide.* Clifton Park, NY: Thomson Delmar Learning.

Heidenthal, P., & Marthaler, M. (2005). *Delegation of nursing care.* Clifton Park, NY: Thomson Delmar Learning.

National Council of State Boards of Nursing. (1997). *The five rights of delegation.* Chicago, IL: Author.

National Council of State Boards of Nursing. (2005). *ANA and NCSBOB Joint Statement of Delegation.* Chicago, IL.

State of Kentucky. (1999). Delegation of nursing tasks. KRS 311A.170, 314.011, 201 KAR 20:400. Retrieved July 2, 2007, from http://www.lrc.state.ky.us/kar/201/020/400.htm.

State of New Jersey. (1999). New Jersey State Board of Nursing fact sheet: decision making model for delegations of selected nursing tasks. N.J.A.C. 13:37-36-2. Retrieved July 2, 2007, from http://www.state.nj.us/lps/ca/nursing/ago1.htm.

Sullivan, E., & Decker, P. (2001). *Effective leadership and management in nursing* (5th ed.). Upper Saddle River, NJ: Prentice Hall.

CHAPTER 4

Evidence-Based Practice

Chapter Objectives

1. Differentiate between research utilization and evidence-based practice.
2. Review the nurse's role in the implementation of evidence-based practice.
3. Identify the hierarchy of evidence.
4. Discuss the critical appraisal process in evaluating evidence.
5. Identify the PICO format of identifying a question.

Definitions

Evidence-based practice Conscientious use of current best practice or research evidence in making clinical decisions

Research evidence Use of findings from a single study or a set of studies for the development of patient care

Randomized clinical trial Effects of an intervention are examined by comparing the treatment group with the nontreatment group; patients are placed in treatment or nontreatment group through random sampling

Nonrandomized clinical trial Same as a randomized clinical trial but patient placement in treatment or nontreatment group depends on study variables, with not every individual having an opportunity for selection

Correlational study Study examining the relationship between or among two or more variables in a single group; it does not examine cause and effect

Observational study Use of structured and unstructured observations to measure study variables

Descriptive study Used to identify and describe variables and examine relationships that exist in a situation; provides an accurate portrayal of the phenomenon of interest

MEDICAL MYTHS AND TRUTHS

Two sentinel publications by the Institute of Medicine—*To Err Is Human* and *Crossing the Quality Chasm* (IOM, 2000; IOM, 2001)—drew attention to quality issues in U.S. health care (see Chapter 10). A major theme of both reports was that although the technology of health care had advanced at lightning speed, the delivery system had not advanced, causing potentially lethal situations in health care. One of the most common situations seen was the increased rate of hospital-acquired infections, and one of the proposed solutions to the improvement of care was the use of evidence-based decision making in health care.

Evidence-based practice requires a shift from the traditional paradigm of clinical practice grounded in pathophysiology and clinical experience to one of the integration of best practice and scientific evidence. This paradigm shift allows for the continuous improvement of practice and a creation of environments that stimulate innovation.

As a new nurse, there will be many times that you ask yourself, "Why do we do it this way?" Or "There must be a better way to do this." For answers to these questions, you must look to the evidence. What does the evidence tell you? What is the best practice, or what is the best way to do this? Some of our standard practices are "sacred cows," meaning they represent "the way it has always been done." For instance, does every patient admitted to your unit need their temperature taken at 7 AM? Perhaps not, but that is just the "way that we do it" or perhaps that was the "best practice" when the policy was implemented. But what does the evidence (scientific data) tell us today? As nurses, it is important that you remain current within your practice area, because the evidence is always changing and growing. Estabrooks (1998) and Pravikoff et al. (2005) found that knowledge sources most frequently used by nurses were school experiences and colleague experience. Assuming that this is the case, a nurse with 15 years of experience may be using "evidence" that is 15 years out of date, and this experienced nurse who is mentoring new nurses may be fostering practice in the new nurse that is 15 years out of date. A colleague of this author once said that "health care was a long history of tradition unimpeded by progress"—the move to evidence-based practice is changing this.

EXAMPLES OF SOME MEDICAL MYTHS

Myth: Patients with musculoskeletal back pain respond best to bed rest followed by a specialized back exercise program (myths from Flaherty, 2007).

Truth:

- Bed rest is not an effective treatment for acute low back pain and may delay recovery. Current advice is to stay active and to continue ordinary activities, which results in a faster return to work, less chronic disability, and fewer recurrent problems (Waddell, 1997).
- Among patients with acute low back pain, continuing ordinary activities within the limits permitted by the pain leads to more rapid recovery than either bed rest or back-mobilizing exercises (Malmivaara, 1995).

Myth: "Figure-of-eight" dressings or similar appliances are the preferred treatment for clavicle fractures.

Truth:

- No statistical difference was found in the speed of recovery when clavicle fractures were treated by either a figure-of-eight bandage or a broad arm sling (Stanley & Norris, 1988).
- Treatment with a simple sling caused less discomfort and perhaps fewer complications than with the figure-of-eight bandage. The functional and cosmetic results of the two methods of treatment were identical and alignment of the healed fractures was unchanged from the initial displacement (Andersen et al., 1987).

Myth: Bed rest is a useful adjunctive therapy.

Truth: A meta-analysis of 39 studies of the use of bed rest versus early mobilization for prevention and treatment of a variety of medical conditions showed bed rest to be at best not beneficial and at worst harmful (Allen, 1999).

Myth: Rectal temperature can be accurately estimated by adding $1°$ C to the temperature measured at the axilla.

Truth: In children and young adults, temperature measured at the axilla does not agree sufficiently with temperature measured at the rectum to be relied on in clinical situations where accurate measurement is important (Craig, 2000).

DECISION-MAKING MODEL

Evidence-based practice is a decision-making model based on the "conscientious, explicit and judicious use of current best practice in making decisions about the care of individual or groups of patients" (Sackett, Rosenberg, Gray, Haynes, & Richardson, 1996). "This practice requires the integration of individual clinical expertise with the best available external clinical evidence from systematic research, available resources, and our patient's unique values and circumstances" (Sackett et al., 1996). This definition requires nurses to carefully and thoroughly integrate evidence into their practice. But how do they do this?

This new paradigm of evidence-based practice requires the development of a clinical inquiry approach. Nurses must ask themselves the following questions and not blindly accept standard practice (Salmon, 2007):

- Why are we doing it this way?
- Is there a better way to do this?
- What is the evidence to support what we are doing?
- What practice guidelines support this practice?
- Would doing *this* be as effective as doing *that*?
- What constitutes best practice?

RESEARCH UTILIZATION

Evidence-based practice differs from research utilization. Research utilization is the process of using research-generated knowledge to make an impact on or a change in existing practices (Burns and Grove, 2007). Evidence-based practice requires synthesizing research study findings to determine best research evidence. Research evidence is a synthesis of high-quality, relevant studies to form a body of empirical knowledge for the selected area of practice. The best research evidence is then integrated with clinical expertise and patient values and needs to deliver quality, cost-effective care (Sackett et al., 2000).

QUESTION FORMULATION

The first thing that you will need to do is to formulate the question. As nurses, we make numerous decisions when caring for our patients. As we make these decisions, we are influenced by a number of factors (Craig & Smyth, 2002):

- Clinical expertise
- Beliefs, attitudes
- Routine (tradition)
- Organizational factors
  - State and federal policies
  - Regulatory factors
  - Funding
  - Time
- Factors related to the patient
  - Clinical circumstances
  - Preferences, beliefs, attitudes, needs

Up-to-date, valid evidence needs to be integrated with these factors to maximize the likelihood of what we want to happen (the outcome). The more explicit the question, the easier it is to run searches through the multiple electronic databases available to nurses (CINAHL, MEDLINE, Cochrane Library). For example, you are interested in determining best practice for change-of-shift reports. If you enter "end-of-shift report" into the search line, you will receive 56 references. If you narrow the search to within the past 5 years, the number of references is cut to 32. A focused question makes your "search strategy" much easier. It is very helpful for any nurse working in a hospital to develop a good relationship with the hospital librarian; he or she will assist you in the gathering of research evidence.

RELIABLE EVIDENCE

Once you have focused your question, you need to select the best evidence. Just because something has been published, albeit in print or on the Internet, does not mean that it is a valid source of evidence. You must first determine the reliability of the source. Your librarian will assist you in this. A research study on urinary catheters funded by the company that makes urinary catheters may not be the most reliable source of evidence; a study supporting their catheter is in the company's best interest. The first question in your critical appraisal of the evidence is whether this study is good enough to use the findings. You will be attempting to determine if the quality of the study that you are reading is good enough for you to use the results in the design of a nursing protocol. You would need to look at the research design, the sample, and the sample size. Obviously, results from a study directed at children may not be appropriate in the design of a protocol addressed at adults. Also, a study with a sample size of 4 will not carry as much strength as will a study with a sample size of 1000. Some research designs are more powerful than others. The fact that some studies are more powerful than others has given rise to the hierarchy of evidence (Peto, 1993). The hierarchy of evidence for questions about effectiveness of an intervention follows (Polit & Beck, 2008, p. 31):

Level 1   a. Systematic review of randomized controlled trials
          b. Systematic review of nonrandomized trials

Level 2   a. Single randomized controlled trial
          b. Single nonrandomized trial

Level 3   Systematic review of correlational/observational studies

Level 4   Single correlational/observational study

Level 5   Systematic review of descriptive/qualitative/physiologic studies

Level 6   Single descriptive/qualitative/physiologic study

Level 7   Opinions of authorities, expert committees

Draw as a triangle.

CRITICAL APPRAISAL

The next question to ask in your critical appraisal is whether the findings are applicable to your setting. The patients used in a study will never be identical to yours but there may be similarities. The following questions

can be asked to determine applicability of the study to your practice area:
- Is it clear what the study is about?
- Is the sample/context adequately described?
- Are my patients/contexts so different that the results will not apply?
- Is the intervention available, or is the change possible in my setting?
- Do the benefits of the change for my patient/context outweigh the costs?
- Are the patients' values and preferences satisfied by change?

Part of this question will be to ask what these results mean for your patients.

POPULATION, INTERVENTION, COMPARISON INTERVENTION, OUTCOME (PICO)

A framework for formulating evidence-based questions is PICO (Population, Intervention, Comparison Intervention, Outcome). Box 4-1 describes the focus of the PICO question.

In health care organizations, there may be many triggers that initiate the need for change. They can be data driven, resulting from performance review data, risk management data, benchmarking data, and financial data. Or they can be knowledge driven, resulting from new research findings, change in regulatory guidelines and standards, or questions from practitioners.

As a nurse manager, your role will be in the promotion and implementation of evidence-based practice in your organization. The Iowa Model of Evidence-Based Practice provides direction for the development of evidence-based practice in a clinical facility (Figure 4-1).

This model of evidence-based practice can be used as a guide for implementing a research-based protocol. The steps in this model are to:
- Synthesize relevant research
- Determine the sufficiency of the research base for use in practice
- Pilot the change in practice
- Institute the change in practice
- Monitor outcomes

SUMMARY

As a new nurse entering the profession, it is imperative that you maintain currency within your profession. Here are some strategies for using research evidence in your own practice:
- Read widely and critically—professionally accountable nurses keep abreast of their practice by reading journals relating to their practice.
- Join a professional organization related to your specialty—many innovations in practice and best practices are shared through professional organizations.
- Attend professional conferences and continuing education seminars.
- Participate in evidence-based projects.

Box 4-1	FOCUS OF THE PICO (POPULATION, INTERVENTION, COMPARISON INTERVENTION, OUTCOME) QUESTION
Patient or Population	Define who or what the question is about. *Tip:* Describe a group of patients similar to yours.
Intervention	Describe which intervention, test, or exposure that you are interested in. An intervention is a planned course of action. An exposure is something that happens such as a fall, anxiety, exposure to house mites, etc. (Bury & Mead, 1998). *Tip:* Describe what it is that you are considering doing or what has happened to the patient.
Comparison intervention (if any)	Describe the alternate intervention. *Tip:* Describe the alternative that can be compared to the intervention.
Outcomes	Define the important outcomes, beneficial or harmful. *Tip:* Define what you are hoping to achieve or avoid.

From Craig, J., and Smyth, R. (2002). *The evidence-based manual practice manual for nurses* (p. 30). Edinburgh: Churchill Livingstone.

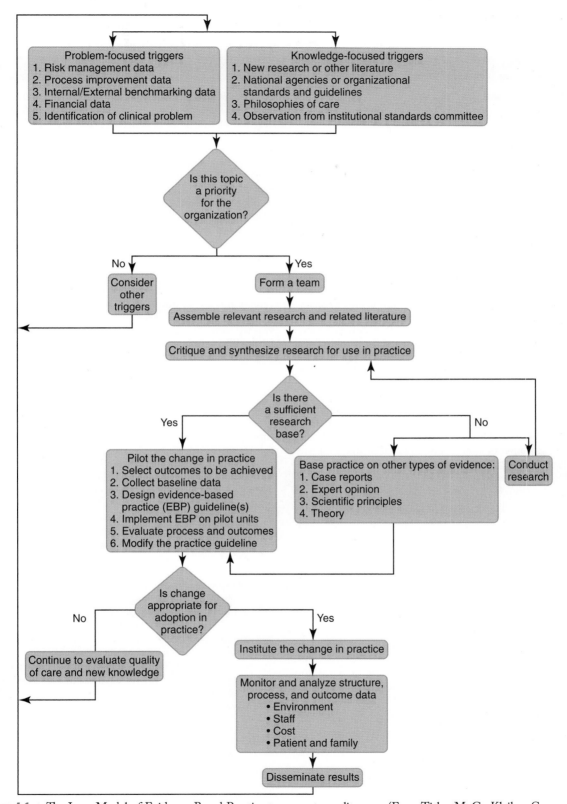

Figure 4-1 • The Iowa Model of Evidence-Based Practice to promote quality care. (From Titler, M. G., Kleiber, C., Steelman, V. J., Rakel, B. A., Budreau, G., Everett, L. Q., et al. [2001]. The Iowa Model of Evidence-Based Practice to promote quality care. *Critical Care Nursing Clinics of North America, 13*[4], 497-509; reprinted from Burns, N., & Grove, S. K. (2007). *Understanding nursing research: building an evidence-based practice,* [p. 514]. St. Louis, MO: Saunders Elsevier.)

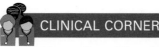

CLINICAL CORNER

Evidence-Based Practice Changes

Vera Usinowicz

The best evidence in patient care often travels a hard, sometimes circuitous, journey before becoming embedded into the practice of nursing care and ritualized. In acknowledging this, our hospital's Nurse Research Council attempts to provide an open forum for bringing evidence-based practice to the council membership for review and to make decisions on implementation, with the final goal of streamlining the process of adoption to dissemination within our facility.

New research and evidence-based practice guidelines issued by national organizations frequently provide triggers to question our current policy and practice. This was just the scenario in June 2008, when a Nurse Research Council member brought an article to the scheduled meeting about evidence-based guidelines for enteral feeding. It was noted in the peer-reviewed article that feeding tube placement should be confirmed only by radiography. This generated a lively discussion within the council about what was our current practice and what was being put forth as the best practice. Fueled by the substantiated findings that 1.4% to 27% of hospitalized patients have enteral tube placements inadvertently placed in the lung, we pursued a further literature search of the evidence and investigated our own standard of practice (Marderstein, Simmons, and Ochoa, 2004).

In our institution, if a certain procedure is already outlined in an approved nursing reference manual, then that manual serves as the guideline for that particular standard of care or procedure. If there is no standard of reference for a related practice, then a policy or procedure will be developed and written. We discovered that the hospital had no specific written policy for insertion and confirmation of placement of enteral feeding tubes, so we looked to our approved nursing reference manuals that we subscribed to—the *Lippincott Manual of Nursing Practice,* 8th Edition, and the *AACN Procedure Manual for Critical Care,* published in 2005. Neither approved nursing reference manual endorsed radiographic confirmation as the only reliable method to confirm enteral feeding tube placement.

The Nurse Research Council members then spent the next month searching the literature to lend strength to the evidence cited in the one peer-reviewed journal article.

In September 2008, our council met and proceeded to assemble the relevant findings from our literature search. We critiqued the literature, synopsized the findings, and weighed the evidence. Would it be sufficient to endorse a change in practice? Yes! We discovered that no other method, including air insufflation, visual inspection, or testing of aspirate for pH or capnography, proved to be a 100% reliable in confirming correct enteral feeding tube placement. Recognizing that requiring the hospital's neonate population to have radiographic confirmation every time a feeding tube is placed would result in multiple x-ray exposures on a daily basis for an infant, our recommendation for implementing the evidence-based practice change was only for our adult patient population.

Our recommendation for radiographic confirmation would require the availability of a physician to read a radiograph 24 hours a day, 7 days a week. Being a nonteaching hospital, without residents or interns, we worked with our radiology department and director of medical administration to ensure that we had the resources to support our proposed practice change. At first, the director was not appreciative of the proposed practice change until he was duly convinced by the presentation and weight of the evidence from our literature search. At the request of the director, we commenced to poll our entire nursing staff as to how many times they inserted enteral feedings tubes to evaluate the feasibility of using the house physician's time to provide the necessary radiographic confirmation. The information from the informal survey was that, on average, between the medical-surgical units and the critical care units, tubes were inserted two to three times a week by nursing staff, certainly not an overwhelming number that would monopolize the time of the house physician staff. With the endorsement of the director of medical administration in December 2008, we set out to develop a policy that would include evidence-based guidelines in the placement and confirmation of enteral feeding tubes in adult patients that would ensure the resource to read radiographs whenever necessary. The recommended evidence-based practice change will be finalized and approved at the necessary committee levels following our shared governance philosophy that we adopted at our hospital, which states that nursing governs its own practice and makes autonomous decisions to provide the best care to our patients.

Reference

Marderstein, E. L., Simmons, R. L., & Ochoa, J. B. (2004). Patient safety: effects of institutional protocols on adverse events related to feeding tube placement in the critically ill. *Journal of the American College of Surgeons*, 199(1), 39-50.

EVIDENCE-BASED PRACTICE

Saline Versus Heparin Flushes

Adapted from Building an evidence-based practice. *In Burns, N., Grove, S. K. (2007).* Understanding nursing research: building an evidence-based practice *(4th ed.) (pp. 515-517). St. Louis, MO: Saunders Elsevier.*

Research Example: Synthesis of Research

Goode and colleagues (1991) conducted a meta-analysis "to estimate the effects of heparin flush and saline flush solutions on maintaining patency, preventing phlebitis, and increasing duration of peripheral heparin locks [peripheral venous catheters]" (p. 324). The meta-analysis was conducted on 17 high-quality studies, which the investigators summarized in a table (Table 14-A). The total sample size for the 17 studies was 4153; the study settings included a variety of medical-surgical and critical care units. The small effect size values (most are less than 0.20) for clotting, phlebitis, and duration indicate that saline flush is as effective as heparin flush in maintaining peripheral venous catheters. Goode and colleagues summarized current knowledge on the use of saline versus heparin flushes:

• It can be concluded that saline is as effective as heparin in maintaining patency, preventing phlebitis, and increasing duration in peripheral heparin locks. Quality of care can be enhanced by using saline as the flush solution, thereby eliminating problems associated with anticoagulant effects and drug incompatibilities. In addition, an estimated yearly savings of $109,100,000 to $218,200,000 U.S. health care dollars could be attained (Goode et al., 1991, p. 324).

These investigators also provided a table (Table 14-B) to present evidence of cost savings from changing to saline.

Based on this review of the evidence, the following patient care protocol was developed.

Evidence-Based Protocol for Irrigating Peripheral Venous Catheters in Adults*

1. Review the medical order for irrigation of the peripheral venous catheter. Order should indicate that the catheter be irrigated with saline (0.9% sodium chloride) (Goode et al., 1991: Randolph et al., 1998).
2. Obtain the saline flush for irrigation from the hospital pharmacy (ASHP, 1994).
3. Wash hands with chlorhexidine, collect equipment for irrigating the peripheral venous catheter, and put on gloves.
4. Evaluate the peripheral venous catheter site every 8 hours for complications of phlebitis. The symptoms of phlebitis include the presence of erythema, tenderness, warmth, and a tender or palpable cord (Goode et al., 1991; Randolph et al., 1998).
5. Cleanse the peripheral venous catheter prior to irrigation with alcohol.
6. Flush the peripheral venous catheter with 1 ml for normal saline every 8 hours if no other medication

is being given through the site (Goode et al., 1991; Randolph et al., 1998). Check the loss of catheter patency by noting any resistance in irrigating with 1 ml of saline or by the inability to administer saline solution within 30 seconds (Geritz, 1992; Shoaf & Oliver, 1992).
7. If a patient is receiving IV medication, administer 1 ml of saline, administer the medication, and follow with 1 ml of saline (Goode et al., 1991; Shoaf & Oliver, 1992).
8. Chart the date and time of the peripheral venous catheter irrigation and the appearance and patency of the catheter site.

*Note: All peripheral venous catheters for pediatric patients must be flushed with heparin flush unless otherwise ordered by physician (Randolph et al., 1998).

References

American Society of Hospital Pharmacists (ASHP). (1994). ASHP therapeutic position statement on the institutional use of 0.9% sodium chloride injection to maintain patency of peripheral indwelling intermittent infusion devices. *American Journal of Hospital Pharmacy, 51*(12), 1572-1574.

Geritz, M. A. (1992). Saline versus heparin in intermittent infuser patency maintenance. *Western Journal of Nursing Research, 14*(2), 131-141.

Goode, C. J., Titler, M., Rakel, B., Ones, D. S. Kleiber, C., Small, S., et al. (1991). A meta-analysis of effects of heparin flush and saline flush: quality and cost implications. *Nursing Research, 40*(6), 324-330.

Randolph, A. G., Cook, D. J., Gonzales, C. A., & Andrew, M. (1998). Benefits of heparin in peripheral venous and arterial catheters: Systematic review and meta-analysis of randomized controlled trials. *British Medical Journal, 316*(7136), 969-975.

Shoaf, J., & Oliver, S. (1992). Efficacy of normal saline injection with and without heparin for maintaining intermittent intravenous site. *Applied Nursing Research, 5*(1), 9-12.

As can be seen by this research example, the change in practice resulted from a critical analysis of research evidence, and the patient care protocol is based on evidence.

Evidence-based practice has been emphasized since the advent of the Institute of Medicine report. Professional organizations and federal agencies have developed many evidence-based guidelines. An excellent source of research publications is the Cochrane Library Collection (available online at http://www.cochrane.org). The Agency for Healthcare Quality and Research (AHRQ) has developed many guidelines relevant to your nursing practice. Some of the practice areas with guidelines are management of acute pain in adults, infants, and children; predication and prevention of pressure ulcers in adults; treatment of depression in primary care; and availability of cardiac rehabilitation services. AHRQ has also developed many tools to assess the quality of care that is provided. Access to the numerous clinical practice guidelines is available at www.ahrq.gov.

Table 14-A　STUDIES INCLUDED IN THE META-ANALYSIS

Study	N	Subject	Assignment	Heparin Dose (U/ml)	Clotting Effect Size (d_c)	Phlebitis Effect Size (d_p)	Duration Effect Size (d_d)
Ashton et al., 1990	16 exp_c	Adult critical care	Random, double blind	10	0.3590	−0.1230	
	16 con_c						
	13 exp_p						
	14 con_p						
Barrett & Lester, 1990	59 experimental	Adult med-surg patients	Nonrandom double-blind	10	−0.1068	−0.4718	
	50 control						
Craig & Anderson, 1991	129 exp	Adult med-surg patients	Random double-blind crossover	10	0.0095	−0.0586	
	145 con						
Cyganski et al., 1987	225 exp	Adult med-surg patients	Nonrandom	10	0.2510		
	196 con						
Donham & Denning, 1987	8 exp_c	Adult critical care	Random, double blind	10	0.0000	0.0548	
	4 con_c						
	7 exp_p						
	5 con_p						
Dunn & Lenihan, 1987	61 experimental	Adult patients	Nonrandom	50	−0.2057	−0.2258	
	51 control						
Epperson, 1984	138 exp	Adult med-surg patients	Random, double blind	10	−0.1176		
	120 con			100	−0.1232		
	138 exp						
	154 con						
Garrelts et al., 1989	131 exp	Adult med-surg patients	Random, double blind	10	−0.1773	0.1057	0.2753
	173 con						
Hamilton et al., 1988	137 exp	Adult patients	Random, double blind	10	−0.0850	−0.1819	−0.0604
	170 con						
Holford et al., 1977	39 experimental	Young adult volunteers	Nonrandom, double blind	3.3, 10, 16.5, 100, 132	0.6545		
	140 control						

Table 14-A STUDIES INCLUDED IN THE META-ANALYSIS—cont'd

Study	N	Subject	Assignment	Heparin Dose (U/ml)	Clotting Effect Size (d_c)	Phlebitis Effect Size (d_p)	Duration Effect Size (d_d)
Kasparek et al., 1988	49 exp	Adult med patients	Random, double blind	10	0.3670	−0.5430	
	50 con						
Lombardi et al., 1988	34 experimental	Pediatric patients (4 wk to 18 yr)	Nonrandom, sequential double blind	10	−0.2324	0.0000	
	40 control						
Miracle et al., 1989	167 exp	Adult med-surg patients	Nonrandom	100	−0.0042		
	441 con						
Shearer, 1987	87 exp	Med-surg patients	Nonrandom	10	−0.1170	−0.0977	
	73 con						
Spann, 1988	15 experimental	Adult telemetry step-down	Nonrandom, double blind	10	−0.3163	−0.3252	
	19 control						
Taylor et al., 1989	369 exp	Adult med-surg patients	Nonrandom, time series	10	0.0308	0.0288	−0.1472
	356 con						
Tuten & Gueldner, 1991	43 exp	Adult med-surg patients	Nonrandom	100	0.0000	0.1662	
	71 con						

Modified from Goode, C. J., Titler, M., Rakel, B., Ones, D. S., Kleiber, C., Small, S., & Triolo, P. K. (1991). A meta-analysis of effects of heparin flush and saline flush: quality and cost implications. *Nursing Research, 40*(6), 325. Copyright © 1991, The American Journal of Nursing Company. Used with permission.

Table 14-B ANNUAL COST SAVINGS FROM CHANGING TO SALINE

Study	Cost Savings	Hospital
Craig & Anderson, 1991	$40,000/yr	525-bed tertiary care hospital
Dunn & Lenihan, 1987	$19,000/yr	530-bed private hospital
Goode et al., 1991 (this study)	$38,000/yr	879-bed tertiary care hospital
Kasparek et al., 1988	$19,000/yr	350-bed private hospital
Lombardi et al., 1988	$20,000-$25,000/yr	52-bed pediatric unit
Schustek, 1984	$20,000/yr	391-bed private hospital
Taylor et al., 1989	$30,000-$40,000/yr	216-bed private hospital

From Goode, C. J., Titler, M., Rakel, B., Ones, D. S., Kleiber, C., Small, S., & Triolo, P. K. (1991). A meta-analysis of effects of heparin flush and saline flush: quality and cost implications. *Nursing Research, 40*(6), 325. Copyright © 1991, The American Journal of Nursing Company. Used with permission.

NCLEX® EXAM QUESTIONS

1. A key component of evidence-based practice is:
   1. traditional practice
   2. organizational commitment
   3. patient preference
   4. nurse ability
2. In the hierarchy of evidence, which of the following has the highest value?
   1. Single correctional studies
   2. Randomized clinical trials
   3. Case study, opinion
   4. Descriptive studies
3. The experienced nurse can do the following to use evidence-based practice in their own practice:
   1. Use textbooks from school for reference.
   2. Maintain membership in alumni organization.
   3. Review professional journals.
   4. Go back to school for an advanced degree.
4. When implementing an evidence-based practice change, the all-important final step is to:
   1. pilot the protocol
   2. monitor the results
   3. publish the study
   4. do a cost-benefit analysis
5. The first step in integrating evidence into practice is to convert the clinical concern into a:
   1. solution
   2. question
   3. decision
   4. goal
6. In the PICO framework for developing the question of concern, "I" stands for:
   1. intervention
   2. interdisciplinary
   3. interrelational
   4. integrity
7. As a nurse, you have just read about a change in intravenous insertion practice that sounds like it would work on your unit. Before suggesting such a change in practice, you need to:
   1. perform a cost-benefit analysis of the new practice
   2. talk with the nurse manager to gain her opinion
   3. conduct a further review of the literature
   4. contact the nursing research committee
8. In reviewing a study for applicability for use on your unit, you need to evaluate the study in terms of:
   1. the sponsoring agency of the study
   2. patient context and assess whether they similar to your unit
   3. whether the sample adequately is described
   4. qualifications of the study authors
9. Which of the following would be a reliable source of information for a change in pediatric practice?
   1. Physician/staff discussion
   2. Editorial in *Pediatric Nursing*
   3. Growth and development charts
   4. Clinical trial results
10. An example of a knowledge trigger for an evidence-based research question is:
    1. patient fall data
    2. database review
    3. benchmark information
    4. research study

Answers: 1. 3   2. 2   3. 3   4. 2   5. 2   6. 1   7. 3   8. 2   9. 4   10. 4

REFERENCES

Allen, C., et al. (1999). Bed rest: a potentially harmful treatment needing more careful evaluation. *Lancet*, *354*(9186), 1229-1233.

Andersen, K., et al. (1987). Treatment of clavicular fractures. Figure-of-eight bandage versus a simple sling. *Acta Orthopaedica Scandinavia*, *58*(1), 71-74.

Burns, N., & Grove, S. (2007). *Understanding nursing research: building an evidence-based practice* (4th ed.). St. Louis, MO: Saunders Elsevier.

Craig, J. V., et al. (2000). Temperature measured at the axilla compared with rectum in children and young people: systematic review. *British Medical Journal*, *320*, 1174-1178.

Craig, J., & Smyth, R. (2002). *The evidence-based manual practice manual for nurses*. Edinburgh: Churchill Livingstone.

Estabrooks, C. (1998). Will evidence-based nursing practice make practice perfect? *Canadian Journal of Nursing Research*, *30*(1), 15-36.

Flaherty, R. Medical mythology. Retrieved August 2, 2007, from http://www.montana.edu/wwwebm/myths.html.

Institute of Medicine. (2000). *To Err is Human: Building a Safer Health Care System*. Washington, DC: National Academy Press.

Institute of Medicine. (2001). *Crossing the Quality Chasm: a New Health System for the 21st Century*. Washington, DC: National Academy Press.

Malmivaara, A., et al. (1995). The treatment of acute low back pain—bed rest, exercises, or ordinary activity? *New England Journal of Medicine, 332*(6), 351-355.

Pravikoff, D., Tanner, A., & Pierce, S. (2005). Readiness of US nurses for evidence based practice. *American Journal of Nursing, 105*(9), 40-51.

Peto, R. (1993). Large scale randomized evidence; large sample trials and overview trials. *Annals of the New York Academy of Science, 703,* 314-340.

Polit, D., & Beck, C. (2008). *Nursing research* (8th ed.). Philadelphia, PA: Lippincott Williams & Wilkins.

Sackett, D., Rosenberg, W., Gray, J., Haynes, R., & Richardson, W. (1996). Evidence based medicine: what it is and what it is not. *British Medical Journal, 312,* 71-72.

Sackett, D. L., Straus, S. E., Richardson, W. C., Rosenberg, W., & Haynes, R. M. (2000). *Evidence-based medicine: how to practice and teach EBM* (2nd ed.). New York: Churchill Livingstone.

Salmon, S. (2007). Advancing evidence based practice. *Orthopaedic Nursing, 26*(2), 118.

Stanley, D., & Norris, S. H. (1988). Recovery following fractures of the clavicle treated conservatively. *Injury, 19*(3), 162-164.

Waddell, G., et al. (1997). Systematic reviews of bed rest and advice to stay active for acute low back pain. *British Journal of General Practice, 47*(423), 647-652.

CHAPTER 5

Management of Emergencies and Disasters

Chapter Objectives

1. Define *environment of care.*
2. Identify hospital safety and security policies and procedures.
3. Define *sentinel event.*
4. Discuss strategies for implementation of proper procedures in the event of a disaster.
5. Identify and evaluate the implementation of all hospital codes.
6. Incorporate management of environment of care in everyday tasks.

Definitions

Accreditation survey (The Joint Commission) An evaluation of an organization to assess its level of compliance with applicable Joint Commission standards and to make determinations regarding its accreditation status

Code A Sudden emergency

Disasters Unforeseen and often sudden events that cause great damage, destruction, and suffering. The disaster is caused by nature or humans

Emergency Any unplanned event that can cause deaths or significant injuries to patients, employees, volunteers, or visitors or can shut down the hospital, disrupt operations, cause physical or environmental damage, or threaten the hospital's financial standing or public image

Emergency management plan Component of an organization's environment of care program designed to manage the consequences of natural disasters or other emergencies that disrupt the organization's ability to provide care and treatment

Hazardous wastes Any solid waste that exhibits any of the characteristics of hazardous waste identified by New Jersey hazardous waste management regulations

Internal emergencies Abnormal conditions that arise within the hospital and require a special response by the hospital

External emergencies Abnormal conditions that arise outside of the hospital and require a special response by the hospital

Evacuation Removal of all people from within the facility to outside of the facility

Material safety data sheets (MSDSs) Written descriptions of each hazardous chemical used in a workplace

THE JOINT COMMISSION STANDARDS

The Joint Commission (TJC) is an organization whose mission is to continuously improve the safety and quality of care provided to the public through the provision of health care accreditation and related services that support performance improvement in health care organizations (TJC, 2007). A TJC survey is an evaluation of an organization to assess its level of compliance with applicable TJC standards and to make determinations regarding its accreditation status. TJC accreditation is a requirement to receive federal funding. The survey includes evaluation of documentation of compliance provided by organization staff; verbal information concerning the implementation of standards or examples of their implementation that will enable a determination of compliance to be made; on-site observations by surveyors; and an opportunity for education and consultation regarding standards compliance and performance improvement (TJC, 2003).

This chapter deals with those TJC requirements that measure an institution's level of performance and compliance with standards of *environment of care* (TJC, 2005). These standards encompass a variety of hospital functions and processes such as the following:

- How the organization manages its safety risks
- How the organization maintains a safe environment
- How the organization identifies and manages its security risks
- How the organization manages hazardous materials and waste risks
- Education that the staff members, students, and volunteers receive as appropriate for work in their particular environment to provide care
- Description of the roles and responsibilities of each staff member, student, and volunteer when dealing with environment of care issues
- How the organization meets the standards of all applicable agencies (Occupational Safety and Health Administration [OSHA], etc.)

As a result of the response to the Hurricane Katrina disaster, there has been increased focus on the total emergency response of all institutions. All health care agencies are required by TJC and the Health Insurance Portability and Accountability Act (HIPAA) to have a detailed emergency management plan in place to deal with natural and other occurrences. The hospital-wide safety committee usually has the responsibility for compliance with environment of care standards. The *environment of care* as defined by TJC as the provision of a safe, functional, supportive, and effective environment for all individuals within the hospital (TJC, 2007). The standards of environment of care require each hospital to develop a plan of care for the following:

- Safety management
- Security management
- Hazardous materials and waste management
- Emergency management
- Fire safety
- Medical equipment management
- Utilities management

EMERGENCY MANAGEMENT PLAN

This hospital plan ensures effective responses to disasters or internal or external emergency conditions affecting the safety of patients. The goal of the emergency management plan is to achieve a safe environment for patients, staff, volunteers, and visitors. Hospitals must meet regulatory compliance guidelines. The plan clearly identifies those individuals responsible in the event of a disaster. Only one appointed individual has the power and authority to implement an evacuation.

Hospitals are required to have available alternate sources of electrical power, safe water, safe medical gas, safe waste disposal, and communications.

The plan should meet the following objectives (OSHA, 2008):

- Pre-emergency drills implementing the emergency management plan
- Practice sessions with other local emergency response organizations using the ICS
- Personnel roles and responsibilities, including who will be in charge of directing the response, training, and communications
- Lines of authority and communication between the incident site and hospital personnel regarding hazards and potential contamination
- Designation of a decontamination team, including emergency department physicians, nurses, aides, and support personnel
- Description of the hospital's system for immediately accessing information on toxic materials
- Evacuation plan and designation of alternate facilities that could provide treatment in case

of contamination of the hospital's emergency department

- Plan for managing emergency treatment of noncontaminated patients
- Decontamination equipment, procedures, and designation of decontamination areas (either indoors or outdoors)
- Hospital staff use of protective personal equipment (PPE) based on hazards present or likely to be present, routes of exposure, degree of contact, and each individual's specific tasks
- Location and quantity of PPE
- Prevention of cross-contamination by airborne substances via the hospital's ventilation system or other means
- Prevention of cross-contamination by hazardous substances that are not airborne (e.g., surface contamination)
- Air monitoring to ensure that the facility is safe for occupancy following treatment of contaminated patients
- Post-emergency critique and follow-up of drills and actual emergencies

Patient, employee, volunteer, and visitor safety is of utmost concern to hospital administration. The emergency management program must be compatible with federal, state, and local laws. Because state laws differ, all policies and procedures must be up to date and reviewed annually or by the time specified for each hospital according to state regulations. Priorities must be clearly defined and outlined.

The hospital president/chief executive officer appoints an individual, usually the hospital safety officer, to be the lead person in the event of an emergency situation. This individual is responsible for the coordination and implementation of the policies and procedures for the emergency management of the hospital. Department heads and managers are responsible for instituting these policies and procedures. Staff members and volunteers are responsible for being aware of these policies by completing new employee orientation and annual competencies regarding the policies and procedures. You will be first exposed to your roles in emergency management during your new employee orientation (Box 5-1). Then, you will be expected to participate in routine drills that allow the safety committee members to evaluate and improve the institution's response to emergency situations.

Box 5-1   NEW EMPLOYEE ORIENTATION

- Specific roles and responsibilities during emergencies
- Patient safety activities and requirements
- Sentinel event review
- Skills and information required during emergencies
- Backup communication services
- Supplies and equipment procurement

EMERGENCY PREPAREDNESS DRILLS

The most common emergency drill that you will participate in will be routine fire drills. All institutions are required to hold fire drills at regulated intervals. A localized fire within an institution is an example of an internal emergency. Other *internal emergencies* include electrical failure, communication failure, and internal security concerns such as infant abductions. Drills mimicking such potential internal disasters will occur routinely in your institution.

Hospitals are often the first responders to emergency situations that occur outside of the hospital. For example, during the 9/11 disaster, all hospitals and potential first responding facilities within the radius of the World Trade Center towers were placed on alert to assist potential victims of the disaster. Such external disaster responses require careful planning and collaboration by all members of the community. This collaboration has resulted in community-wide external disaster drills that mimic the wide variety of potential threats to the community. The federal agency that oversees disaster management is the Federal Emergency Management Agency (FEMA).

The purposes of these drills are to evaluate and improve the response of all agencies and to determine what changes need to be made to the emergency response plan. Your role will be to participate in such drills and to assist in the evaluation of response and the creations of improvements to the plan. Some institutions have named these plans "all-hazards disaster plans." *All-hazards* is a general term that describes all types of natural and terrorist events such as biological accidents or disasters, chemical spills or exposure, conventional disasters caused by weapons, radiological or nuclear exposures, bombings, agricultural contamination, and cyber viruses (Box 5-2).

Box 5-2   ALL-HAZARDS DISASTERS

Biological accident or disaster	An incident involving a natural or deliberate outbreak of a pathogen affecting large numbers of adults and children
Chemical spills or exposures	Exposure to hazardous chemically toxic materials that may produce a wide range of adverse health effects
Conventional disaster, bombings	A catastrophic event caused by the use of weapons such as bombs, missiles, grenades, etc.
Radiological/nuclear exposures	A radiological or nuclear emergency that may result from accidents occurring within a facility or from external sources involving vehicles transporting radioactive materials or caused by terrorism events involving nuclear weapons or radiologically contaminated conventional weapons
Cyber viruses	A catastrophic event affecting large numbers of people and lasting more than a few hours that affects the ability to use information technology
Agricultural contamination	An event involving deliberate introduction of an animal or plant disease with the intent of generating fear, causing economic losses, and undermining stability

Modified from Inova Health System (2001a, 2001b, 2001c).

TOPOFF 2 INITIATIVE

Top Officials 2 (TOPOFF 2) was a congressionally mandated, national terrorism exercise that was designed to identify vulnerabilities in the nation's domestic incident management capability by exercising the plans, policies, procedures, systems, and facilities of federal, state, and local response organizations against a series of integrated terrorist threats and acts in separate regions of the country.

TOPOFF 2 was the largest and most comprehensive terrorism response exercise ever conducted in the United States. The exercise scenario, which was played out from May 12 to May 16, 2003, depicted a fictitious, foreign terrorist organization that detonated a simulated radiological dispersal device (RDD) in Seattle, Washington, and released the pneumonic plague *(Yersinia pestis)* in several Chicago metropolitan area locations. There was also significant preexercise intelligence play, a cyber attack, and credible terrorism threats against other locations. These exercises brought together top government officials from 25 federal, state, and local agencies and departments and the Canadian government to test the domestic incident management in response to weapons of mass destruction (WMD) terrorist attacks in the United States.

NATIONAL RESPONSE FRAMEWORK

The National Response Plan was replaced by the National Response Framework effective March 22,

2008. This plan establishes a comprehensive all-hazards approach to enhance the ability of the United States to manage domestic incidents. The plan incorporates best practices and procedures from incident management disciplines such as homeland security, emergency management, law enforcement, firefighting, public works, public health, responder and recovery worker health and safety, emergency medical services, and the private sector, which integrates them into a unified structure. It forms the basis of how the federal government coordinates with state, local, and tribal governments and the private sector during incidents. It establishes protocols to help (Department of Homeland Security, 2007):

- Save lives and protect the health and safety of the public, responders, and recovery workers
- Ensure the security of the homeland
- Prevent an imminent incident, including acts of terrorism
- Protect and restore critical infrastructure and key resources
- Conduct law enforcement investigations to resolve the incident, apprehend the perpetrators, and collect and preserve evidence for prosecution and/ or attribution
- Protect property and mitigate damages and impacts to individuals, communities, and the environment
- Facilitate recovery of individuals, families, businesses, governments, and the environment

HAZARDOUS MATERIALS AND WASTE

While hospitals are often perceived as safe environments, there are a variety of chemicals, energy sources, and waste products that can cause damage to the individual and the environment if not dealt with properly. Hospitals are required to have specific plans and processes for the use and disposal of such hazardous materials. Examples of hazardous waste commonly used within health care agencies are

- Diagnostic radioisotopes
- Oxygen and other combustible gases
- Surgical and other medical waste
- Chemotherapeutic agents
- Needles, syringes, and surgical equipment
- Cleaning fluids
- Energy sources, such as lasers and radiation

Hospitals must have a program in place for the safe management of hazardous materials and waste. The goal is to achieve a safe environment for patients, employees, volunteers, and visitors. The use of hazardous materials and the management of hazardous waste must be monitored and reviewed to ensure regulatory compliance throughout the hospital.

Federal Agencies for Environment of Care Issues (Box 5-3) provide information on bloodborne pathogens, radioactive waste, infectious waste, workplace safety, and national patient safety goals.

The plan should meet the following objectives:
- Identify, use, store, and dispose of hazardous materials.
- Identify, use, store, and dispose of universal waste.
- Identify specific policies and procedures.
- Provide a mechanism to reduce risk of exposure to hazardous materials and waste.
- Provide a mechanism to prevent accidents involving hazardous materials and waste.
- Develop a plan for new employee orientation and annual competencies in regard to hazardous materials and waste disposal.
- Comply with all local, state, federal, and other regulatory agencies.
- Minimize workers' compensation accidents.
- Provide to hospital administrators an annual report on the performance and effectiveness of the plan.

All adverse events that occur with hazardous materials must follow the procedure established by the employing agency. It is important that you know the policies that will affect your workplace safety as well as your patients. Documentation of all education, compliance, adverse events, and process improvement is usually the charge of the hospital-wide safety committee (Box 5-4).

Before the purchase of any new hazardous material or product, the hospital must evaluate the product for safety and proper use, storage, and disposal. A material safety data sheet (MSDS) must be provided to the hos-

---

Box 5-3   FEDERAL AGENCIES FOR ENVIRONMENT OF CARE ISSUES

Agency	Category
Occupational Safety and Health Administration (OSHA)	Bloodborne pathogens: blood and blood-soaked items, workplace safety
Nuclear Regulatory Commission (NRC)	Radioactive waste
Centers for Disease Control and Prevention (CDC)	Infectious waste
National Institute for Occupational Safety and Health (NIOSH)	Workplace safety
Environmental Protection Agency (EPA)	Workplace safety
The Joint Commission (TJC)	National patient safety goals

Box 5-4   SAFETY COMMITTEE REPORTS

- Employee exposure
- Hazardous waste incidents
- Annual reports
- Chemical spills
- Blood spills
- Recycling events/incidents
- Personal protective equipment usage
- Air quality concerns
- Regulatory deficiencies
- Hazardous surveillance results
- Universal waste monitoring results
- Record review
- Specific area evaluation (areas with hazardous materials)
- Storage space
- Material safety data sheets (sample sheet)
- Training records
- Safety policies and procedures
- Exposure records
- Waste disposal records

pital from the vendor of the material. MSDSs are standardized sheets that inform the user of the following:

- Chemical product and name
- Composition of and information on ingredients
- Hazards information
- First aid measures
- Fire fighting measures
- Accidental release measures
- Exposure controls, personal protection
- Physical and chemical properties
- Stability and reactivity
- Toxicological information
- Ecological information
- Disposal considerations
- Transport information
- Regulatory information

MSDSs are available to all members of the hospital community through a standardized communication method determined by the individual facility (Figure 5-1).

An MSDS is a written description of each hazardous chemical used in a workplace. MSDSs are the primary source of information about workplace chemicals for employers and workers. Each MSDS contains comprehensive technical information about a particular substance and explains the risks, precautions, and potential solutions related to hazardous chemicals, both during normal work and in emergency situations. The MSDS is at the heart of OSHA's Hazard Communication standard (Safety.BRL.com, 2007).

A large part of the hazardous material within a hospital falls under the category of regulated medical waste; Table 5-1 lists the seven classes of such waste.

FIRE SAFETY

Hospitals must provide a systemwide program for the safety of human life during a fire.

The plan should meet the following objectives:

- Protect patients, employees, volunteers, visitors, and property from fire and combustion
- Identify and maintain all fire protection safety standards.
- Ensure that fire alarm systems, fire detection systems, and fire extinguishers are inspected, tested, and maintained in accordance with requirements.
- Ensure that deficiencies, failures, and errors are reported and investigated.
- Ensure that a fire plan exists.
- Ensure that fire drills are held in accordance with regulatory agencies.
- Ensure that incident reports are completed in the event of a hospital fire.
- Ensure that employees receive initial employment and annual education and competencies in fire safety.

The RACE (Rescue, Alarm, Contain, Extinguish) fire plan is used by an employee who is the first individual to arrive at the scene of a fire (Box 5-5).

Text continued on p. 65

Box 5-5	RACE FIRE PLAN
R—Rescue	Rescue anyone in immediate danger from the fire. Close door to fire origin.
A—Alarm	Pull fire alarm box lever. Announce "Code Red" and exact location twice.
C—Contain	Contain fire. Close all doors and windows.
E—Extinguish	Attempt to extinguish small fire.

Adapted from http://www.safety.duke.edu/FireSafety/SSFP/Plans/SiteSpecific%20Fire%20Plan%20Part%20II%20%20Duke%20Hospital.pdf. Accessed December 27, 2009.

Table 5-1 REGULATED MEDICAL WASTE MANAGEMENT CATEGORIES

Waste Class	Item	Example	Disposal Method
1	Cultures and stocks	Live attenuated vaccine	Sharps container
2	Pathological wastes	Body fluids	Down drain
3	Human blood/products	Saturated gauze	Red bags
4	Sharps	Needles	Sharps container Waste management company
5	Animal waste	Body	Waste management company
6	Isolation waste	Smallpox virus	Waste management company
7	Unused sharps	Needle	Sharps container

Adapted from http://www.state.nj.us/dep/dshw/resource/26sch03a.pdf. Accessed December 27, 2009.

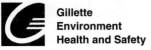

**Gillette
Environment
Health and Safety**

37 A Street
Needham, MA 02492
Tel 781.292.8151

MATERIAL SAFETY DATA SHEET

NAME: **DURACELL ALKALINE BATTERIES**
CAS NO: Not applicable   Effective Date: 6/25/2004   Rev: 8

A. — IDENTIFICATION

Composition* (1% or greater)	%	Formula:	Mixture
Manganese Dioxide (1313-13-9)	35-40	Molecular Weight:	NA
Zinc (7440-66-6)	10-25		
Potassium Hydroxide (35%) (1310-58-3)	5-10		
Graphite, natural (7782-42-5) or	1-5		
synthetic (7440-44-0)			

Synonyms: Alkaline Manganese Dioxide Batteries
MN1300 (D): MN1400 (C): MN1500 (AA) MN2400 (AAA): MX1300 (D): MX1400 (C): MX1500 (AA): MX2400 (AAA); MX2500 (AAA); MX1604 (9V);

MN908 (Lantern 6V); MN918 (Lantern 4.5V); MN1604 (9V); MN9100 (N), MN1203 (4.5V); 5K69 (Flatpack); 7K67 (Flatpaack) (J) and batteries comprised of these cells.

B. — PHYSICAL DATA

Boiling Point		Melting Point		Freezing Point	
NA °F	NA °C	NA °F	NA °C	NA °F	NA °C

Specific Gravity (H2O=1)	Vapor Density (air=1)	Vapor Pressure @_____ °F
NA	NA	NA mm Hg

Evaporation (_____ Ether _____ =1)	Saturation in Air (by volume @ _____ °F)	Autoignition Temperature _____ °F _____ °C
NA	NA	NA

% Volatiles	Solubility in Water	
NA	NA	pH NA

Appearance/Color   Copper top battery.   Contents dark in color.

Flash Point and Test Method(s)   NA

Flammable Limits in Air
  (% by volume)   Lower _____ NA _____ %   Upper _____ NA _____ %

C. — REACTIVITY

Stability	[X] stable	[ ] unstable	Polymerization	[ ] may occur	[X] will not occur

Conditions to Avoid	Conditions to Avoid
Do not heat, crush, disassemble, short circuit or recharge.	Not applicable

Incompatible Materials	Hazardous Decomposition Products
Contents incompatible with strong oxidizing agents.	Thermal degradation may produce hazardous fumes of zinc and manganese; hydrogen gas; caustic vapors of potassium hydroxide and other toxic by-products.

Footnotes   NA = Not Available
Please note: Some Duracell alkaline batteries contain the Duracell Power Check™ battery energy gauge which is a small conductive strip located underneath the PVC battery label that indicates the amount of charge in the battery. It is composed of minute quantities of conductive materials. Due to the small quantity of materials and their solid form, a health or environmental risk is unlikely.

Figure 5-1 • Material safety data sheets. (With permission from Business & Legal Reports, Inc.)

D. — HEALTH HAZARD DATA

Occupational Exposure Limits (PELs, TLVs, etc.)
8-Hour TWAs: Manganese Dioxide (as Mn) - 5 mg/m3 (Ceiling) (OSHA); 0.2 mg/m3 (ACGIH/Duracell)
           Potassium Hydroxide - 2 mg/m3 (Ceiling) (ACGIH)
             Graphite (all kinds except fibrous)-2 mg/ m3 (ACGIH); (synthetic)-15 mg/m3 (total, OSHA);
                       5 mg/m3 (respirable, OSHA)

These levels are not anticipated under normal consumer use conditions.

Warning Signals

Not applicable

Routes/Effects of Exposure
These chemicals and metals are contained in a sealed can. For consumer use, adequate hazard warnings are included on both the package and on the battery. Potential for exposure should not exist unless the battery leaks, is exposed to high temperatures or is mechanically, physically, or electrically abused. Contains concentrated (35%) potassium hydroxide, which is caustic. Anticipated potential leakage of potassium hydroxide is 2 to 20 ml, depending on battery size. A similar amount of zinc/zinc oxide may also leak.

1. Inhalation   Respiratory (and eye) irritation may occur if fumes are released due to heat or an abundance of leaking batteries.

2. Ingestion   Not anticipated due to size of batteries; choking may occur with the smaller AAA and AAAA batteries. Irritation, including caustic burns/injury, may occur following exposure to a leaking battery.

3. Skin   a. Contact
               Irritation, including caustic burns/injury, may occur following exposure to a leaking battery.

               b. Absorption
               Not anticipated

4. Eye Contact   Irritation, including caustic burns/injury, may occur following exposure to a leaking battery.

5. Other   Not applicable

E. — ENVIRONMENTAL IMPACT

1. Applicable Regulations -   All ingredients listed in TSCA inventory.

2. DOT Hazard Class -   Not applicable

3. DOT Shipping Name -   Not applicable
                         Please note: These batteries are not regulated by U. S. DOT or international agencies as hazardous materials or dangerous goods when shipped. Duracell uses the article name 'Alkaline Batteries - Non-hazardous' on all domestic and international bills of lading.

Environmental Effects
These batteries pass the U. S. EPA's Toxicity Characteristic Leaching Procedure and therefore, may be disposed of with normal waste.

Figure 5-1 • cont'd

F. — EXPOSURE CONTROL METHODS

Engineering Controls
General ventilation under normal use conditions.

Eye Protection
None under normal use conditions. Wear safety glasses when handling leaking batteries.

Skin Protection
None under normal use conditions. Use neoprene, rubber or latex gloves when handling leaking batteries.

Respiratory Protection
None under normal use conditions.

Other
Keep batteries away from small children.

G. — WORK PRACTICES

Handling and Storage
Store at room temperature. Avoid mechanical or electrical abuse. DO NOT short or install incorrectly. Batteries may explode, pyrolize or vent if disassembled, crushed, recharged or exposed to high temperatures. Install batteries in accordance with equipment instructions. Do not mix battery systems, such as alkaline and zinc carbon, in the same equipment. Replace all batteries in equipment at the same time. Do not carry batteries loose in pocket or bag. Do not remove battery tester or battery label.

Normal Clean Up
Not applicable

Waste Disposal Methods
Individual consumers may dispose of spent (used) batteries with household trash. Duracell does not recommend that spent batteries be accumulated (quantities of five gallons or more should be disposed of in a secure landfill), in accordance with appropriate federal, state and local regulations. Do not incinerate, since batteries may explode at excessive temperatures.

Figure 5-1 • cont'd

H. — EMERGENCY PROCEDURES

Steps to be taken if material is released to the environment or spilled in the work area
Notify safety personnel of large spills. Caustic potassium hydroxide may be released from leaking or ruptured batteries. Avoid eye or skin contact and inhalation of vapors. Increase ventilation. Clean-up personnel should wear appropriate protective gear.

Fire and Explosion Hazard	Extinguishing Media
Batteries may burst and release hazardous decomposition products when exposed to a fire situation. See Sec. C.	As appropriate for surrounding area.

Firefighting Procedures
Use self-contained breathing apparatus and full protective gear.

I. — FIRST AID AND MEDICAL EMERGENCY PROCEDURES

Eyes
Not anticipated. If battery is leaking and material contacts eyes, flush with copious amounts of clear, tepid water for 30 minutes. Contact physician at once.

Skin
Not anticipated. If battery is leaking, irrigate exposed skin with copious amounts of clear, tepid water for at least 15 minutes. If irritation, injury or pain persists, consult a physician.

Inhalation
Not anticipated. If battery is leaking, contents may be irritating to respiratory passages. Remove to fresh air. Contact physician if irritation persists.

Ingestion
Not anticipated. Rinse the mouth and surrounding area with clear, tepid water for at least 15 minutes. Consult a physician immediately for treatment and to rule out involvement of the esophagus and other tissues.

Notes to Physician
1) The primary acutely toxic ingredient is concentrated (35%) potassium hydroxide.
2) Anticipated potential leakage of potassium hydroxide is 2-20 ml, depending on battery size.
3) This MSDS does not include or address the small button cell batteries, which can be ingested.

This MSDS covers the following discontinued product numbers: DAC100, 105,110,116-118,123-124, 130, 200, 610,810, 820,918

The information contained in the Material Safety Data Sheet is based on data considered to be accurate, however, no warranty is expressed or implied regarding the accuracy of the data or the results to be obtained from the use thereof.

Figure 5-1 • cont'd

MEDICAL EQUIPMENT

The wide variety of equipment used by most hospitals also must be monitored for proper functioning, calibration, and potential recalls. Intravenous pumps that deliver medication need to be routinely checked to ensure that calibration of medication delivery is accurate. Blood pressure monitors also need to be checked for proper functioning. Implantable devices such as pacemakers need to be carefully tracked by hospitals in case of a product recall. Such recalls can also apply to artificial joints, cardiac monitors, or any device used in patient care. The Safe Medical Device Act of 1990 (public law 101-629) established a reporting system to the manufacturer to report adverse effects of such devices (FDA, 1991). It is your responsibility to make sure that all device maintenance is completed and that defective devices are immediately reported to the appropriate department. If you deal with implantable patient equipment, you must follow the required documentation process of your institution.

A medical device plan should meet the following objectives:
- Establish criteria for identifying, evaluating, and taking inventory of medical equipment.
- Test and ensure safe operation of equipment.
- Perform timely repair and service to defective equipment.
- Monitor and act on any medical equipment recalls.
- Monitor and record any incidents with the use of medical equipment.
- Assess and minimize risks associated with the use of medical equipment.

Equipment management written criteria should include but is not limited to the following:
- Equipment function
- Physical risks associated with the use of equipment
- Equipment maintenance requirements
- Equipment incident history

All employees using new equipment should have departmental orientation for use of the equipment as well as annual competencies on proper use of the equipment.

Departmental in-service education should include but is not limited to the following:
- Capabilities, limitations, and special applications of equipment use
- Basic operating and safety procedures for equipment use
- Emergency procedures in the event of equipment failure
- Information and skills necessary to perform assigned maintenance responsibilities
- Processes for reporting medical equipment management problems, failures, and user errors

SECURITY PLAN

Everyone assumes that hospitals are havens of safety, yet because they are open to the public on a 24-hours-a-day/7-days-a-week basis, there are potential workplace security concerns that plague hospitals. A security plan is necessary to protect both the patients and staff. This plan ensures that the hospital provides for a safe and secure physical environment for patients, employees, visitors, and volunteers and maintains protection of equipment and property.

The plan should meet the following objectives:
- Respond to incidents of potential harm or personal dangers to patients, employees, visitors, and volunteers.
- Conduct security risk assessments.
- Report and investigate all security incidents involving patients, employees, visitors, and volunteers.
- Provide identification for patients, employees, visitors, and volunteers.
- Control security-sensitive areas.
- Control vehicular movement on hospital grounds, including parking lot.
- Provide security orientation and education about staff responsibilities for patient care.
- Develop a plan for ongoing monitoring.

Issues commonly dealt with by the security plan include infant abduction from maternal/child units, potential patient suicides, hostage situations, unruly visitors or employees, crimes committed within the facility, and others.

Table 5-2 lists various institutional responses to emergency "codes" commonly associated with environment of care issues; all of these plans report all activities and plans to the larger hospital-wide safety committee.

Table 5-2	EMERGENCY CODES ASSOCIATED WITH ENVIRONMENT OF CARE ISSUES		
Event	**Description**	**Initial Response**	**Secondary Response**
Fire—code red	Fire/smoke/smells like something burning	Dial emergency in-house number; announce "code red" R—Rescue A—Activate alarm C—Contain fire E—Extinguish	To extinguish: P—Pull pin A—Aim hose S—Squeeze handle S—Sweep side to side
Patient abduction—code amber	Patient is missing or is known to be abducted	Give patient information to operator. Notify police. Guard exits.	Decide if code should be called. Assemble alert team. Stop access exit. Seal off units. Maintain patient confidentiality. Support parent/guardian. Suspend visiting hours.
Bomb threat—code yellow	Notification of a bomb on campus, usually by an outside caller	Obtain as much information as possible. Do not interrupt. Refer to bomb threat checklist in hospital telephone directory.	Call police, hospital security, and administrative offices. Report all information. Cooperate with authorities.
Security emergency—code gray	Situations that require immediate presence of a supervisor	Dial emergency in-house number; announce code and location. Members of security, psychology, and engineering will arrive.	All other personnel will clear the area and keep hallways clear.
Hostage situation—code silver	An individual is being held against her or his will by an armed perpetrator	Clear the area to avoid escalation. Report to supervisor and others in charge of response.	Personnel unable to be cleared of the area will remain concealed until further instructions are received. Coordinate with authorities.
Incident hazardous materials spill—code orange	Small spill presenting no hazard to trained staff or environment	Trained staff cleans spill wearing appropriate personal protection equipment and decontamination equipment.	Dispose of material appropriately.
Emergency hazardous materials spill—code orange	Any spill that may present a hazard to people or the environment or when effects are not known	Evacuate and isolate spill area. Notify supervisor. Assist contaminated victims in decontamination process if you can do so safely.	Immediately seek and coordinate appropriate medical treatment for decontaminated victim.
Unusual incident disaster—code triage	Disaster not covered by other plans	Clear area—notify supervisor.	Follow instructions from hospital leader.
Evacuation relocation of patients—code triage	Event where the hospital becomes uninhabitable	Relocate patients to safe place inside the hospital. Prepare for transport. Prioritize the severity of patients' needs.	Call local hospitals for accommodations. Transport via local rescue squad. Ensure proper transfer of patient information.

Note: Colors of codes are not universal; follow your institution's naming device.

SAFETY COMMITTEE

The hospital-wide safety committee meets between 6 and 12 times per year. The agenda items include but are not limited to safety management, security management, hazardous materials and waste management, emergency management, life safety, medical equipment management, and utilities management.

The safety plan should include but is not limited to the following:

- Develop and implement an organization-wide safety management program.
- Review written policies and procedures related to safety both inside and outside the institution.
- Assist in the development of safety rules and practices.
- Manage the hospital's ongoing monitoring of performance.
- Monitor an incident/injury reporting system.
- Maintain a network for continued safety-related information exchange.
- Establish monitoring guidelines.
- Coordinate and monitor the hazard surveillance program.
- Establish reliability and validity of statistics, records, and reports.
- Establish committee goals and objectives.
- Evaluate the effectiveness of all safety-related programs, including
  - Safety management
  - Security management
  - Emergency management
  - Hazardous materials and waste
  - Life safety
  - Medical equipment
  - Utilities

SAFETY COMMITTEE REPORTS

- Occurrence
- Assessment/surveillance
- Notices
- Drills
- Annual evaluations of programs
- Annual reports
- Periodic monitoring

REPORTS

- Building and building grounds
- Information collection and evaluation

- Biomedical and utilities
- Safety and security
- Hazardous surveillance
- Infection control
- Performance improvement
- Risk management
- Employee incidents
- Grounds and equipment
- Hazardous materials
- Regulatory audit
- Exposure monitoring
- Life safety
- Emergency management

DEPARTMENT MANAGERS' RESPONSIBILITIES

- Maintain plans.
- Ensure plan compliance.
- Clearly define staff responsibilities.
- Ensure staff attendance at educational sessions.
- Maintain current records of education and training.
- Supervise staff to comply with all safety standards.
- Know your role and employees' role in safety plan.
- Correct unsafe practices.
- Educate staff on location of fire equipment and oxygen shut-off valves.
- Provide safety officer with potential hazards in your area.
- Provide information to new employees on:
  - Staff/employee safety
  - Infection control
  - OSHA bloodborne pathogens/tuberculosis exposure plans
  - MSDSs
  - Hazardous materials/waste disposal
  - Incident reporting
  - Fire/disaster assignment
  - Emergency codes

INCIDENT REPORTS

- Personal injuries
- Damages to or loss of personal or hospital property
- Occupational injuries
- Potential safety hazard

Your role in the management of a safe environment of care is based on a multitude of regulatory requirements and individual response to the overall safety of your workplace. It is imperative that you are aware of the hazards of the workplace for both you and your patients. Also, as a health care professional, you need to be prepared to react to the unexpected and to collaborate with all members of the health care team and community in the creation of a safe environment for your patients and yourself.

When an incident occurs, most hospitals require that an incident report be completed within 24 hours of the incident. Also, some hospitals use a computer-based incident report system with prompts to ensure the report is concise and accurate. See Figure 5-2 for a downtime event report.

SUMMARY

The management of the processes that have an impact on the safety and the actual environment where the care takes place is crucial to the achievement of patient and staff outcomes. Effective management of the environment of care reduces hazards and risks, prevents accidents and injuries, maintains safe conditions for all patients and staff, and maintains an environment that is conducive to care. The nurse needs to participate in the processes and activities that make the environment safe and effective. The nurse manager needs to identify and communicate the conditions of the care environment so that resources are used to continually ensure the safety of the hospital.

CLINICAL CORNER

The Watson Room at St. Joseph's Regional Medical Center: Caring for Yourself in Times of Stress, Emergencies, Disasters, and "Bad Days"
Joy Espejo

The Watson Room is named after the nursing theorist Jean Watson. This is a quiet space created for nurses to use before, during, or after their shift to achieve personal satisfaction in their work. We know that nurses face tremendous challenges each day, and especially in times of emergency and potential disaster. But, rarely, do we as nurses acknowledge this stress and the need to "de-stress."

The purpose of the Watson Room is to allow nurses to center on self and engage in refocusing, destressing, and rejuvenating in a Zen-like environment. Nurses are greeted with the scent of lavender, tranquil music, gently flowing waterfalls, healing tree of stones, Buddha board, and soft drapery gathered toward the massage seat. Representing the 10 caritas or caring factors of Watson's Caring Theory, the Caring Mosaic artwork is made of medicine caps and materials nurses use every day. These aesthetic enhancements and harmonious interplay of complementary and alternative therapies for nurses give an instant sense of relaxation. This will, in turn, create and sustain a caring and healing environment for the patients, families, and staff.

Creating the Watson Room was the decision of the Shared Governance Council working on the 14 Forces of Magnetism, Watson Caring Theory, relationship-based care delivery model, and healthy work environment to achieve our vision for excellence in patient care. This council is comprised of staff nurses who meet monthly to shape our professional practice at St. Joseph's.

Believing in our commitment to a culture of excellence, a small space used as a consultation room was donated to us by the chief of surgery and trauma. A staff nurse from medical ICU engaged staff nurses, maintenance staff, patient care associates, nurse managers, directors of nursing, and the chief nurse officer to help with the design and transformation of the room.

The effects of personal satisfaction derived from the Watson Room can be echoed from the positive comments of nursing staff. Good patient care outcomes result from destressing and refocusing. Caring and healing for the patient, families, and the staff in a healthy work environment take place when the nurses are nurtured first.

> Thank-you note from Dorothy Salerno, RN, Post Anesthesia Care Unit (PACU) Staff Nurse, St. Joseph's Regional Medical Center, Paterson, NJ

> Dear Mary Ann Hozak, RN   11/21/08

I wanted to say thank you for the Watson Room. Last year my Father passed away on Hospice at Lyons V.A. Hospital. I was comforted by a lovely nurse and soothing music and with my immediate family. We at St. Joseph's did not have our Watson Room up and ready at the time of my father's illness.

This past month my mother became seriously ill and wanted to stay at her home for her final days. Even though we had 24-hour care, it was different and difficult being both the daughter and the nurse.

Continued

LISA MO MEDICAL CENTER

DOWNTIME EVENT REPORT

The following form should be completed when electronic Event Report Downtime System is not available. Once Event Report Downtime System has been restored, this information will be transferred electronically and this form will be destroyed. Complete all fields below.

Individual Affected

Check all that apply:

____ Inpatient   ____ Outpatient   ____ Parent/guardian/relative   ____ Employee   ____ Volunteer   ____ Visitor

Name _____ Medical Record # _____

Address _____

Unit _____ DOB ___ / ___ / ___ Diagnosis _____

Type of Incident

____ Airway management   ____ Treatment   ____ Restraint
____ Blood or blood products   ____ Safety   ____ Skin
____ Diagnosis   ____ Privacy   ____ Laboratory test
____ Diagnostic test   ____ IV Line   ____ Tubing
____ Fall   ____ Medication   ____ Security

Incident Report

Date of Incident: _____

_____

Exact Location: _____

_____

All Departments involved: _____

_____

Services involved: _____

_____

Figure 5-2 ● Downtime event report.

Specific Details

Incident type: _____

Contributing factors: _____

Specific Actions Taken

Name of physician called and time physician examined patient _____

Name of family member called and time called _____

Name of nursing supervisor and time called _____

Severity Level Reported

A Potential harm   B No harm   C Temporary harm   D Permanent harm   E Death

Description of Incident _____

_____

_____

Injury Details

Degree of Injury: _____ Type of Injury: _____

Body Part: _____

Equipment Involved _____

_____

_____

Notification (Please identify all the individuals that were notified of the incident.)

Name/Location: _____

Date: _____ Time: _____

Name/Location: _____

Date: _____ Time: _____

Figure 5-2 • cont'd

CLINICAL CORNER—cont'd

I sought solace at the beautiful Watson Room.

My coworkers also helped me with a kind word, a soft touch, or a helping hand in relieving me of work responsibilities so I could care for my mother.

The PACU nurses are truly Magnet nurses. The combination of aroma therapy, massage therapy chair, soft soothing music, and the sound of running water along with the kindness of my coworkers helped relieve my overwhelming stress and strain during this difficult time. Slowly as I return to work with less personal stress, the Watson Room will allow me to refocus and show more empathy and attention to my patients.

The Watson Room fostered a caring and healing environment for me. I hope all St. Joseph's nurses take advantage and the time to visit the Watson Room.

Sincerely,

Dorothy Salerno, RN

EVIDENCE-BASED PRACTICE

Influences on Nurse Perception of Hospital Unit Safety Climate: an HLM Approach

Ramanujam, R., Abrahamson, K., & Anderson, J. (2007). Influences on nurse perception of hospital unit safety climate: an HLM approach. *Modified from Purdue University e-Pubs. Retrieved April 16, 2009 from http://docs.lib.purdue.edu/ rche_rp/34/.*

Patient safety is a critical issue in health care. Unfortunately, due to the demands for both safety and efficiency, conflicts exist within the health care environment. Nurses are expected to be agents of caring and protection while managing high workloads. In attempting to negotiate the safety/efficiency dichotomy, nurses may inadvertently be jeopardizing patient safety.

It is believed that nurses play a crucial role in patient safety and that many of the most serious medical errors are preventable. It is for this reason that further examination of registered nurse perceptions of patient safety is warranted.

Direct care nurses who struggle with the dichotomy of patient safety and efficiency traditionally have not had the power and position to direct organizational processes. However, they have previously identified some inadequate work environment issues that have resulted in errors or near misses

- The inability of a nurse to access necessary information or materials
- Lack of available support from qualified coworkers is a major source of stress

Unlike the aviation industry, which embraces a more collective approach to safety, those in health care are less likely to acknowledge the universal potential of human error. They are also significantly more likely to think their organization handles error poorly. This study seeks to determine the influence that a hospital unit's overall level of nurse education and experience has on individual nurse perceptions of their patients' opportunity to receive safe care.

These perceptions of patient safety may provide invaluable information regarding improving the safety of hospitalized patients. Previous literature finds that nurses who are well supported by qualified coworkers report lower levels of work-related distress. Therefore, it is predicted that individual nurse perceptions of patient safety will be increased on units with more highly qualified nurses.

The results of this study showed that there was statistically significant data to confirm previous research, which stated that providing nurses with coworkers who are able to offer collegial support improves the nurse's perception of his or her workplace environment. This helps to support the conclusion that factors that have been shown to decrease workplace distress such as collegial support may also contribute to improving patient safety. These results highlight the potential importance of collegial support in nursing but do not support the assumption that nurses with more education or those working full-time have a positive effect on individual registered nurse perception of patient safety.

Previous work has also found that the addition of informational technology such as electronic medical records, decision support, and error reporting systems to the hospital setting reduces medical errors. However, an adequate reduction in medical errors has not been achieved through technology upgrades alone. The present analysis indicates a combination of social and technological modifications may best provide nurses with the environments needed to reduce error.

NCLEX® EXAM QUESTIONS

1. RACE stands for:
   1. rescue, alarm, contain, extinguish
   2. rescue, act, confine, extinguish
   3. react, alert, contain, extinguish
   4. remove, alarm, contain, extinguish
2. An example of an internal disaster would be:
   1. a tornado that does not affect the hospital
   2. flooding of a street near the hospital
   3. a tree falling onto a patient unit
   4. a hurricane in the next town
3. An example of the need for an incident report is:
   1. a medication error
   2. a patient fall
   3. injury to employee
   4. all of the above
4. You are the charge nurse. One of your employees had a splash to the face from a cleaning agent. What is the FIRST thing you would do?
   1. Take the employee to the eye wash station and rinse his or her eyes for 15 minutes.
   2. Call 911 immediately.
   3. Take the employee to the emergency department of the hospital.
   4. Send the employee to a private physician for care.
5. When you walk into the pantry, you see a bag of popcorn on fire in the microwave oven. What is the FIRST thing you would do?
   1. Go to the pull station and pull the alarm lever.
   2. Go to a telephone and tell the operator to call "code red."
   3. Call the fire department directly from your unit.
   4. Call the nursing supervisor.
6. All of the following is on the materials safety data sheet EXCEPT:
   1. price of item
   2. contents of item
   3. instructions in event of chemical spill onto skin
   4. none of the above
7. You are the nurse in charge of the unit. What would you do if a fire is called in the unit directly below yours?
   1. Report to that unit to see if they need assistance.
   2. Make sure all employees are accounted for.
   3. Have all nurses wait at the nurses' station for instructions.
   4. Make sure all patients are accounted for.
8. A feeding pump is defective. What should you do?
   1. Place a defective sticker on it and inform materials management.
   2. Tell the nursing supervisor.
   3. There is no need to do anything.
   4. Call the manufacturing company to replace it.
9. The Joint Commission is an agency that strives to:
   1. ensure employees are paid properly
   2. improve the safety and quality of patient care
   3. decrease the number of "near misses"
   4. decrease the number of incident reports at a facility
10. An example of an external disaster is a:
    1. tornado
    2. hurricane
    3. plane crash into the hospital parking lot
    4. all of the above

Answers: 1. 1   2. 3   3. 4   4. 1   5. 1   6. 1   7. 2   8. 1   9. 2   10. 4

REFERENCES

Department of Homeland Security. (2007). National response framework. Retrieved June 19, 2007, from http://www.dhs.gov/xprepresp/committees/editorial_0566.shtm.

Inova Health System. (2001a). *All-hazards disaster preparedness plan. Annex B*. Falls Church, VA: Inova Health System.

Inova Health System. (2001b). *All-hazards disaster preparedness plan. Annex C*. Falls Church, VA: Inova Health System.

Inova Health System. (2001c). *All-hazards disaster preparedness plan. Annex R*. Falls Church, VA: Inova Health System.

Joint Commission on Accreditation of Healthcare Organizations. (2003). *Comprehensive accreditation manual*. Oakbrook Terrace, IL: Author.

Joint Commission. (2007). *Comprehensive accreditation manual*. Oakbrook Terrace, IL: Author.

Occupational Safety and Health Administration (OSHA). (2008). *Hospitals and community emergency response*. OSHA 3152-3R. Washington, D.C.: U.S. Department of Labor.

Ramanujam, R., Abrahamson, K., & Anderson, J. (2007). Influences on nurse perception of hospital unit safety climate: an HLM approach. Purdue University e-Pubs. Retrieved April 16, 2009, from http://docs.lib.purdue. edu/rche_rp/34/.

Safety.BRL.com. MSDS training, regulations, analysis, news, and tools. Retrieved June 19, 2007, from http://safety.blr. com/topics.aspx?topic=124.

U.S. Food and Drug Administration (FDA). (1991). The Safe Medical Devices Act of 1990. *Federal Register*, *56*(66), 14111-14113.

Leadership

The following section deals with the payment, regulatory, and ethical issues that you will confront as a nurse manager. The health care environment is much more than the patient care environment. Everything that you do as a nurse is influenced by the decisions of the payors, the economic realities, the many regulatory and certifying agencies, and the moral decision making of the patient and family.

As a nurse leader, you will be asked to advocate for the patient and family. You will want to do everything possible for the patient, but your actions will be constrained by the reimbursement services allowed for the patient and family. Many of the patients who you see will be in good health, but many citizens are disabled, sick, and in need of service. Sadly, many Americans today do not have health care insurance, and many who do have limited coverage. How many individuals will access care depends on their type of insurance and health coverage. This coverage will also influence how many people use health care. As a nurse, you will need to be able to balance the many conflicting variables of need for care, payment for care, and availability of care.

The care environment is also heavily regulated on local, state, and national levels. Compliance with the rules of the regulators is imperative for agencies. If agencies do not comply, they become ineligible for reimbursement; thus, the nurse needs to be knowledgeable of all of the regulations that have the potential to influence patient care and the delivery of patient care.

Knowledge of each of these areas forms a basis for some of the leadership competencies of the new nurse. As you develop your management skills, you will need to take into account many variables beyond what you have already learned as a nurse. You will need to broaden your knowledge base to include knowledge of the larger health care environment.

Last, there will be many decisions that will result in ethical dilemmas for the nurse manager. Personal and professional values serve as a baseline for many of these decisions, but ethical decision making will be evidenced in many of the decisions and some of the policies of the organization. This section will also discuss ethical decision making and how it relates to management practices in the highly regulated health care environment.

CHAPTER 6

Health Care

Chapter Objectives

1. Define *health care*.
2. Identify factors influencing today's health care system.
3. Discuss the economic realities of U.S. health care.
4. Identify the major forms of reimbursement for health care.
5. Describe the U.S. health care system.

Definitions

Health State of complete physical, social, and mental well-being; not merely the absence of disease or infirmity, as defined by the World Health Organization (2008). Health is a resource for everyday life, not the object of living. It is a positive concept emphasizing social and personal resources as well as physical capabilities.

Health care system All of the structures, organizations, and services designed to deliver professional health and wellness services to consumers

Health care network Refers to interconnected units that are owned by the institution or have cooperative agreements with other institutions to provide a full spectrum of wellness and illness services

Health Maintenance Organization (HMO) Geographically organized system that provides an agreed-on package of health maintenance and treatment services

Medicare Health insurance program for people aged 65 and older or under age 65 with certain disabilities or any age with end-stage renal disease

Medicaid Joint federal and state assistance program designed to pay for medical long-term care assistance for individuals and families with low income and limited resources

Private agencies Private agencies have voluntary governing bodies. They are not administered or governed by the U.S. government. Private agencies are required to meet state licensing requirements and regulations related to the area of their governing authorities. Private agencies are for profit or not for profit.

For-profit organizations Organizations with stated financial structures that include profit goals and tax liabilities

Not-for-profit organizations Organizations with financial structures that project financial goals with particular tax and legislative protection or shelters

Preferred provider organization (PPO) Managed care company that contracts with health care providers (both physicians and hospitals) and payers (self-insured employers, insurance companies, or managed care organizations) to provide health care services to a defined population for predetermined fixed fees

Centers for Medicare & Medicaid Services (CMS) Formerly known as the Health Care

Financing Administration, the federal agency that administers Medicare, Medicaid, State Children's Health Insurance Program (SCHIP), and several other health-related programs

Managed care Linkage between the financing and delivery of services in such a way as to permit payers to exercise control over the delivery of services

Continuum of care Matching an individual's ongoing needs with the appropriate level and type of medical, psychological, health, or social care or service within an organization or across multiple organizations

Veterans Health Administration The mission of the Veterans Healthcare System is to serve the needs of America's veterans by providing primary care, specialized care, and related medical and social support services. To accomplish this mission, the VHA needs to be a comprehensive, integrated health care system that provides excellence in health care value, excellence in service as defined by its customers, and excellence in education and research, and needs to be an organization characterized by exceptional accountability and by being an employer of choice

World Health Organization (WHO) Specialized agency of the United Nations (UN) that acts as a coordinating authority on international public health. Established in April 1948 and headquartered in Geneva, Switzerland, the agency inherited the mandate and resources of its predecessor, the Health Organization, which had been an agency of the League of Nations.

HEALTH

With the advent of health care delivery services organized under hospitals and care-giving facilities in the early nineteenth century, there has been movement toward standardizing care and financial practices within these institutions. It was not until the early twentieth century that hospitals began a pay-for-service financial plan. In this arrangement, the patient pays for services received. Insurance companies paid for the services rendered by most institutions. As the cost of health care in the United States rose exponentially, insurers began exploring more cost-effective ways to pay for health care. This has resulted in the health care plans, insurance plans, and federal plans that exist today. This change in reimbursement for health care services has dramatically affected all aspects of health care delivery in the United States driven by changes in Medicare reimbursement.

This has also affected the way nursing care is provided. For example, today, patients who are hospitalized have a much higher acuity than they did 20 years ago. Today, the norm is for many patients to be treated at home or in ambulatory care settings; only the critically ill remain in the hospital. Nursing has been expected to meet these challenges both in acute care and in home care. Today there are more ambulatory services, shorter inpatient stays, and an increase in care for chronic illnesses. The greatest challenge facing the U.S.

health care system is the high cost of care and services. Technology enables the survival of premature infants weighing 2499 g or less. Some of the infants are kept alive with life support, which may include ventilators and/or feeding tubes. These infants may have a lifetime connection with pediatricians, nurses, specialists, and therapists. Many of them are placed in early intervention programs, whereby the nurses and therapists visit the child and family in the home setting. Once these "preemies" are 3 years old, they are placed in preschool programs for the handicapped. This is just one isolated example of the trend of health care in the United States. Health care in the United States is paramount, but at what expense? At an insurmountable expense. So … not only are the elderly living longer, the preemies are kept alive on life support. Individuals in severe motor vehicle accidents are air lifted to trauma centers and kept alive. What is the cost to the families and to the nation? The costs effect employers, health care providers, the government, and the public sector.

FACTORS THAT INFLUENCE THE FINANCIAL BURDEN OF HEALTH CARE IN THE UNITED STATES

There are numerous factors that influence the continuing financial burden of health care within the United States.

DEMOGRAPHIC INFLUENCES

The United States is culturally diverse. There is a continuous influx of people from all countries of the world. It is crucial for the U.S. health care system to deliver culturally competent care. The United States spends more on health care per capita than any other industrialized Western nation, but the United States has disproportionately more people without access to appropriate health care (Yoder-Wise, 2006, p. 277).

Steep population growth and an aging population will increase the need for health care services. The U.S. population aged 65 years and over is predicted to reach 82 million in 2050, a 137% increase over 1999. Between 2011 and 2030, the number of elderly could rise from 40.4 million (13% of the population) to 70.3 million (20% of the population) as "baby boomers" begin turning 65 (U.S. Census Bureau, 2000; http://www.census.gov/).

Economic interests shape the evolution of technology and health care. The types of healthcare services delivered continue to be limited by multiple factors, most notably cost constraints (Wywialowski, 2004, p. 33).

UNINSURED INDIVIDUALS

It is estimated that 45 million Americans do not have access to health insurance. One reason is that their place of employment does not provide health care coverage; another reason is that they cannot afford the high cost of health care. The uninsured and underinsured populations affect hospitals as well as the communities in which health care is sought.

This places an added burden on the facilities to provide "charity care." When a patient who is uninsured receives care, the cost of the care trickles down to other payers, to the government, or to private insurance companies. This added cost is then passed down to the customers and to taxpayers. In the end, the uninsured population affects everyone, not just the uninsured. Bankruptcy in the United States has had a direct correlation to medical expenses and depleted savings.

MEDICAL TECHNOLOGY

The expansion of medical technology and specialty medicine also affects the economics of health care. For example, diagnostic and therapeutic techniques such as magnetic resonance imaging, organ transplantation, and electronic medical records enhance the capabilities of health care.

HEALTH CARE PAYMENT SOURCES

There are rising expectations about the value of health care services in the United States. It is the cultural norm in America that we will all receive the highest quality of health care at all times. To this end, the United States spends a great deal of money on health care services. The people of the United States are covered by Medicare, Medicaid, insurance companies, and managed care companies, and 16.3% of the U.S. population is not insured (Kelly-Heidenthal, 2003, p. 5).

The United States continues to rely on a free-market approach to health care with the private sector providing insurance coverage (through employers) and the federal sector providing for some individuals who are unable to pay. Health care is paid for by four sources: government (36%), private insurance companies (41%), individuals (19%), and other, primarily philanthropy (4%) (Yoder-Wise, 2007, p. 222).

Medical insurance began in 1847 with payments made to offset income loss that resulted after an accident. Blue Cross Blue Shield originated the reimbursement of general health costs in the 1930s. The private health care industry has changed dramatically with the advent of managed care. In the private sector, the following five types of organizations fund health care costs:

- Traditional insurance companies, which includes Blue Cross Blue Shield for profit commercial insurance companies
- Preferred provider organizations (PPOs), which act as brokers between insurers and health care providers
- Health maintenance organizations (HMOs), which are independent prepayment plans
- Point of service (POS) plans, which combined features of classic HMOs with client choice characteristics of PPOs
- Self-funded plans in which the employer takes on the role of insurer

PRIVATE INSURANCE

The majority of insured Americans received health care insurance through their place of employment. The focus of such coverage has moved from the straight fee-for-services rendered model to managed health care. Managed health care organizations provide for both the delivery and the financing of health care for their members. The principal force behind the movement away from fee-for-service was the belief that health care costs can be controlled by "managing" the way in which health care is delivered and used.

The foundation of the managed care organization is the primary care provider (PCP). The PCP can be a physician or a nurse practitioner. This provider serves as the gatekeeper to coordinate and manage the patient's use of resources and referrals and protects the patient from unnecessary overtreatment.

HMOs deliver comprehensive health maintenance and treatment services for a group of enrolled individuals. Several models of the HMO structure have evolved. The group model is where practitioners employed by the insurer spend all their time caring for patients of that particular HMO. An example of this model is the Kaiser-Permanente Health Care System. Another model is Independent Practice Associations (IPAs) where independent practitioners (not employed by the HMO) provide care for HMO members and are reimbursed for that care. Practitioners in an IPA contract may be restricted to caring only for members enrolled in that IPA, but some contracts allow practitioners to provide for nonmembers as well. In a network model, HMOs contract with individual practitioners and practitioner groups for both primary and specialty services. In a capitation system, each provider receives a flat annual fee for each patient regardless of how often services are used. Box 6-1 provides various types of HMOs.

Box 6-1	TYPES OF HEALTH MAINTENANCE ORGANIZATIONS (HMOs)
Staff model	Self-contained organization
	Providers are employees of the HMO
Group model	Contractual agreement with multispecialty physician groups to deliver care for group
Network model	Contractual agreements with physician practice groups
Independent practice association	Contractual agreements with a wide variety of care providers
	Members have greater choice
PPO	Network of providers that provides care to group

Modified from Grohar-Murray, M. E., & DiCroce, H. R. (2003). *Leadership and management in nursing* (p. 11). 3rd ed. Upper Saddle River, NJ: Prentice Hall.

POINT OF SERVICE PLANS

POS plans evolved in response to patient concerns about their lack of choice in choosing providers in the previously mentioned plans. These plans allow members to pay additional fees to use providers outside of the individual network.

PPOs agree to deliver services to members for a fee-for-service negotiated price. Members must receive care exclusively from within the PPO or incur additional costs. To control costs, the health care agency must receive preauthorization from the PPO for a member to be hospitalized and second opinions are required before all major procedures.

U.S. GOVERNMENT

The federal government oversees plans that assist the elderly, the disabled, and some uninsured individuals.

MEDICAID

Medicaid is a joint federal and state assistance program designed to pay for medical long-term care assistance for individuals and families with low income and limited resources. Medicaid is available only to certain low-income individuals and families who fit into an eligibility group that is recognized by federal and state law. Medicaid sends payments directly to health care providers. Medicaid went into effect in 1967 and is known as Title XIX of the Social Security Administration. Each state sets its own guidelines regarding eligibility and services. These may include age, disabilities, income, financial resources (e.g., bank accounts, real property, or other items that can be sold for cash), and citizenship status, and whether the individual is a U.S. citizen or a lawfully admitted immigrant. There are special rules for those who live in nursing homes and for disabled children living at home. Children may be eligible for coverage if they are U.S. citizens or lawfully admitted immigrants. Eligibility for children is based on the child's status, not the parents'.

STATE CHILDREN'S HEALTH INSURANCE PROGRAM (SCHIP)

Of all developed countries, the United States has the highest proportion of uninsured individuals. The lack of health insurance is greatest for blacks and Hispanics, younger Americans 18 to 34, and men more than women. Most of the uninsured have at least one family member who is working full-time but they do not obtain coverage because the cost of premiums is high. A plan that targets uninsured children who are not eligible for Medicaid established State Children's Health Insurance Program (SCHIP). These programs were implemented at the state level to provide insurance for all children.

MEDICARE

Medicare is the government's largest health care financing program. In 2003, Medicare paid out more than $277 million to 40 million elderly and disabled people (CBO, 2003). Medicare is the name given to a health insurance program administered by the U.S. government, covering people who are either aged 65 and over or who meet other special criteria. There have been numerous changes to the Medicare system since its introduction. Many of these changes have been attempts to deal with the high cost of Medicare expenditures.

Administration of Federal Insurers

The Centers for Medicare & Medicaid Services (CMS), a component of the Department of Health and Human Services (HHS), administers Medicare, Medicaid, and SCHIP. The Social Security Administration is responsible for determining Medicare eligibility and processing premium payments for the Medicare program.

Benefits

The "Original Medicare" program has two parts: Part A (Hospital Insurance) and Part B (Medical Insurance). Only a few special cases exist where prescription drugs are covered by Original Medicare, but as of January 2006, Medicare Part D provides more comprehensive drug coverage. Medicare Advantage plans are another way for beneficiaries to receive their Part A, B, and D benefits.

Part A: Hospital Insurance
Part A covers hospital stays. It also will pay for stays in a skilled nursing facility if certain criteria are met:
1. The hospital admission must be at least 3 days, 3 midnights, not counting the discharge date.
2. The nursing home admission must be for a condition diagnosed during the hospital stay or for the main cause of hospital stay. For instance, a hospital stay for broken hip and then nursing home stay for physical therapy would be covered.

3. If the patient is not receiving rehabilitation but has some other ailment that requires skilled nursing supervision, then the nursing home condition would be covered.
4. The care being rendered by the nursing home must be skilled. Medicare Part A does not pay for custodial, nonskilled, or long-term care activities, including activities of daily living (ADLs) such as personal hygiene, cooking, cleaning, etc.

The maximum length of stay that Medicare Part A will cover in a skilled nursing facility per diagnosis is 100 days. The first 20 days would be paid for in full by Medicare with the remaining 80 days requiring a co-payment (as of 2007, $124.00 per day). Many insurance companies have a provision for skilled nursing care in the policies they sell.

If a beneficiary uses some portion of their Part A benefit and then goes at least 60 days without receiving skilled services, the 100-day clock is reset and they qualify for a new 100-day benefit period.

Part A is financed by taxes paid by employers and working individuals. Medicare Part A (Hospital Insurance) helps cover inpatient care in hospitals, including critical access hospitals and skilled nursing facilities (not custodial or long-term care). It also helps cover hospice care and some home health care. Beneficiaries must meet certain conditions to get these benefits.

Part B: Medical Insurance
Part B medical insurance helps pay for some services and products not covered by Part A, generally on an outpatient basis. Part B is optional and may be deferred if the beneficiary or his or her spouse is still actively working. There is a lifetime penalty (10% per year) imposed for not taking Part B if not actively working.

Part B coverage includes physician and nursing services, radiographs, laboratory and diagnostic tests, influenza and pneumonia vaccinations, blood transfusions, renal dialysis, outpatient hospital procedures, limited ambulance transportation, immunosuppressive drugs for organ transplant recipients, chemotherapy, hormonal treatments such as Lupron, and other outpatient medical treatments administered in a physician's office. Medication administration is covered under Part B only if it is administered by the physician during an office visit.

Part B also helps with durable medical equipment (DME), including canes, walkers, wheelchairs, and mobility scooters for those with mobility impairments.

Prosthetic devices such as artificial limbs and breast prostheses following mastectomy, as well as one pair of eyeglasses following cataract surgery, and oxygen for home use are also covered. As with all Medicare benefits, Part B coverage is subject to medical necessity. Complex rules are used to manage the benefit, and advisories are periodically issued that describe coverage criteria. On the national level, these advisories are issued by CMS and are known as national coverage determinations (MCDs). Local coverage determinations (LCDs) only apply within the multistate area managed by a specific regional Medicare Part B contractor, and local medical review policies (LMRPs) were superseded by LCDs in 2003.

Part B Medical Insurance is a supplementary voluntary medical insurance financed by general tax revenues and by required premium contributions. Medicare Part B (Medical Insurance) helps cover physicians' services and outpatient care. These may include:

- Outpatient surgery
- Diagnostic tests
- Radiology and pathology services
- Emergency services
- Outpatient rehabilitation services
- Renal dialysis
- Medical equipment and supplies
- Preventive services (mammography)

Part C: Medicare Advantage Plans

With the passage of the Balanced Budget Act of 1997, Medicare beneficiaries were given the option to receive their Medicare benefits through private health insurance plans, instead of through the Original Medicare plan (Parts A and B). These programs were known as "Medicare+Choice" or "Part C" plans. Pursuant to the Medicare Prescription Drug, Improvement, and Modernization Act of 2003, the compensation and business practices changed for insurers that offer these plans, and "Medicare+Choice" plans became known as "Medicare Advantage" (MA) plans. In addition to offering comparable coverage to Part A and Part B, Medicare Advantage plans may also offer Part D coverage.

Part D: Prescription Drug Plans

Medicare Part D went into effect on January 1, 2006. Anyone with Part A or B is eligible for Part D. It was made possible by the passage of the Medicare Prescription Drug, Improvement, and Modernization Act in 2003. To receive this benefit, a person with Medicare must enroll in a stand-alone prescription drug plan (PDP) or MA plan with prescription drug coverage (MA-PD). These plans are approved and regulated by the Medicare program but are actually designed and administered by private health insurance companies. Unlike Original Medicare (Parts A and B), Part D coverage is not standardized. Plans choose which drugs (or even classes of drugs) they wish to cover and at what level (or tier) they wish to cover it and are free to choose not to cover some drugs at what level (or tier) they wish to cover it and are free to choose not to cover some drugs at all. The exception to this is drugs that Medicare specifically excludes from coverage, including but not limited to benzodiazepines, cough suppressants, and barbiturates. Plans that cover excluded drugs are not allowed to pass those costs on to Medicare, and plans are required to repay CMS if they are found to have billed Medicare in these cases.

The national health insurance program is for persons aged 65 and older, some disabled persons, and persons with end-stage renal disease.

PRESCRIPTION DRUG COVERAGE

Most people will pay a monthly premium for this coverage. Starting January 1, 2006, new Medicare prescription drug coverage will be available to everyone with Medicare. Everyone with Medicare can get this coverage, which may help lower prescription drug costs and help protect against higher costs in the future. Medicare prescription drug coverage is insurance.

Private companies provide the coverage. Beneficiaries choose the drug plan and pay a monthly premium. Like other insurance, if a beneficiary decides not to enroll in a drug plan when they are first eligible, they may pay a penalty if they choose to join later.

HOSPICE

In 1983, Medicare added hospice benefits for the last 6 months of life to cover services for the terminally ill patient. An organized program consists of services provided and coordinated by an interdisciplinary team at a frequency appropriate to meet the needs of individuals who are diagnosed with terminal illnesses and have a limited life span. Hospice workers view death as a normal part of the life cycle. Hospice emphasizes living the remaining months of life as fully and as comfortably as possible.

The hospice specializes in palliative management of pain and other physical symptoms, meeting the psychosocial and spiritual needs of the individual and the individual's family or other primary care person(s). The program also includes a continuum of interdisciplinary team services across all settings where hospice care is provided, the availability of 24-hour access to care, utilization of volunteers, and bereavement care to the survivors, as needed, for an appropriate period of time.

CHARITY CARE ASSISTANCE

As an example, the New Jersey Hospital Care Payment Assistance Program (Charity Care Assistance) provides free or reduced-charge care to patients who receive inpatient and outpatient services or care in an acute care hospital throughout New Jersey. Hospital assistance and reduced charge care are available only for necessary hospital care.

Hospital care payment assistance is available to New Jersey residents who

- Have no health coverage or have coverage that pays only for part of the bill and
- Are ineligible for any private or government-sponsored coverage and
- Meet both the listed income and assets eligibility criteria

The reimbursement for charity care varies from state to state, so it is important to be aware of the charity care regulations at your workplace. Income criteria that are related to the percentage of hospital charge to be paid by patients are listed in Box 6-2.

TYPES OF HEALTH CARE SERVICES

With the continuing focus on the cost effectiveness of delivery of care, health care has moved from the acute care hospital to a full continuum of services within the community and the hospital. Twenty years ago, it was not uncommon for a community hospital to attempt to provide all services for a majority of patients. Length of stays were long and expensive. As the cost improvement model advanced, health care services have been divided into primary, secondary, and tertiary centers of care.

Health promotion and disease prevention are a focus of many HMOs. Practitioner's offices provide many health maintenance activities, as do community centers for education and health assessment.

There are three types of health care services: primary, secondary, and tertiary care (Box 6-3). Primary care is health maintenance that decreases the risk for disease; secondary care encourages disease prevention through early intervention; and tertiary care is long-term care.

Many diagnostic services such as colonoscopies are now being provided in ambulatory care settings and physician's offices. Many surgical procedures are also now being provided in ambulatory care settings. Secondary and tertiary care is provided in a number of settings across the health care continuum. Health care is provided by the types of agencies and facilities listed in Box 6-4.

It is important for you as a nurse to realize that different levels of care are paid for at differing rates by

---

Box 6-2   INCOME CRITERIA FOR HEALTH AND HUMAN SERVICES POVERTY INCOME GUIDELINES

Income as a Percentage of HHS Poverty Income Guidelines	Percentage of Charge Paid by Patient
≤200%	0%
>200% but ≤225%	20%
>225% but ≤250%	40%
>250% but ≤275%	60%
>275% but ≤300%	80%
>300%	100%

From New Jersey Hospital Care Payment Assistance Fact Sheet. (January 2006). Retrieved July 17, 2007, from http://www.spannj.org/keychanges/ccfactsh.pdf.

Box 6-3   TYPES OF HEALTH CARE SERVICES

Type of Care	Description	Examples
Primary	Decreases risk for disease	Immunizations
	Health maintenance	Nutrition counseling
Secondary	Disease prevention through early intervention	Surgery
Tertiary	Long-term care	Durable medical equipment
		Education

Box 6-4   AGENCIES AND FACILITIES THAT PROVIDE HEALTH CARE

Health Care Facility	Examples
Acute care	Hospitalization for episode of illness
	Example: patient suffering an acute myocardial infarction
Subacute care	Continued hospitalization after initial acute stage has passed
	Example: patient requiring long-term ventilatory assistance
Long-term care	Continued hospitalization after stabilization of chronic long-term condition
	Example: patient in end-stage Alzheimer disease
Residential care	Living facilities for patients in need of basic support
	Example: group home for individual with mental retardation
Assisted living	Living facilities with an option of basic support
	Example: 85-year-old independent patient with occasional falls
Ambulatory care	Diagnostic testing screenings
	Low-acuity surgery
	Example: same-day operations
Rehabilitation	Postinjury focus on restoration of function
	Example: patient with spinal cord injury learning activities of daily living
Home health care	Posthospitalization support within the home
	Example: post congestive heart failure patient requiring medication and dietary follow-up
Hospice services • Inpatient • Outpatient	Care of the dying patient and family
	Example: in-home care for dying patient
Health care centers	Full range of preventative health care services
	Example: federally qualified health care center
Local health departments	Preventative health services in support of *Healthy People 2010*
	Examples: blood pressure screenings, immunizations
Urgent care centers	Treatment of nonurgent injuries
	Examples: physical examinations and first aid

both private and federal insurers. This differentiation in financial reimbursement for these services results in "type-specific" staffing, standards of care, and services rendered. Each type of service also has to meet differing accreditation requirements (see Chapter 7).

FOR-PROFIT AND NOT-FOR-PROFIT HEALTH CARE AGENCIES

While the majority of the health care facilities in the United States function as not-for-profit agencies, there is a movement toward hospitals becoming for-profit institutions. An example of a for-profit entity would be a physician opening his or her own same-day surgery center. There are examples of hospitals that have become for-profit institutions where the profit is funneled back to either the hospital or an overseeing corporation.

With health care costs continuing to escalate, it will be important for you as a nurse to be aware of the economic forces that affect your day-to-day nursing care.

VETERANS HEALTH ADMINISTRATION

The goal of the Veterans Health Administration (VHA) is to provide excellence in patient care, veterans' benefits, and customer satisfaction. The VHA strives for high-quality, prompt, and seamless service to U.S. veterans. Of the 25 million veterans currently alive, nearly three of every four served during a war or an official period of hostility. About a quarter of the nation's population—approximately 70 million people —are potentially eligible for VA benefits and services because they are veterans or family members or survivors of veterans.

SUMMARY

Health care has undergone many changes in the past 10 years. The rapid pace of change shows no signs of abating, and it is important for the nurse to be aware of the rules and regulations of payment, reimbursement, and the various types of health care systems and care available to patients and their families. The nurse usually is the advocate for the care that the patient receives and works with the case manager to determine the level of services necessary for the patient. Sadly, the reimbursement method often dictates much of the care available to the patient, so it is imperative for the nurse to be aware of all of the ramifications of the payers, so that appropriate care can be planned and implemented for the duration of the patient's need.

CLINICAL CORNER

APN Role in Core Measures

Mary Jo Assi

In 2004, the advanced practice nurse (APN) team of The Valley Hospital was asked to participate in development of new strategies to meet organizational goals related to core measures improvement.

Once mobilized, the APN team first endeavored to learn core measure requirements in detail. The quality assurance (QA) staff, all nurses and experts in this arena, provided the education needed. Stakeholders for the change process were identified in a joint collaboration between the APN group and QA staff that included physician department chairs and champions for core measures and staff and administrators from medical records, pharmacy, infection control and information systems, including the nursing informatics liaison to that department. In addition, emergency department staff, administrators, and physicians were included as key participants.

Work focus and strategies developed by the APN team included the following:

1. Tools and methods to identify 100% of patients who meet core measure criteria for acute myocardial infarction, heart failure, and pneumonia on admission and identification of patients undergoing surgery that meet Surgical Care Improvement Project (SCIP) criteria
2. Development of user-friendly systems and framework to improve evidence-based care of a time-sensitive nature to 100% of patients identified
3. Development of systems for prospective review of core measure care elements to ensure completion before patient discharge from the hospital
4. Method for retrospective analysis of all charts of failed procedures to identify and track what element(s) failed and why
5. Implementation of APN-led multidisciplinary monthly forum for development and evaluation of systems to improve care for each of the four core measures in conjunction with current outcomes results

6. Ongoing education for nursing staff regarding elements of core measures, particularly those for which nursing is directly accountable, and best practice clinical care for patients

The subsequent recruitment of two APN clinical quality specialists has proved a key factor to improve our core measure scores. In general, the role was envisioned and executed to incorporate the clinical expert/leader, educator, and system change agent aspects inherent in the educational preparation of this group of nursing professionals. Both positions have leadership responsibility and accountability for the following:

- Prospective monitoring of admitted patients with known or suspected diagnosis of acute myocardial infarction, heart failure, or pneumonia and for patients undergoing surgical procedures that meet SCIP criteria
- Core measure monthly meetings
- Oversight of analysis, development, and revision of systems to achieve goals
- Retrospective chart review of all failed core measure scores and communication/resolution in collaboration with QA staff for any area of disagreement
- Interface with key physician champions and departments to align systems and work to meet goals, particularly where nursing and medicine share responsibility for one or more elements of a given measure

The evolution of these two oversight positions allowed our unit-based APNs to shift their focus to collaborate with nursing managers and staff to implement other key strategies such as daily rounds on inpatient units to monitor clinical care for all patients. Specific questions related to core measure elements are included as appropriate to patient diagnosis or problem. While the initial impetus for this change in practice was improvement in core measure scores, the benefit realized for participants and patients has far exceeded the original goal.

EVIDENCE-BASED PRACTICE

Nurse Staffing and Reimbursement

The Joint Commission. (2008). One size does not fit all: meeting the needs of diverse populations. *Retrieved November 14, 2008, from http://www.jointcommission.org/NR/rdonlyres/ 5AA54D85-0879-4C29-B517-1241365581AF/0/ One_Size_Report_One_Pager.pdf*

A cross-sectional qualitative study funded by The California Endowment, *Hospitals, Language and Culture: A Snapshot of the Nation* (HLC) sought to explore how 60 hospitals across the United States addressed the need to provide quality health care to culturally and linguistically diverse patient populations. The study's most recent report, *One Size Does Not Fit All: Meeting the Health Care Needs of Diverse Populations,* is designed to assist hospitals in developing and employing practices for meeting diverse patient needs which are identified as unique for each organization. The report suggests that each hospital bring people together from across the organization to identify the needs of their patient population and evaluate how

well these needs are being met, assess current practices through sharing of experiences, barriers, and gaps, and develop a system for continuous assessment, monitoring, and evaluation. Cultural and language needs should be considered and a range of practices implemented in a systemic manner to align organizational resources with patient needs. The framework is presented in a thematic fashion derived from current practices in hospitals that are successful at providing services to diverse populations. The four themes are: Building a Foundation, Collecting and Using Data to Improve Services, Accommodating the Needs of Specific Populations, and Establishing Internal and External Collaborations. A self-assessment tool is provided for organizations to use as the process of assessment and evaluation is begun. As part of The Joint Commission's Patient Safety Initiatives, hospitals and health care organizations are encouraged to tailor initiatives to the needs of their diverse populations with the goal of providing the highest quality care to every patient served.

NCLEX® EXAM QUESTIONS

1. As a nurse, you are aware that The World Health Organization defines *health* as:
   1. a state of complete physical, mental, and social well-being and not merely the absence of disease or infirmity
   2. a state of well-being with absence of disease
   3. a state of well-being
   4. absence of disease or infirmity
2. As a nurse, you are aware that Medicare is a:
   1. health insurance program for people aged 65 and older or under age 65 with certain disabilities or any age with end-stage renal disease
   2. health insurance program for people aged 66 and older
   3. joint federal and state assistance program designed to pay for medical long-term care assistance for individuals and families with low income and limited resources
   4. state assistance program designed to pay for medical long-term care assistance for individuals and families with low income and limited resources

3. When questioned by a patient about Medicaid benefits, as a nurse you are aware that Medicaid is a:
   1. health insurance program for people aged 65 and older or under age 65 with certain disabilities or any age with end-stage renal disease
   2. joint federal and state assistance program designed to pay for medical long-term care assistance for individuals and families with low income and limited resources
   3. health insurance program for people age 66 and older
   4. joint federal and state assistance program designed to pay for medical long-term care assistance for individuals and families regardless of income
4. You are the nurse caring for a 54-year-old woman who has just been diagnosed with end-stage pancreatic cancer. Along with the social worker, you are discussing hospice programs with her. Which of the following will be explained to the patient?

NCLEX® EXAM QUESTIONS—cont'd

1. Hospice programs are hospital based only.
2. Hospice programs allow patients to die with dignity at home or in a facility.
3. Hospice programs are for adults over the age of 66 only.
4. Hospice programs are for those patients who will die within 1 year of diagnosis.

5. You are completing the discharge plan for a patient who has Medicare Part B. You will inform the patient that this part of her Medicare coverage plan pays for:
   1. prescription medications
   2. a new ramp for her wheelchair access
   3. surgical procedures as an outpatient
   4. durable medical equipment

6. Your patient is being transferred to a subacute facility tomorrow. In planning for this transfer, you are aware that subacute care would provide services for patients with the following condition:
   1. long-term ventilator dependency
   2. newly diagnosed cancer requiring chemotherapy
   3. a condition in which the patient will die within 2 weeks
   4. breastfeeding difficulty for a first-time mother

7. One type of health care delivery system is a health maintenance organization (HMO). You are aware that:
   1. this type of a system delivers comprehensive health maintenance and treatment services for a group of enrolled individuals.
   2. there is only one independent model of HMO

3. there is only a group model where practitioners employed by the insurer spend all their time caring for patients of that particular HMO
4. HMOs are part of Medicare Part C

8. The health care system includes all of the following EXCEPT:
   1. structures to deliver professional health and wellness
   2. organizations to deliver professional health and wellness
   3. services to deliver professional health and wellness
   4. structures and organizations to deliver chronic care only

9. You are caring for an adolescent who has sustained a severe spinal cord injury and is paralyzed from the waist down. The physician has written an order for transfer to a rehabilitation facility. Along with the case manager, you will inform the patient and family that the:
   1. family is responsible for full payment for the rehabilitation facility
   2. patient and family will be given the name of one facility only
   3. family can visit the facility before transfer
   4. choice of facility is up to the physician

10. A chronic hemodialysis patient would have his or her bills paid for by:
    1. Medicare Part A
    2. Medicare Part B
    3. Medicare Parts A and B
    4. Medicare Part C

Answers: 1. 1   2. 1   3. 2   4. 2   5. 4   6. 1   7. 1   8. 4   9. 3   10. 2

REFERENCES

Grohar-Murray, M. E., & DiCroce, H. R. (2003). *Leadership and management in nursing* (3rd ed.). Upper Saddle River, NJ: Prentice Hall.

Kelly-Heidenthal, P. (2003). *Nursing leadership and management*. Clifton Park, NY: Delmar Thompson Learning.

New Jersey Hospital Care Payment Assistance Program (Charity Care Assistance). Retrieved April 16, 2009, from www.nj.gov/health/cc/documents/ccfactsh.pdf.

U.S. Census Bureau. (2000). Retrieved from http://www.census.gov/.

Veterans Health Administration. (2008). Retrieved March 17, 2008, from http://www.va.gov/about_va/.

Veterans Health Administration. (2008). Health care. Retrieved March 17, 2008, from http://www1.va.gov/health/AboutVHA.asp.

World Health Organization. (1998). Health education and promotion. Retrieved July 31, 2007, from http://www.who.int/about/en/.

World Health Organization. (2008). Health. Retrieved March 17, 2008, from http://en.wikipedia.org/wiki/Health.

Wywialowski, E. F. (2004). *Managing client care* (3rd ed.). St. Louis, MO: Mosby.

Yoder-Wise, P. S. (2006). *Beyond leading and managing nursing administration for the future*. St. Louis, MO: Mosby.

Yoder-Wise, P. S. (2007). *Leading and managing in nursing* (4th ed.). St. Louis, MO: Mosby.

CHAPTER 7

Health Care Regulatory and Certifying Agencies

Chapter Objectives

1. Identify health care regulatory and certifying agencies.
2. Explain the nurse's role in relation to hospital surveys.
3. Define *The Joint Commission*.
4. Define *accreditation*.
5. Discuss strategies for implementation of proper procedures for an upcoming hospital survey.
6. Discuss strategies for implementation of proper procedures using appropriate regulatory and certifying agency guidelines.

Definitions

Accreditation Determination by an accrediting body that an eligible health care organization complies with applicable standards of The Joint Commission

American Osteopathic Association (AOA) Osteopathic accreditation program that ensures osteopathic students receive their training with the provision of high-quality patient care

Centers for Disease Control and Prevention (CDC) Agency charged with the promotion of health and quality of life by preventing and controlling disease, injury, and disability; has created multiple infection control standards that are now part of standard Joint Commission accreditation

Compliance To act in accordance with stated requirements, such as standards. Levels of compliance include noncompliance, partial compliance, and substantial compliance

The Joint Commission (TJC) Accreditation organization that strives to continuously improve the safety and quality of care provided to the public through the provision of health care accreditation and related services that support performance improvement in health care organizations

National Institute for Occupational Safety and Health (NIOSH) Federal agency responsible for conducting research and making recommendations for the prevention of work-related injury and illness. NIOSH is part of the CDC within the U.S. Department of Health and Human Services

Occupational Safety and Health Administration (OSHA) U.S. Department of Labor agency that ensures the safety and health of America's workers by setting and enforcing standards; providing training, outreach, and education; establishing partnerships; and encouraging continual improvement in workplace safety and health

State departments of health and human services Foster accessible and high-quality health and senior services to help all people to achieve optimal health, dignity, and independence in an attempt to prevent disease, promote, and protect well-being at all life stages and encourage informed choices that enrich quality of life for individuals and communities.

U.S. Department of Health and Human Services (USDHHS) U.S. government's principal agency for protecting the health of all Americans and providing essential human services, especially for those who are least able to help themselves

REGULATORY AGENCIES

Health care organizations work with a myriad of accrediting and regulatory agencies so that optimum standards of care and delivery of care can be met. Regulatory agencies are charged by federal and state governments to:

- Set standards for the operation of health care organizations
- Ensure compliance with federal and state regulations developed by government administrative agencies
- Investigate and make judgments regarding complaints brought by consumers of the services and the public

Licensing of health care agencies to maintain practice occurs through state departments of health. State departments of health usually oversee outcomes of care within health care facilities, investigate consumer complaints, and deal with issues of importance to the public health. These agencies monitor basic compliance with the specific health care regulations of that state. Compliance with regulatory standards on both national and state levels is mandatory, and fines can be leveled against organizations for noncompliance.

Accreditation agencies evaluate health care organization against a set of standards that have been validated against best practice. Accreditation is voluntary.

ACCREDITATION

Accreditation agencies were initially founded to set a minimum of standard of care. As they have matured, their missions have expanded to "continuously improve the safety and quality of care provided to public" (The Joint Commission, 2009). They have moved from compliance agencies to agencies that hope to drive improvement and quality of care.

Accrediting agencies move beyond basic compliance and look to the continuous improvement of operational systems critical to patient care and safety. While accreditation is listed as a voluntary process, federal reimbursement of health care is dependent on accreditation.

THE JOINT COMMISSION

The mission of The Joint Commission (previously known as the Joint Commission on Accreditation of Healthcare Organizations) is to continuously improve the safety and quality of care provided to the public through the provision of health care accreditation and related services that support performance improvement in health care organizations. The Joint Commission evaluates and accredits more than 15,000 health care organizations and programs in the United States. An independent, not-for-profit organization, The Joint Commission is the nation's predominant standards-setting and accrediting body in health care. Since 1951, The Joint Commission has maintained state-of-the-art standards that focus on improving the quality and safety of care provided by health care organizations. The Joint Commission's comprehensive accreditation process evaluates an organization's compliance with these standards and other accreditation requirements.

The Joint Commission's evaluation and accreditation services are provided for the following types of organizations:

- General, psychiatric, children's, and rehabilitation hospitals
- Critical access hospitals
- Health care networks, including managed care plans, preferred provider organizations, integrated delivery networks, and managed behavioral health care organizations
- Home care organizations, including those that provide home health services, personal care and support services, home infusion and other pharmacy services, durable medical equipment services, and hospice services
- Nursing homes and other long-term care facilities, including subacute care programs, dementia special care programs, and long-term care pharmacies
- Assisted living facilities that provide or coordinate personal services, 24-hour supervision and assistance (scheduled and unscheduled), activities, and health-related services

- Behavioral health care organizations, including those that provide mental health and addiction services, and services to persons with developmental disabilities of various ages, in various organized service settings
- Ambulatory care providers, such as outpatient surgery facilities, rehabilitation centers, infusion centers, group practices, and office-based surgery
- Clinical laboratories, including independent or free-standing laboratories, blood transfusion and donor centers, and public health laboratories

Accreditation by The Joint Commission is recognized nationwide as a symbol of quality that reflects an organization's commitment to meeting certain performance standards. To earn and maintain The Joint Commission's Gold Seal of Approval, an organization must undergo an on-site survey conducted by The Joint Comission at least every 3 years. Laboratories must be surveyed every 2 years.

BENEFITS OF JOINT COMMISSION ACCREDITATION

There are many benefits to accreditation, but those specific to health care accreditation include:

- Leads to improved patient care
- Demonstrates the organization's commitment to safety and quality
- Offers an educational on-site survey experience
- Supports and enhances safety and quality improvement efforts
- Strengthens and supports recruitment and retention efforts
- May substitute for federal certification surveys for Medicare and Medicaid
- Helps secure managed care contracts
- Facilitates the organization's business strategies
- Provides a competitive advantage
- Enhances the organization's image to the public, purchasers, and payers
- Fulfills licensure requirements in many states
- Recognized by insurers and other third parties
- Strengthens community confidence

STANDARDS AND PERFORMANCE MEASUREMENT

The Joint Commission standards address the organization's level of performance in key functional areas, such as patient rights, patient treatment, and infection control, and the standards focus not simply on an orga-

---

Box 7-1   THE JOINT COMMISSION HOSPITAL ACCREDITATION STANDARDS OVERVIEW

Patient-Focused Functions
- Ethics, rights, and responsibilities
- Provision of care, treatment, and services
- Medication management
- Surveillance, prevention, and control of infection

Organization-Focused Functions
- Improving organization performance
- Leadership
- Management of the environment of care
- Management of human resources
- Management of information

Structures with Functions
- Medical staff
- Nursing

© Copyright 2007, The Joint Commission. JC Hospital Accreditation Standards 2007 Manual.

---

nization's ability to provide safe, high-quality care but also on its actual performance. Standards set forth performance expectations for activities that affect the safety and quality of patient care. If an organization does the right things and does them well, there is a strong likelihood that its patients will experience good outcomes. The Joint Commission develops its standards in consultation with health care experts, providers, measurement experts, purchasers, and consumers. See Box 7-1 for an overview of The Joint Commission's Hospital Accreditation Standards.

There are also disease-specific certifications such as The Joint Commission's certificate of distinction for primary stroke centers. This certification program was developed in collaboration with the American Stroke Association. Other disease-specific certifications of The Joint Commission include those for asthma, heart failure, and trauma. Disease-specific care certifications focus on:

- Creating an organized comprehensive approach to disease-specific performance improvement
- Using comparative data to evaluate disease-specific program processes and patient outcomes
- Evaluating the patients' perception of care quality
- Maintaining data quality and integrity

The Joint Commission survey is considered a "rite of passage" for any new nurse manager. Before 2008, the survey would occur every 3 years and was announced.

Box 7-2   THE JOINT COMMISSION'S SHARED VISIONS—NEW PATHWAYS

Shared Visions—New Pathways includes the following changes in the accreditation process
- A substantial consolidation of the standards was undertaken to reduce the paperwork and documentation burden associated with the accreditation process. The intent of this change is to increase the organization's focus on patient safety and health care quality by improving the clarity and relevance of the remaining standards.
- A midcycle, periodic performance review (PPR) is now required, during which the organization must evaluate its compliance with TJC standards. If noncompliance is noted, a plan of action must be developed and reported. Validation of PPR findings and corrections will be reviewed by TJC during the organization's next on-site survey.
- A priority focus process (PFP) is used to design each organization's on-site survey. The PFP uses

the organization's core measures data, previous recommendations, demographic data related to clinical service groups, complaints, sentinel event information, and MedPar data to design a survey that is relevant to that organization's patient safety and health care quality issues.
- On-site evaluation is now focused on compliance to the standards in relation to the care experiences of actual patients in the facility. This process is known as the tracer methodology.
- Individual organizational performance reports have been revised to provide "Quality Reports," which include specific organizational performance information.
- Surveyors actively seek the engagement of physicians and other direct caregivers during the accreditation process.

From Yoder-Wise, P. S. (2006). *Beyond leading and managing nursing administration for the future.* St. Louis, MO: Mosby, 2006:381.

On the eve of the announced visit, there would be much preparation and energy invested in the satisfactory completion of the survey. In 2008, The Joint Commission started making unannounced visits. This change requires that all health care institutions be in a state of "constant readiness." Changes in The Joint Commission accreditation process are summarized in Box 7-2.

The importance of the nurse's role in ensuring patient safety and delivering quality care is emphasized through key nursing activities such as:
- Influencing improved design of care processes
- Creating a nonpunitive environment to enhance error reporting
- Participating in error reporting and analysis

The importance of the nurse's position is further elaborated by her or his leadership role in complying with the necessary standards for medication management, infection control, pain management, and the environment of care.

As a nurse, daily adherence to the standards is of the utmost importance. During a site visit from the accrediting agencies, you will be asked to participate in interviews or team meetings with representatives from the accrediting bodies.

One of the most common standards of The Joint Commission that affects nursing care deals with the management of pain. The standard includes the following:

- Documentation of assessment of pain
- Documentation of the relief of pain
- Use of therapeutics to manage pain
- Assessment of use of therapeutics

Your documentation of this standard will be reviewed for compliance with the standard. Under this standard, organizations will be required to (The Joint Commission, February 2001):
- Recognize patients' rights to assessment and management of pain
- Assess the nature and intensity of pain in all patients
- Establish safe medication prescription and ordering procedures
- Ensure staff competency and orient new staff in pain assessment and management
- Monitor patients postprocedurally and reassess patient problems appropriately
- Educate patients on the role of pain management in treatment
- Address patients' needs for symptom management in the discharge planning process
- Collect data to monitor performance

The Joint Commission's surveyors measure an institution's compliance through:
- Interviews with patients, families, and clinical staff
- Review of policies, procedures, protocols, and practices for effective pain management

- Review of clinical records
- Educational materials for patients, family, and staff
- Statement of patient rights or other statements reflecting the organization's commitment to effective pain management

It is important for you to remember that you may be interviewed and your patient charts may be reviewed and evaluated by the team.

THE AMERICAN OSTEOPATHIC ASSOCIATION

The American Osteopathic Association (AOA) is a recognized alternative to certification by the Centers for Medicare & Medicaid Services (CMS) or accreditation by The Joint Commission. This accrediting agency deals primarily with osteopathic hospitals. The Medicare conditions of participation require that hospitals be accredited by an organization with "deeming authority."

OTHER ACCREDITING AGENCIES

There are also specialty certifications for specialty care units, and you may be asked to participate in these evaluations.

- American College of Surgeons Commission on Cancer—Accrediting agency that evaluates cancer treatment in hospitals and outpatient and freestanding facilities. In addition to participating in a TJC and state licensing survey, you may also be asked to participate in a specialty survey such as this depending on your area of practice or expertise.
- Commission on Accreditation of Rehabilitation Facilities (CARF)—Accrediting agency that evaluates hospital-based or freestanding medical rehabilitation, employment, and community services
- Community Health Accreditation Program (CHAP)—Evaluates home care and community health organizations
- Accreditation Association for Ambulatory Health Care (AAAHC)—Evaluates ambulatory surgery centers, medical and dental group practices, diagnostic imaging centers, and student health centers
- American Association for Accreditation of Ambulatory Surgery Facilities (AAAASF)—Accreditation of ambulatory surgery settings
- Commission of Accreditation of Ambulance Services (CAAS)—Accreditation of medical transportation services
- National Commission for Correctional Health Care (NCCHC)—Accreditation of U.S. prisons, jails, and juvenile detention facilities
- National Committee for Quality Assurance (NCQA)—Accreditation and evaluation of quality management systems and managed care organizations

EDUCATIONAL ACCREDITATION

If your hospital participates in education of health care personnel, nurses, and physicians, you will also be exposed to visits by the accrediting agencies used by the schools working with your hospital. The schools are usually responsible for the compliance with standards in these situations. You role will be to respond to the role of the students in the provision of care on your unit. Examples of such agencies include National League of Nursing Accrediting Association (NLNAC), the Commission on Collegiate Nursing Education (nursing college accreditation), the Liaison Committee on Medical Education (medical schools), and the Commission on Accreditation in Physical Therapy.

REGULATORY AGENCIES

In addition to these accrediting agencies, there are multiple regulatory and advisory agencies that have an impact on standards of health care. As discussed in Chapter 6, agencies such as the Occupational Safety and Health Administration (OSHA) regulate the manner in which a hospital implements workplace safety standards. These standards then become part of The Joint Commission's management of the environment of care standard. The Centers for Disease Control and Prevention (CDC), an agency charged with the promotion of health and quality of life through the prevention and control of disease, injury, and disability, has created multiple infection control standards that are now part of standard TJC accreditation by The Joint Commission as well as the practice standards of most hospitals. The Food and Drug Administration (FDA) is a federal agency that regulates drugs, medical devices, and radiation-emitting products. These regulations also form the basis of the medication management standard of The Joint Commission.

LICENSING BODIES

Health care organizations are licensed to perform services by the state department of health. Most state departments of health:

- Regulate a wide range of health care settings for quality of care, such as hospitals, nursing homes, assisted living residences, ambulatory care centers, home health care, medical day care, and others
- Investigates complaints received from consumers and other state and federal agencies
- Provides consumer information in the form of report cards and other performance information

You may be called to assist hospital administrators regarding complaints lodged with the state department of health.

GOVERNMENT AGENCIES

There are a number of government agencies that will provide oversight for some of the functions within health care. Examples of these agencies follow.

OCCUPATIONAL SAFETY AND HEALTH ADMINISTRATION

OSHA's mission is to ensure the safety and health of America's workers by setting and enforcing standards; providing training, outreach, and education; establishing partnerships; and encouraging continual improvement in workplace safety and health.

The staff establishes protective standards, enforces those standards, and reaches out to employers and employees through technical assistance and consultation programs. An example of an OSHA guideline of importance to nursing was the September 12, 2005, OSHA guideline for the recommendation to minimize patient lifting to prevent health care musculoskeletal injuries. OSHA recommended that:

- Manual lifting of residents be minimized in all cases and eliminated when feasible.

THE U.S. DEPARTMENT OF HEALTH AND HUMAN SERVICES

The U.S. Department of Health and Human Services (USDHHS) provides more than 300 programs covering a wide spectrum of activities; examples follow (HHS, 2007).

- Health and social science research
- Preventing disease, including immunization services
- Assuring food and drug safety
- Medicare (health insurance for elderly and disabled Americans) and Medicaid (health insurance for low-income people)
- Health information technology
- Financial assistance and services for low-income families
- Improving maternal and infant health
- Head Start (preschool education and services)
- Faith-based and community initiatives
- Prevention of child abuse and domestic violence
- Substance abuse treatment and prevention
- Services for older Americans, including home-delivered meals
- Comprehensive health services for Native Americans
- Medical preparedness for emergencies, including potential terrorism.

CENTERS FOR DISEASE CONTROL AND PREVENTION

The CDC, an agency within the DHHS, is charged with the promotion of health and quality of life by preventing and controlling disease, injury, and disability. The CDC seeks to accomplish its mission by working with partners throughout the nation and the world to

- Monitor health
- Detect and investigate health problems
- Conduct research to enhance prevention
- Develop and advocate sound public health policies
- Implement prevention strategies
- Promote healthy behaviors
- Foster safe and healthful environments
- Provide leadership and training

You will come in contact with the CDC in the development of policies and in the possible investigation of disease outbreaks.

Other agencies with health care oversight are known by the acronyms detailed in Table 7-1.

OTHER GROUPS RECOGNIZING HEALTH CARE PERFORMANCE AND EXCELLENCE

In this time of heated hospital competition, many institutions are attempting to differentiate their performance from the norm through recognition in other

Table 7-1	GLOSSARY OF ACRONYMS
Acronym	**Full Name**
AAAASF	American Association for Accreditation of Ambulatory Surgery Facilities
AAAHC	Accreditation Association for Ambulatory Health Care
AAHCC	American Accreditation Health Care Commission
ACHC	Accreditation Commission for Health Care, Inc.
ACR	American College of Radiology
ACS-CoC	American College of Surgeons Commission on Cancer
ALS	American Lithotripsy Society
AOA	The American Osteopathic Association
CAAS	Commission on Accreditation of Ambulance Services
CAP	College of American Pathologists Commission on Inspections and Accreditation
CARF	Commission on Accreditation of Rehabilitation Facilities
CCAC	Continuing Care Accreditation Commission
CDC	Centers for Disease Control and Prevention
CHAP	Community Health Accreditation Program, Inc.
CMS	Centers for Medicare & Medicaid Services
COA	Council on Accreditation
COLA	Commission on Office Laboratory Accreditation for Blood Banks and Transfusion Services
DHHS	U.S. Department of Health and Human Services
FDA	U.S. Food and Drug Administration
FEMA	Federal Emergency Management Agency
HAP	Hospital Accreditation Program
NCCHC	National Commission for Correctional Health Care
NIOSH	The National Institute for Occupational Safety and Health
OSHA	Occupational Safety and Health Administration
TJC	The Joint Commission
URAC	Utilization Review Accreditation Commission

Modified from George Mason University. (2007). Accreditation agencies in United States. Retrieved July 6, 2007, from http://gunston.gmu.edu/healthscience/547/MajorAccreditationAgencies.asp.

areas of performance. Such levels of recognition demonstrate excellence beyond accreditation, regulatory, and licensing areas.

- The most significant group, in terms of nursing performance, is the American Nurses Credentialing Center (ANCC), which oversees the Magnet Award. The Magnet Award is the highest level of recognition that the ANCC can award to organized nursing services in the national and international arena. Through this award, the ANCC recognizes nursing-sensitive outcomes as a predictor of quality of patient care and values the retention and recruitment of highly competent nurses (ANCC, 2008).
- The Malcolm Baldrige Award for Performance Excellence recognizes health care institutions that

demonstrate performance excellence across all areas of the organization. The requirements for excellence must exist in seven categories: Leadership, Strategic Planning, Customer and Market Knowledge, Information Management, Workforce Focus, Process Management, and Results (Baldrige National Quality Program, 2008).

- *U.S. News and World Report* annually ranks the "best hospitals in the U.S." This ranking rates hospitals across the nation in terms of breadth of expertise and quality. In 2007, 5462 hospitals were screened. Just 173 made it to the rankings, and 18 made it to the honor role (*U.S. News and World Report,* 2007). Of the hospitals listed in the 2007 rankings, 7 of the top 10 were also Magnet Hospitals.

- J. D. Power and Associates recognizes hospitals for service excellence. The firm's Distinguished Hospital Program expands the traditional evaluation of quality by recognizing hospitals that achieve a notable level of satisfaction with services that are provided. This program helps consumers identify hospitals that provide outstanding service excellence and may serve as a competitive advantage when consumers are looking for service excellence (J. D. Power and Associates, 2008).

SUMMARY

It is important to realize the integration of regulation, accrediting standards, and licensing requirements forms a major part of the health care accreditation in the United States. As with all regulatory and accrediting bodies, there are multiple standards for each regulation or level of accreditation. As a nurse, it is your responsibility to understand your role in the accreditation process, your role in the adherence to regulatory standards, and your role in meeting accreditation standards. While many of the accreditations are "voluntary," hospitals cannot receive reimbursement unless they are accredited. The accreditation process validates the effectiveness and safety of the care being rendered. Also, in this era of highly competitive hospitals, the levels and amounts of accreditation may be a way of marketing the excellence of one particular hospital compared with another.

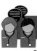

CLINICAL CORNER

Accreditation Readiness

Joan Brennan

AtlantiCare Regional Medical Center (ARMC) is a 600-bed, two-hospital campus located in southeastern New Jersey. In addition to the two hospitals, ARMC also has a large free-standing clinic, a special care center, three outpatient services sites, and two psychiatric acute partial hospitalization programs under the hospital licenses. Survey preparation applies to all these sites. Preparation for the accreditation process of The Joint Commission can be a challenge in such an environment.

ARMC's approach to survey readiness is to develop and implement a Survey Readiness Plan that integrates the requirements and standards of multiple regulatory agencies. This includes The Joint Commission, Centers for Medicare and Medicaid Services (CMS), and the New Jersey Department of Health and Senior Services (NJDHSS). This plan addresses processes to maintain survey readiness at all times, as well as the process to respond when surveyors present at ARMC for any one of the myriad of potential surveys related to our business.

The plan is designed to assign accountability to all staff so they are "survey ready" at all times. On an annual basis, the Survey Readiness Plan is reviewed and approved by senior leaders. The plan is in alignment with the organization's strategic goal of continual survey readiness, thereby ensuring a continued prioritization.

Providing a structure for survey readiness is The Joint Commission task force. The task force is composed of ARMC leaders who take ownership for standards within each of their assigned Joint Commission chapters as well as any associated CMS or NJDHSS regulations. The role of the task force leader is to provide internal expertise on standards interpretation, policy and procedure development, and deployment. The task force leaders collaborate with ARMC committees, councils, educators, directors, managers, and staff to ensure structures, processes, and practices comply with all regulatory requirements. The role of the task force leaders provides the opportunity to have an accurate and consistent interpretation in an efficient manner. Task force leaders receive regular reports from the Veterans Health Administration's Quality Council related to recent survey findings from hospitals within the collaborative. The task force leaders also assemble and regularly update all related survey documents in the primary campus for ready access when surveyors arrive.

Supporting the deployment of the Survey Readiness Plan are multiple staff and leader resources organized to implement appropriate practice consistent with policies and procedures. For example, unit based "Champions" in all departments educate and mentor staff, then monitor compliance, and work with their managers to improve performance.

EVIDENCE-BASED PRACTICE

The Magnet Hospital Concept

From McClure, M. (July/August 2005). Magnet hospitals: insights and issues. The pull of magnetism. Nursing Administration Quarterly, 29, *198-201; Aiken, L., Smith, H., & Lake, E. (1994). Lower mortality among a set of hospitals known for good nursing care.* Medical Care, 32, *771-787.*

The Magnet Hospital concept is more than 20 years old. It arose in the 1980s out of concern for nursing workforce issues. The American Academy of Nursing appointed a task force, which recognized that acute care facilities were experiencing serious problems in their ability to attract and retain registered nurses. It seemed that there was a lot of information and publicity about what was "wrong" out there but no one had ever explored what variables went into making successful settings. It was clear, though, that there were a number of thriving organizations that were not experiencing these problems. The task force undertook a national study that was later published as a monograph titled "Magnet Hospital Attraction and Retention of Professional Nurses." This research enabled other institutions to emulate these settings of excellence.

The Magnet Hospital program that is known today is an outgrowth of the studies that have been completed over the past two decades. The program is one of the most important efforts to date that has been made to recognize positive work environments within health care.

The success of the program also represents a burden. It is an enormous responsibility to mount an effort that is specifically designed to recognize excellence. Appropriate criteria must be objective and measurable, and validity and reliability must be maintained when the stakes are so high.

Nurse administrators should be aware of some insights and issues that were gained through experience with the American Nurses Credentialing Center (ANCC) Magnet Recognition Program. First, Magnet Hospitals demonstrate that their corporate structures were completely supportive of nursing and of quality patient care. The culture permeated the entire institution. It was palpable! These were good places for employees to work (not just nurses), and they were good places for patients to receive care. Excellence is a characteristic of the organization, and everyone connected with it reaps the benefits of that environment. Hospitals that succeed in attaining Magnet status always do so with the involvement of every single department and discipline.

The question for today's Magnet program is, "Should most attain Magnet status or should it remain within reach of only the best?" Excellence is by definition rare; therefore, it is not something every institution should be expected to achieve. However, the concepts involved in the program are useful to others. The fact is that every patient care setting can develop ideas and goals from studying the Magnet Hospital criteria.

The Magnet designation attained by successful institutions was often viewed as a journey where the travelers felt proud and energized in having the opportunity to share the variety of positive going on in their work environments.

Finally, one interesting characteristic that seems to pertain to all Magnet Hospitals is that of personnel stability. It has also been noted by Magnet site observers that these organizations have large numbers of long-term employees. Loyalty is a two-way street. This means that hospitals that enjoy stability among their staff members are equally loyal in return, which demonstrates the extent to which they value the contributions, that these seasoned individuals make to the organization. This is the very essence of Magnetism.

NCLEX® EXAM QUESTIONS

1. A benefit of accreditation by The Joint Commission is that it:
   1. leads to improved patient care and demonstrates the organization's commitment to safety and quality
   2. allows for increased financial gain through Medicare and Medicaid reimbursement and offers employee assistance programs
   3. influences the improved design of care processes, creating a nonpunitive environment to enhance error reporting and allow participate in error reporting and analysis
   4. offers an educational off-site survey experience
2. As a nurse, your documentation of patient pain assessment will be reviewed for The Joint Commission standard compliance. Under this

Continued

standard, organizations are required to provide proof that nurses:

1. recognize patients' right to assessment and management of pain and assessment of the nature and intensity of pain
2. demonstrate a safe medication pass with the surveyors
3. provide medication documentation from the past 10 years
4. provide The Joint Commission with the pharmacy orders from the past 7 years

3. The Joint Commission's evaluation and accreditation services are provided for the following types of organizations:
1. state department of health and town senior housing services
2. physicians' offices and freestanding laboratory service agencies
3. home hemodialysis and peritoneal dialysis programs
4. critical access hospitals, home care organizations, and nursing homes

4. The U.S. Department of Health and Human Services (USDHHS) is the most important federal actor in health care. What are some of the other federal agencies with major health services roles?
1. Department of Veterans Affairs
2. Department of the Treasury and Taxation
3. Department of Corrections and Law
4. Department of Agriculture and Taxation

5. The mission of the USDHHS is to:
1. protect and promote the health and social and economic well-being of legal immigrants by helping them and their families develop and maintain productive and independent lives
2. support legal immigrants both financially and legally
3. protect and promote the health and social and economic well-being of Americans by helping them and their families develop and maintain productive and independent lives
4. deport all illegal immigrants to their countries in an effort to maintain alliances with those countries

6. The Joint Commission disease-specific care certifications focus on all of the following EXCEPT:
1. maintaining data quality and integrity
2. evaluating patient's perception of care quality

3. using comparative data to evaluate disease-specific program process and patient outcome
4. keeping statistics and data on all negative health care outcomes

7. An example of what the Centers for Disease Control and Prevention (CDC) would evaluate is a(n):
1. toxic spill on a state highway
2. outbreak of rubella in a school
3. flu shot clinic at a pharmaceutical company
4. outbreak of respiratory syncytial virus in a neonatal intensive care unit

8. OSHA has provided guidelines for minimizing patient lifting to prevent health care musculoskeletal injuries. Within these guidelines, OSHA recommends that:
1. patients be allowed to decide whether safe lifting equipment should be used when transferring out of bed
2. manual lifting of residents be minimized and eliminated when feasible
3. only specific types of lifting equipment be used, such as a ceiling-mounted patient lift with a sling
4. institutions should be allowed to decide based on patient population whether safe lifting equipment should be used

9. The National Institute for Occupational Safety and Health (NIOSH) is the:
1. agency that works closely with The Joint Commission and hospital accreditation
2. local agency that coordinates patient care and patient services
3. state agency that is part of the Centers for Disease Control and Prevention (CDC) in the U.S. Department of Health and Human Services
4. federal agency responsible for conducting research and making recommendations for the prevention of work-related injury and illness

10. What agency provides national and world leadership to prevent work-related illnesses and injuries and conducts a range of efforts in the area of research, guidance, information, and service?
1. The Centers for Disease Control and Prevention (CDC)
2. National Institute for Occupational Safety and Health (NIOSH)
3. The Joint Commission (TJC)
4. Centers for Medicare & Medicaid Services (CMS)

Answers: 1. 1   2. 1   3. 4   4. 1   5. 3   6. 4   7. 2   8. 2   9. 4   10. 2

REFERENCES

American Nurses Credentialing Center (ANCC). (2008). Retrieved July 23, 2008, from http://www.nursecredentialing.org/Magnet/ProgramOverview.aspx.

Baldrige National Quality Program (2008). *Health care criteria for performance excellence*. Gaithersburg, MD: Baldrige National Quality Program.

J. D. Powers and Associates. (2008). Turning information into action. Retrieved July 23, 2008, from http://www.jdpower.com/corporate/healthcare/hospital.aspx.

Joint Commission (2001). Pain assessment and management, Feb 2001, 8, 10; Oct 2001, 4, 11. *Perspectives*.

Joint Commission (2009). The Joint Commission Mission–related commitments. January 1, 2009. Retrieved May 5, 2009, from http://www.jointcommission.org/AboutUs/mission_commitments.htm

OSHA guideline. Retrieved March 17, 2007, from http://www.osha.gov/ergonomics/guidelines/nursinghome/final_nh_guidelines.html.

U.S. Department of Health and Human Services. HHS.gov. HHS: What we do. Retrieved August 7, 2007, from http://www.hhs.gov/about/whatwedo.html/.

U.S. News and World Report. (2007). Retrieved July 23, 2008, from http://health.usnews.com/sections/health/besthospitals.

Yoder-Wise, P. S. (2006). *Beyond leading and managing nursing administration for the future*. St. Louis, MO: Mosby.

WEBSITES

http://www.state.nj.us/health/
http://www.osha.gov/oshinfo/mission.html
http://www.cdc.gov/niosh/
http://www.osha.gov/oshinfo/mission.html
http://gunston.gmu.edu/healthscience/547/MajorAccreditationAgencies.asp
http://www.hhs.gov/about/whatwedo.html
http://www.osha.gov/ergonomics/guidelines/nursinghome/final_nh_guidelines.html

CHAPTER 8

Ethical Issues in Patient Care

Chapter Objectives

1. Differentiate between *ethics* and *bioethics*.
2. Identify ethical dilemmas in nursing.
3. Discuss the role of the nurse in advance directives.
4. Review the principles of ethical decision making.

5. Identify interventions designed to protect patients' rights.
6. Discuss the responsibility of the ethics committee.

Definitions

Autonomy Provides for the privilege of self-determination in deciding what happens to one's body in health care

Bioethics Ethics specific to health care

Ethics Science that deals with the principles of right and wrong and of good and bad, and governs our relationships with others; is based on personal beliefs and values

Beneficence Duty to do good to others; to maintain a balance between benefits and harm; to provide all patients, including terminally ill, with caring attention; and to treat every patient with respect and courtesy. Requires that care providers contribute to the health and welfare of the patient and not merely attempt to avoid harm to the patient or client

Institutional review board (IRB) Group that has been formally designated to approve, monitor, and review biomedical and behavioral research involving humans with the alleged aim to protect the rights and welfare of the subjects. This group performs critical oversight functions for research conducted on human subjects that are scientific, ethical, and regulatory. Research review panels that determine the legal and ethical protection of subjects participating in medical research

Nonmaleficence Principle of doing no harm: observe safety rules and precautions and keep skills up to date. Prohibits deliberate harm and demands weighing risks with the benefits of treatment (Grohar-Murray & DiCroce, 2003)

Justice Principle of fairness in which an individual receives what is due, owed, or legitimately claimed: treat all parties equally, regardless of economic or social background, and learn state's and organization's laws for reporting abuse. Requires that individuals be given what they deserve or can legitimately claim

Morality Behavior in accordance with custom or tradition and usually reflects personal or religious beliefs (DeLaune & Ladner, 2002)

ETHICAL DECISION MAKING

Today's nurses are in the public eye in the discussion of many different ethical issues and dilemmas, such as technology that maintains life for severely premature infants, technology that advances the life of severely brain-damaged patients, stem cell research, the issues of what constitutes brain death, transplant and donor programs, and end-of-life decisions. Concern for ethics has also moved beyond the clinical arenas to the business of health care, with the potential for Medicare fraud, suspect business decision making, and the protection of patient information. Ethical decision making will have an impact on your clinical professional role, your leadership role, and your research role.

Ethical decision making is required when there is an ethical dilemma. *Ethical dilemmas* occur when there is a conflict between two or more ethical principles.

Common Ethical Principles and Their Rules

1. Beneficence—Duty to do good and to protect the patient's welfare. An example is carefully adhering to infection control principles for all patients.
2. Nonmaleficence—Principle of doing no harm. Nurses who maintain their skills are practicing the principle of "doing no harm."
3. Justice—Principle of fairness in which an individual receives what is owed. All patients receiving the same level of culturally competent care is an example.
4. Autonomy—Respect for individual liberty and the person's right to self-determination. Informed consent is an example of adherence to the principle of autonomy.
5. Fidelity—Duty to keep one's word. Senior leaders adhering to all contracts is an example of leadership fidelity.
6. Respect for others—Right of people to make their own decisions, such as not telling a patient what he "should do" but allowing him to make his own decision.
7. Veracity—Obligation to tell the truth. As a professional, this would be a requirement to admit mistakes promptly or to not lie to a patient about bad news (list adapted from Little, 2003, p. 469).

Such a conflict comes into place with the conflict between (a) the principle of autonomy (the duty to respect the patient's choice) and the duty to do only what the patient wants and (b) the principle of beneficence (the duty to protect the patient's welfare) and the duty to do only what the patient needs. An example would be the conflict that arises when a patient refuses dialysis that will prolong her life. Another example would be the situation where the family does not want their frail elderly mother given the news that her grandson has been hospitalized with a life-threatening injury. The conflict here is between veracity and self-respect. The decision of what to do is guided by beneficence. Often, there is no correct decision. There are many questions that arise in clinical care, such as the following (Schroeder, 1995):

- When do we refrain from using technology?
- When do we stop using technology, once it is started?
- Who is entitled to technology? Those who can pay? Those who are uninsured? Everyone, no matter what?

In addition to the clinical situations that cause ethical conflicts, nurses and health care personnel bring their own values and beliefs into the dilemma. There are times where the beliefs of the health care personnel are the dilemma. An individual with a strong religious belief in the sanctity of life may have ethical conflicts about DNR (do-not-resuscitate) orders or abortions. It is important be aware of your beliefs and to not let them interfere with the legal and professional requirements of your position. If you have beliefs that will prevent you from performing some of the requirements of your position, it is necessary to inform your supervisor, so that the patient needs can always be met.

TRADITIONAL ETHICAL THEORIES

The study of ethics has resulted in different theories that are used to guide decision making. Box 8-1 provides traditional ethical theories.

As a nurse, you will be guided by ethical theories and your own personal values and beliefs and professional expectations (ANA, 2001; ICN, 2009). The fundamental values of nursing are expressed in the Code of Ethics for Nurses. They are the values, such as respect for patient autonomy, acting in the patient's best interest, and maintaining professional competence, that all nurses commit to uphold when they enter the profession.

Box 8-1   TRADITIONAL ETHICAL THEORIES

Utilitarianism
- Decisions based on what will provide the greatest good for the greatest number of people
- For example, the decision to force people with pulmonary tuberculosis into treatment is ethical, according to this theory, because it protects the greater population from infection

Teleology (or consequentialist theory)
- Value of a situation is determined by its consequences
- Thus the outcome, not the action itself, is what counts; sometimes referred to as the "all's well that ends well" ethical approach

Deontology (or formalism)
- An act is good only if it springs from good will
- This ethical theory does not allow for actions based on the concept of "the end justifies the means" (Little, 2003)

Kelly-Heidenthal, P. (2004). *Essentials of nursing leadership and management.* Clifton Park, NY: Thomson Delmar Learning.

AMERICAN NURSES ASSOCIATION'S CODE OF ETHICS FOR NURSES

Nurses must always act as patient advocates on a daily basis. The American Nurses Association (ANA) House of Delegates approved the most recent *Code of Ethics for Nurses* at its June 30, 2001, meeting in Washington, DC. In July 2001, the Congress of Nursing Practice and Economics voted to accept the new language of the interpretive statements (Tomey, 2004).

Revised Code of Ethics for Nurses with Interpretive Statements

1. The nurse, in all professional relationships, practices with compassion and respect for the inherent dignity, worth and uniqueness of every individual, unrestricted by considerations of social or economic status, personal attributes, or the nature of health problems.
2. The nurse's primary commitment is to the patient, whether an individual, family, group, or community.
3. The nurse promotes, advocates for, and strives to protect the health, safety, and rights of the patient.
4. The nurse is responsible and accountable for individual nursing practice and determines the appropriate delegation of tasks consistent with the nurse's obligation to provide optimum patient care.
5. The nurse owes the same duties to self as to others, including the responsibility to preserve integrity and safety, to maintain competence, and to continue personal and professional growth.
6. The nurse participates in establishing, maintaining, and improving health care environments and conditions of employment conducive to the provision of quality health care and consistent with the values of the profession through individual and collective action.
7. The nurse participates in the advancement of the profession through contributions to practice, education, administration, and knowledge development.
8. The nurse collaborates with other health professionals and the public in promoting community, national, and international efforts to meet health needs.
9. The profession of nursing, as represented by associations and their members, is responsible for articulating nursing values, for maintaining the integrity of the profession and its practice, and for shaping social policy (ANA, 2001).

INTERNATIONAL COUNCIL OF NURSES' INTERNATIONAL CODE OF ETHICS FOR NURSES

The International Council of Nurses' (ICN) International Code of Ethics for Nurses, most recently revised in 2006, is a guide for action based on social values and needs. The code has served as the standard for nurses worldwide since it was first adopted in 1953. The code is regularly reviewed and revised in response to the realities of nursing and health care in a changing society. The code makes it clear that inherent in nursing is respect for human rights, including the right to life, to dignity, and to be treated with respect. The ICN International Code of Ethics for Nurses guides nurses in everyday choices and supports their refusal to participate in activities that conflict with caring and healing.

International Council of Nurses' International Code of Ethics for Nurses

1. Nurses and people

The nurse's primary professional responsibility is to people requiring nursing care. In providing care, the nurse promotes an environment in which the human rights, values, customs and spiritual beliefs of the individual, family and community are respected. The nurse ensures that the individual receives sufficient information on which to base consent for care and related treatment. The nurse holds in confidence personal information and uses judgment in sharing this information.

The nurse shares with society the responsibility for initiating and supporting action to meet the health and social needs of the public, in particular those of vulnerable populations. The nurse also shares responsibility to sustain and protect the natural environment from depletion, pollution, degradation and destruction.

2. Nurses and practice

The nurse carries personal responsibility and accountability for nursing, practice, and for maintaining competence by continual learning. The nurse maintains a standard of personal health such that the ability to provide care is not compromised. The nurse uses judgment regarding individual competence when accepting and delegating responsibility.

The nurse at all times maintains standards of personal conduct which reflect well on the profession and enhance public confidence. The nurse in providing care, ensures that uses of technology and scientific advances are compatible with the safety, dignity and rights of people.

3. Nurses and the profession

The nurse assumes the major role in determining and implementing acceptable standards of clinical nursing practice, management, research and education. The nurse is active in developing a core of research-based professional knowledge.

The nurse, acting through the professional organization, participates in creating and maintaining equitable social and economic working conditions in nursing.

4. Nurses and coworkers

The nurse sustains a cooperative relationship with coworkers in nursing and other fields. The nurse takes appropriate action to safeguard individuals when their care is endangered by a coworker or any other person (ICN, 2006; copyright © 2006).

One mark of a profession is the establishment of determination of ethical behavior for its members. In addition to the ANA and ICN codes, specialty nursing organizations and hospitals have developed codes of ethical behavior.

To assist you in dealing with the complex ethical issues that exist, hospitals have formed ethics committees. These committees are interdisciplinary and include representatives from clinical nursing, administration, medicine, social work, pharmacy, legal, and clergy. The work of ethics committees lies in three areas (Agich and Younger, 1991; Dalgo and Anderson, 1995):

- Education (seminars and workshops for committee members)
- Policy and guideline recommendations (specific hospital policies)
- Case review (analyze patient cases and provide clear options)

As a nurse, you have the right to call on the ethics committee for a referral. Cases are often referred to the ethics committee for discussion. Issues commonly addressed by ethics committees are end-of-life issues, organ donation, and futility-of-care issues.

END-OF-LIFE ISSUES

End-of-life issues frequently revolve around the issue of advance directives. An advance directive is an end-of-life decision made by a patient in advance of the actual need. Many individuals confuse an advance directive with a DNR order, but they are not the same.

An *advance directive* instructs health care personnel on the patient's desires for care in certain circumstances. An advance directive, sometimes called a "living will," is a set of instructions documenting a person's wishes about medical care intended to sustain life. It is used if a patient becomes terminally ill, incapacitated, or unable to communicate or make decisions. Everyone has the right to accept or refuse medical care. A living will protects the patient's rights and removes the burden for making decisions from family, friends, and physicians. The ethical dilemma exists if the patient's family refuses to allow the advance directive to be used or if a health care professional refuses the directives. The legal issues regarding advance directives are presented in Chapter 18.

ORGAN DONATION

Although organ donation is a personal choice, there may be times when an ethical dilemma may ensue with carrying out this wish. For example, if a person has decided to be an organ donor and has made this clear on his or her driver's license, at the time of death, the family may strongly disagree with this decision.

Some states have mandated that a request be made for organ or tissue donation at the time of a patient's death. Some families may feel this is a way for their loved one to remain alive in some way; other family members feel just the opposite and are opposed to the idea. Organ donation cards can be completed and placed in your wallet with your driver's license. Mine, for example, stipulates that certain organs can be used for organ donation, excluding my skin. I have made my wishes known to my husband that, in the event of an accident, I wish to have my organs donated.

In hospitals where organ transplantations are done, there usually is a full-time organ donation coordinator. Nurses may be called on to request organ donations if the facility where you are employed charges nurses with this responsibility. Again, the nurse should be very direct in making these requests so there are no miscommunications, saying, for example, "Have you considered organ donation for your loved one?"

Written consent and hospital policies and procedures must be strictly followed. There is no cost to the donor family. The usual funeral expenses still apply.

Organ donation list:
- Skin
- Corneas
- Bone
- Kidney
- Heart
- Liver
- Pancreas

UNITED STATES ORGAN DONOR LISTS

Waiting list candidates	98,194	As of March 10, 2008
Transplants January–December 2007	28,354	As of March 7, 2008
Donors January–December 2007	14,395	As of March 7, 2008

Based on Organ Procurement and Transplantation Network (OPTN) data. http://www.optn.org/. Retrieved March 17, 2008, from http://www.organdonor.gov/.

THE NEW JERSEY ORGAN AND TISSUE SHARING NETWORK

New Jersey Organ and Tissue Sharing Network (NJ Sharing Network) is a nonprofit, federally certified, state-approved organ procurement organization (OPO). An OPO is a program that acquires and coordinates placement of donated organs for patients on national transplant waiting lists. NJ Sharing Network is responsible for the recovery of organs and tissue for New Jersey residents currently awaiting transplantation and is part of the national recovery system.

In 1987, three New Jersey organ procurement programs merged into one, and NJ Sharing Network was formed. From its inception, NJ Sharing Network has set out to educate the general public as to the life-saving benefits of transplantation with the goal of increasing the number of organ donors. Government policy has also helped donation. The federal conditions of participation for organ donation, adopted in 1998, require hospitals to refer all deaths to OPOs for evaluation and to work collaboratively with the OPO on an approach for consent (New Jersey Sharing Network, 2007a).

- Today, there are close to 90,000 Americans registered with the United Network for Organ Sharing on transplant waiting lists.
- Every year, an estimated 6000 people die while waiting for organ transplants.
- In 1988, 4080 people donated organs after death. In 2004, that number nearly doubled to 7150.
- Organ donation occurred in only 0.0025% of all deaths in the United States.
- One individual who donates after death can provide organs, corneas, skin, bone, and tissue for 50 or more people in need.
- In 2004, there were 27,033 organ transplantations performed in the United States.
- An estimated 220,000 Americans are treated with transplanted bone and tissue each year. Tissues include tendons and ligaments, skin used to treat burns, heart valves, and eye corneas.
- About 46,000 cornea transplants are performed annually, with more than 5000 people waiting for donated corneas.
- The greatest number of children who need organ transplants are waiting for kidney donations. Approximately 13% of patients on the national kidney waiting list are children younger than 18 years; almost 1% are age 5 or younger.

- Almost 44% of people waiting for organ transplants are between the ages of 18 and 49 years.
- By gender, 57% of Americans waiting for donated organs are male, and 43% are female.
- African Americans, who represent 27% of the national population, receive more than 40% of all kidney transplants. Because of specific medical conditions, including diabetes and high blood pressure, African Americans have a disproportionately high rate of end-stage renal disease (kidney failure). There are currently more than 24,000 African Americans waiting for kidney or kidney–pancreas transplants nationwide.
- Survival rates for organ recipients continue to rise. The 1-year survival rate for kidney recipients is 95%; for heart recipients, 85%; for liver recipients, 77%; and for pancreas recipients, almost 77%. Between 1996 and 2001, 1-year survival rates for lung recipients increased by almost 34%.
- There is no cost to be an organ and tissue donor. Donation is a gift (list from New Jersey Sharing Network, 2007b).

RELIGIOUS VIEWS

The following are the views of various religious groups on organ donation and transplantation (American Council on Transplantation, 2007).

African Methodist Episcopal (AME) and African Methodist Episcopal Zion (AME Zion)

Organ and tissue donation is viewed as an act of neighborly love and charity by these denominations. These groups encourage all members to support donation as a way of helping others.

Amish

The Amish will consent to transplantation if they know that it is for the health and welfare of the recipient. They would be reluctant to donate their organs if the outcome was known to be questionable; however, nothing in the Amish understanding of the Bible forbids them from using modern medical services.

Baptists

Organ and tissue donation is advocated as an act of charity. In 1988, the Southern Baptist Convention passed a resolution supporting donation as a way to alleviate suffering and have compassion for the needs of others.

Buddhists

Buddhists believe that organ and tissue donation is a matter of individual conscience.

Catholics

Catholics view organ donation as an act of charity, fraternal love, and self-sacrifice. Transplants are ethically and morally acceptable to the Vatican.

The Church of Christ Scientist

The Church of Christ Scientist takes no specific position on transplants or organ donation as distinct from other medical or surgical procedures. Church members usually rely on spiritual rather than medical means of healing. They are free to choose the form of medical treatment they desire, including organ transplantation. The decision of organ donation is left to the individual.

Hindus

Hindus are not prohibited by religious law from donating; it is considered an individual decision.

Jehovah's Witnesses

Jehovah's Witnesses do not encourage organ donation but believe it is a matter for individual conscience according to the Watch Tower and Tract Society, the legal corporation for the religion. The group does not oppose donating or receiving organs; however, all organs and tissue must be completely drained of blood before transplantation.

Judaism

Judaism teaches that saving a human life takes precedence over maintaining the sanctity of the human body.

Latter-Day Saints (Mormons)

Latter-Day Saints (Mormons) are not prohibited by religious law from donating their organs or receiving transplants, according to church leaders. The decision is a personal one.

Mennonites

Mennonites have no prohibition against organ donation and transplantation. Church officials state such decisions are individual ones.

Moslems

The Moslem Religious Council initially rejected organ donation by followers of Islam in 1983, but it has since reversed its position provided that donors consent in writing in advance. The organs and tissues of Moslem donors must be transplanted immediately and not be stored in organ banks.

Protestants

Protestantism encourages and endorses organ donation. Protestants respect the individual's conscience and a person's right to make decisions regarding his or her own body.

Quakers

Quakers do not oppose organ donation and transplantation. The decision, they say, is an individual one.

Seventh-Day Adventists

Seventh-Day Adventist officials have stated organ donation and transplantation to be acceptable practices for members. The decision is an individual one.

FUTILITY OF CARE

Often, there arise ethical dilemmas in patient care situations where there are concerns about the futility of care. The ethical conflict arises when the principle of beneficence ("do not harm") is called into question. Will further treatment benefit the patient? This is a time where a consultation with the ethics committee may be appropriate.

Some hospitals are offering a more humane approach to the DNR request. Families often misinterpret the DNR order as an order to do nothing. The intent of the order is to "allow a natural death" (AND). It is also important to understand that a decision not to receive "aggressive medical treatment" is not the same as withholding all medical care. A patient can still receive antibiotics, nutrition, pain medication, and other interventions when the goal of treatment becomes comfort rather than cure. This is called palliative care, and its primary focus is helping the patient remain as comfortable as possible.

THE JOINT COMMISSION STATEMENT ON PATIENT RIGHTS AND ORGANIZATIONAL ETHICS

The Joint Commission statement on patient rights and organization ethics states that patients have a funda-mental right to considerate care that safeguards their personal dignity and respects their cultural, psychosocial, and spiritual values. These values often influence patients' perception of care and illness. Understanding and respecting these values guide the nurse in meeting the patients' care needs and preferences (Joint Commission on Accreditation of Healthcare Organizations, 2003).

A hospital's behavior toward its patients and its business practices has a significant impact on the patient's experience of and response to care. Thus, access, treatment, respect, and conduct affect patient rights. Access to hospital care is a major ethical issue in health care. Does a hospital have the right to refuse to care for a patient who does not have adequate insurance?

As a manager, you will be responsible for setting the ethical tone on your unit and guaranteeing that all patient rights are respected. You will also have to practice ethically in all leadership and managerial actions. This will mean protecting the rights of your staff and providing a professional work environment. Staff members need to be able to work in an environment where they are free to report issues of concern. Hospitals have created departments of corporate compliance to oversee the reporting, documentation, and continued improvement of areas of organizational ethical concern. Senior leaders of the organization are responsible for safe stewardship of the organization in both business practices and all areas of clinical care.

The Joint Commission guides the hospital in the setting of a framework for ethical practice (Box 8-2).

Hospitals are legally and ethically obligated to uphold the following patient rights to:
- Participate in treatment decisions.
- Provide informed consent to treatment.
- Receive considerate and respectful care.
- Review records.
- Be informed of hospital policies.
- Expect reasonable and appropriate continuity of care after hospitalization.

The Patient Care Partnership of the American Hospital Association replaced what was originally named the Patients' Bill of Rights (Box 8-3). The partnership informs patients about what they should expect during their hospital stay with regard to their rights and responsibilities.

Box 8-2 THE JOINT COMMISSION FRAMEWORK FOR PATIENT CARE AND ORGANIZATIONAL ETHICAL ISSUES

- The patient's right to reasonable access to care
- The patient's right to care that is considerate and respectful of his or her personal values and beliefs
- The patient's right to be informed about and participate in decisions regarding his or her care
- The patient's right to participate in ethical questions that arise in the course of his or her care, including issues of conflict resolution, withholding resuscitative services, forgoing or withdrawal of life-sustaining treatment, and participation in investigational studies or clinical trials
- The patient's right to security and personal privacy and confidentiality of information
- The issue of designating a decision maker in case the patient is incapable of understanding a proposed treatment or procedure or is unable to communicate his or her wishes regarding care
- The hospital's method of informing the patient of these issues identified
- The hospital's method of educating staff about patient rights and their role in supporting those rights
- The patient's right to access protective services

From The Joint Commission (2007).

Box 8-3 PATIENT BILL OF RIGHTS

The American Hospital Association's Patient Care Partnership states that the patient has the following rights:

The Patient Care Partnership: Understanding Expectations, Rights, and Responsibilities

High-quality hospital care

Patients have the right to be provided with the care needed, with skill, compassion, and respect.

A clean and safe environment

There are hospital policies and procedures in place to ensure that patients have an environment free from errors, abuse, and neglect.

Involvement in your care

Patients are entitled to be made aware of the benefits and risks of treatments, whether treatments are experimental or part of a research study, what can be expected from treatment and any long-term effects it might have on quality of life, what should be done after discharge, the financial consequences of uncovered services or out-of-network providers. Patients should inform health care providers of any past illnesses, surgeries, hospital admissions, allergies, all medications and dietary supplements taken. Patients should also inform health care providers of any health care goals and values or spiritual beliefs that are important to the well-being of the patient. It should be made clear who the power of attorney is, if the patient has a living will, or advance directives in place.

Protection of your privacy

Patients' privacy must be protected at all times once in the health care system. Patients will receive a Notice of Privacy Practices that describes the specific hospital privacy plan and means of accomplishing this.

Help when leaving the hospital

The hospital personnel will identify sources of follow-up care such as home care or ordering equipment needed for home.

Help with your billing claims

The hospital billing department will file health care claims and assist the patient with any questions regarding the bill and patient coverage.

Adapted March 17, 2008, from http://www.aha.org/aha/content/2003/pdf/pcp_english_030730.pdf.

RESEARCH

As a nurse, you will participate in clinical research during your career. It is important that the ethical requirements of research are well understood and part of your work. Hospitals and other workplaces participating in research involving human subjects have institutional review boards (IRBs) that set guidelines for the research and approve all research studies that occur in the institution. While the regulations for IRBs are federal law (U.S. Code of Federal Regulations, Department of Health and Human Services [DHHS] Title 45 Part 46, entitled *Protection of Human Subjects*, as well as the U.S. Food and Drug Administration [FDA] Title 21, Part 50 and Title 21 Part 56), they have arisen in light of ethical violations of the rights of patients.

The IRB's primary concerns are to determine that:

- The rights and welfare of the human subjects are protected adequately.

- The risks to subjects are outweighed by the potential benefits of the research.
- The selection of subjects is equitable.
- Informed consent will be obtained and documented.

SUMMARY

As a nurse, you will be confronted with ethical dilemmas throughout your career. The nature of these dilemmas will change as science and technology advances. It is important, however, to recognize that as a nurse and nurse leader, you are responsible for:

- Creating an ethically principled environment
- Upholding standards of conduct established by the profession

- Being committed to bringing about any changes needed
- Being dedicated to ethical principles
- Role modeling the ethical behavior of those working under your supervision; this governs
  - Interactions with people requiring nursing care
  - Responsibility for maintaining competence in nursing practice
  - Responsibility for meeting health needs of the public
  - Maintaining cooperative relationships with members of the interdisciplinary health care team
  - Determining and implementing desirable standards of nursing practice and education (ICN International Code of Ethics for Nurses, cited in Little, 2003, and Carroll, 2006)

 ## CLINICAL CORNER

Role of the Nurse on the Ethics Committee
Mary Frey

Sally Gadow, PhD, RN, a scholar in health care ethics, wrote that "care is the supreme covenant between the nurse and the patient and that care is the moral basis for the nurse-patient relationship" (Fletcher, Lombardo, Marshall, and Miller, 1997, p. 292). As nurses, we see patients as a "whole." Often we are the first to point out when health care providers are not following a patient's wishes. Nursing professionals offer unique perspectives; their prolonged contact with the patients can serve as insight to those on the committees who may not know the patients.

As a nurse serving on the Ethics Committee, I have the moral responsibility to ensure the best ethical decisions are made for the patients in the institution. I see myself as the best advocate for the patient; I can educate the committee about the patient and caregiver needs. I am responsible to follow the same basic clinical ethical principles of respecting patient autonomy, beneficence, nonmalificence, and justice as are all Ethics Committee members. Any nurse has the ability to request an Ethics Consult whenever one of these principles has not been followed.

In the decision making of the committee, the needs of the patient should be a primary consideration—the role of the nurse is to preserve and protect the patient's autonomy, dignity, and rights. For example: The nurse has reviewed a patient's advance directive and knows what his wishes are. She then overhears a conversa-

tion between the physician and the surrogate about insertion of a feeding tube. The patient is suffering from dementia and is no longer able to speak for himself. The physician is telling the surrogate that the feeding tube is necessary: "Do you want your loved one to starve to death?" Of course, the surrogate feels he wants to do everything for his loved one; however, the advance directive clearly states the patient would not want artificial food or hydration. The nurse has a responsibility to point out the patient's advance directive and discuss his wishes with both the physician and the surrogate. If a decision cannot be made, then the nurse needs to request an ethics consult.

At the committee meetings, be an active listener, and hear all views. Remain current in education and literature, and apply that knowledge to each case presented. Advocate for the patient/surrogate, who may not have any medical knowledge. In turn, educate the patient/surrogate about what you have learned at the committee. Challenge physicians; be prepared to defend that which you believe to be ethically appropriate. Seek the evidence to support what you propose, and remain professional, not emotional.

Many cases brought to the ethics committee are of a very sensitive nature. Nurses need to know what their resources are. Do you need to reach out to Legal? Psychiatry? Social work? Pastoral care? Administration? Chief medical officer? Nurses have a plethora of resources available; learn how to use them. If these resources are not usually available on your ethics committee, bring them in ad hoc on a case-by-case need.

Fletcher, J. C., Lombardo, P. A., Marshall, M. F., & Miller, F. G. (1997). *Introduction to Clinical Ethics.* 2nd ed. Hagerstown, MD: University Publishing Group.

EVIDENCE-BASED PRACTICE

Allow Natural Death: A More Humane Approach to Discussing End-of-Life Directives.

From Knox, C., and Vereb, J. (2005). Allow natural death: a more humane approach to discussing end-of-life directives. Journal of Emergency Nursing, 31, *560-561; and Stecher, J. (2008). Allow natural death vs. do not resuscitate.* American Journal of Nursing, 108, *11.*

End-of-life directives and discussions about do not resuscitate (DNR), do not intubate (DNI), and comfort measure only (CMO) are all too familiar to today's health care professionals. While these are everyday terms for these professionals, these can be very frightening and confusing concepts for families and patients who may not fully understand what they mean. The harsh tone suggested by a "do not" statement implies to families that nothing will be done to care for their loved one or, worse, that the patient might be allowed to suffer, magnifying feelings of guilt and despair that may already be felt. Across the United States, a move is happening to eliminate the current DNR terminology and replace it with a gentler and kinder resuscitation status term, "allow natural death" (AND). Begun by Reverend Chuck Meyer in 2000, AND is meant to ensure that only comfort measures are provided. While many health care professionals find it difficult to explain what

a DNR order means to a patient's level of care, an AND order acknowledges that a person is dying and that the dying process will be allowed to occur as comfortably as possible including the withdrawal of nutrition and hydration. DNR and AND are not really different in theory but the AND language has been found more suitable for patients and families and suggests the prevention of unintentional pain, indicates what *will* be done for the patient, and simply allows a natural death. The AND approach has been suggested to be seen as a positive choice in a patient's care versus an end resort as many DNRs are found to be. In addition, an AND approach emphasizes a palliative approach and encourages earlier conversations about end-of-life when a patient might be able to participate and assist family members in making these very difficult decisions. Baptist Hospital East in Louisville, Kentucky, has adopted the AND language and expanded it to be more easily understood by patients and families. Three levels of care have been defined and the staff feel that the language is easier to use and more effective and that patients understand it better. In the long run, it is families who must live with the decision they make for their loved one and they need to be at peace with their decisions.

NCLEX® EXAM QUESTIONS

1. An example that would necessitate the use of an institutional review board (IRB) is a:
   1. study involving humans including children
   2. study involving animals
   3. study not involving humans or children
   4. study involving humans excluding children
2. You are the nurse in the operating room in which a kidney transplantation is about to take place. It is the responsibility of the _____ to check that the organ donor and recipient are correct.
   1. physician and registered nurse
   2. transferring facility
   3. organ procurement manager
   4. accepting facility
3. You are the nurse caring for a patient who is brain dead and ventilator dependent. The physician has decided it would be in the best interest of the patient to discontinue the ventilator. One example of is a need for an ethics committee decision would be if this comatose patient:

1. does not have advance directives
2. has a living will
3. cannot breathe without the ventilator
4. has advance directive and next of kin

4. The Organ Procurement and Transplantation Network (OPTN) is a(n) _____ network.
   1. state
   2. local
   3. national
   4. international
5. You are the nurse in the operating room. The next patient you will be caring for is a 16-year-old girl who will be undergoing a termination of pregnancy. You do not wish to stay in the operating room for this procedure. What is the first thing you should do?
   1. This should have been discussed earlier with your immediate supervisor.
   2. You must stay in the room because this is your assignment.

3. Tell the surgeon you do not agree with this procedure.
4. Stay in the operating room and discuss it later with supervisor.

6. The difference between *bioethics* and *ethics* is:
   1. bioethics is specific to health care; ethics deals with the principles of right and wrong
   2. bioethics is specific to health care; ethics deals with the principles of right and wrong, good and bad
   3. bioethics is specific to health care; ethics deals with the principles of right and wrong, good and bad with no issues of beliefs and values
   4. bioethics is specific to health care, the science that deals with the principles of right and wrong, good and bad, and governs our relationships with others and that is based on personal beliefs and values

7. The Patient Care Partnership of the American Hospital Association replaced what was originally named the:
   1. Patient's Bill of Rights
   2. Patient's advance directives
   3. Patient's living will
   4. Patient's power of attorney

8. You are caring for a terminally ill child. The family has requested an ethics committee meeting regarding a DNR. As a nurse you are aware that the prime functions of the ethics meeting include:
   1. education, policy and guideline recommendations, and case review
   2. education, specific patient decision making, and DNR orders
   3. policy and guideline recommendations, advance directive orders, and case review
   4. termination of life support, hospice care, and education

9. The fundamental values of nursing that all nurses commit to uphold when they enter the profession are expressed in the Code of Ethics for Nurses. They include:
   1. respect for patient autonomy, acting in the hospital's best interest, and maintaining professional competence
   2. respect for patient autonomy, acting in the patient's best interest, and maintaining your nursing license
   3. respect for families, acting in the patient's best interest, and maintaining professional competence
   4. respect for patient autonomy, acting in the patient's best interest, and maintaining professional competence

10. Hospitals are legally and ethically obligated to uphold patient rights, which include the right to:
    1. review records; family can also review records
    2. participate in treatment decisions and to provide consent to treatment
    3. be informed of hospital bylaws and hospital attorneys' names and telephone numbers
    4. expect reasonable care after hospitalization

Answers: 1. 1   2. 1   3. 1   4. 3   5. 1   6. 4   7. 1   8. 1   9. 4   10. 2

REFERENCES

Agich, G. J., & Younger, S. J. (1991). For experts only? Access to hospital ethics committees. *Hastings Center Report*, 21(5), 17-25.

American Council on Transplantation. (2007). Retrieved August 2, 2007, from http://www.sharenj.org/religiou. htm.

American Nurses Association, *Code of ethics for nurses with interpretive statements*. Silver Spring, MD: American Nurses Publishing, 2001. Retrieved August 1, 2007, from http://www.nursingworld.org/ethics/chcode.htm.

Carroll, P. (2006). *Nursing leadership and management: a practical guide*. Clifton Park, NY: Delmar Thomson Learning.

Dalgo, J. T., & Anderson, F. (1995). Notes from the field: developing a hospital ethics committee. *Nursing Management*, 26(9), 104-106.

DeLaune, S. C., & Ladner, P. K. (2002). *Fundamentals of nursing*. Clifton Park, NJ: Delmar Thomson Learning.

Grohar-Murray, M. E., & DiCroce, H. (2003). *Leadership and management in nursing*. 3rd ed. Upper Saddle River, NJ: Prentice Hall.

International Council of Nurses (ICN). (2006). The ICN Code of Ethics. Geneva, Switzerland.

International Council of Nurses (ICN). (2009). Web site. Retrieved April 17, 2009, from http://www.icn.ch/ icncode.pdf; http://www.icn.ch/ethics.htm.

Joint Commission on Accreditation of Healthcare Organizations. (2003). *Comprehensive Accreditation Manual.* Oakbrook Terrace, IL: Author.

Kelly-Heidenthal, P. (2004). *Essentials of nursing leadership and management* (p. 295). Clifton Park, NY: Thomson Delmar Learning.

Little, C. (2003). Ethical dimensions of patient care. In P. Kelly-Heidenthal (Ed.), *Nursing leadership and management* (pp. 266-279). Clifton Park, NY: Thomson Delmar Learning.

New Jersey Sharing Network. (2007a). Retrieved August 2, 2007, from http://www.sharenj.org/.

New Jersey Sharing Network. (2007b). Retrieved August 2, 2007, from http://www.sharenj.org/fastfacts.htm.

Schroeder, S. (1995). Cost containment in US healthcare. *Academic Medicine, 70*, 861-866.

Stecher, J. (2008). Allow natural death vs. do not resuscitate. *American Journal of Nursing, 108*, 11.

The Joint Commission. (2007). *Comprehensive Accreditation Manual.* Oakbrook Terrace, IL: Author.

Tomey, A. M. (2004). *Guide to nursing management and leadership* (p. 75), 7th ed. St. Louis, MO: Mosby.

WEB SITES

http://nursingworld.org/; http://www.nursingworld.org
http://www.jointcommission.org/
http://www.optn.org/
http://www.organdonor.gov/
http://www.ncsbn.org

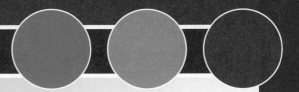

CHAPTER 9

Developing Management Skills

Objectives

1. Discuss the role of the manager.
2. Review the different management levels in nursing.
3. Identify differences between a nurse manager and a nurse executive.
4. Differentiate between the various types of competencies of client care managers.
5. Compare the nursing process and the management process.
6. Discuss activities used by the nurse manager to support the nursing and management processes.
7. Identify the day-to-day activities of the care manager.

Definitions

First-level manager Manager responsible for supervising nonmanagerial personnel and day-to-day activities of specific work units

Middle-level manager Manager who supervises first-level managers within a specified area and is responsible for the people and activities within those areas; generally acts as liaison between first-level and upper-level management

Upper-level manager Top level to whom middle manager reports; primarily responsible for establishing organizational goals and strategic plans for entire division of nursing

Management Process of coordinating actions and allocating resources to achieve organizational goals

LEADER VERSUS MANAGER

As you advance in your nursing proficiency, you will eventually take over some managerial tasks. You may even be asked to become a nurse manager. Just because you take on some managerial tasks does not necessarily make you a nurse manager rather than just a nurse performing some managerial tasks. Also, just because you are an excellent clinical nurse does not mean that you will become an excellent manager. In some organizations, the only promotion opportunities occur through progression to management. If you do not see yourself in such a role, it will be important for you to work in an organization that also has promotion opportunities for nurses who remain at the bedside. The competencies of a nurse manager need to be developed, and the process of manager development occurs through education, mentorship, and professional growth. As discussed in Chapter 1, management is not synonymous with leadership, although management is a part of leadership.

As stated in Chapter 1, *management* and *leadership* are different. To review (Bennis, 1994, p. 45):

- The manager administers; the leader innovates.
- The manager maintains; the leader develops.

- The manager focuses on systems and structure; the leader focuses on people.
- The manager relies on control; the leader inspires trust.
- The manager has a short-range view; the leader has a long-range perspective.
- The manager asks how and when; the leader asks what and why.
- The manager has his or her eye on the bottom line; the leader has his or her eye on the horizon.
- The manager imitates; the leader originates.
- The manager accepts the status quo; the leader challenges it.
- The manager is the classic good soldier; the leader is his or her own person.
- The manager does things right; the leader does the right thing.

Management is a complex process of coordinating and directing the actions of others to accomplish an organization's objectives. It also involves the assignment of resources to these groups so that the objectives can be met. It is achieved through six functions: planning, staffing, organizing, directing, controlling, and decision making (Carroll, 2006).

Planning determines what needs to be done. This may refer to what needs to be done for a single shift or for a longer period, such as the year. *Staffing* refers to the selection and assignment of specific people to accomplish the tasks (see Chapter 3 for discussion on delegation). Organizing is the process of coordinating all resources to meet the goals. *Organizing* is a fluid activity requiring knowledge of the organization and people and having the ability to alter the plan, staffing and organization if the goals are not being met. *Directing* deals with the skills necessary to motivate the staff to accomplish the assigned tasks. In this activity, you need to be able to provide the proper resources, set clear goals, and foster a work environment that encourages goal achievement. *Controlling* is accomplished through the setting of professional standards, compliance with standards of performance, and the ability to lead a staff to excellence. Last, *decision making* is the result of these five actions. According to Sullivan and Decker (2001), the key steps of decision making are (1) identification of the problem, (2) establishment of criteria that can evaluate potential solutions to the problem, (3) seeking alternative solutions, and (4) selection of the best alternative based on the organizational mission, vision, strategic objectives, and available resources.

COMPARING THE NURSING PROCESS WITH THE MANAGEMENT PROCESS

The nursing process focuses on assessing, analyzing, planning, implementing, and evaluating. The management process is used to meet client needs in an efficient and effective manner with available resources. The management process consists of five phases: identification of needs, identification of resources, planning, organizing and direction, and controlling.

LEVELS OF MANAGEMENT

There are levels of patient care management in most institutions. The organizational structure of the organization will determine the titles and the span of authority of the various levels of patient care management (Box 9-1).

FIRST LEVEL

The first-level manager, also known as a first-line manger, nurse manager, or head nurse, is responsible for supervising the work or nonmanagerial personnel and the day-to-day activities of a specific work unit or units (Box 9-2). This manager is responsible for the units on a 24-hours-a-day/7-days-a-week basis.

Key tasks for a first-line nurse manager may include the following (adapted from Carroll, 2006, p. 32):
- Preparation of orientation schedule in collaboration with nursing education department
- Submission of time schedules for nursing shifts

Box 9-1	THREE LEVELS OF MANAGEMENT ARE USED IN NURSING
First	Nurse manager
Middle	Director
Upper	Executive

From Sullivan, E. J., & Decker, P. J. (2005). *Effective leadership and management in nursing* (pp. 60-61). 6th ed. Upper Saddle River, NJ: Pearson/Prentice Hall.

Box 9-2   FIRST-LEVEL MANAGER RESPONSIBILITIES

- Clinical nursing practice
- Patient care delivery
- Use of human, fiscal, and other resources
- Personnel development
- Compliance with regulatory and professional standards
- Fostering interdisciplinary, collaborative relationships
- Strategic planning

From American Organization of Nurse Executives. (1992). The role and functions of the hospital nurse manager. In: *American Hospital Association advisory*. Chicago: American Hospital Association.

Box 9-3   MIDDLE-LEVEL MANAGER RESPONSIBILITIES

- People and activities within the departments they supervise
- Liaison between upper management and first-level manager

From American Organization of Nurse Executives (1992). The role and functions of the hospital nurse manager. In: *American Hospital Association advisory*. Chicago: American Hospital Association.

- Staff assignments for patient care during shifts
- Making budget recommendations to the middle and upper levels of management. These budget needs are made based on unit needs and patient acuity (see Chapter 14)
- Calculating the amount of staff needed per shift, per day, etc. This will also include the alteration of staffing plans based on emergencies, sick calls, and changes in patient acuity
- Making daily patient rounds
- Conducting staff meetings
- Conducting employment reviews, including counseling reports and termination
- Interviewing potential staff members (this is often done in conjunction with middle management)
- Participating in performance improvement activities; review of unit performance on CORE measures, National Patient Safety Goals, and other unit-based performance indicators
- Setting goals with individual staff and for patient care areas
- Maintaining current knowledge of the profession

MIDDLE LEVEL

The middle-level manager, also known as supervisor, director, or assistant or associate director of nursing, supervises a number of first-level managers. These managers usually are within the same specialty or the same geographic location. They may spend more time planning, evaluating, and coordinating and less time

with direct patient care supervision than the first-line manager (Box 9-3). They are responsible for the people and activities within the departments they supervise on a 24-hours-a-day/7-days-a-week basis.

Key tasks that the middle level manager may perform include the following (adapted from Carroll, 2006, p. 33):

- *Assessment:* Observe whether unit policies and objectives are meeting the needs of the patients and staff.
- *Planning:* Set short-term and long-term goals for patient care; revise as needed.
- *Organization:* Put plans in action via delegation and committee work.
- *Control:* Analyze results of action plans, make changes as necessary, facilitate the growth of staff, and communicate changes and opportunities to upper-level staff and to staff reporting to manager.

UPPER LEVEL

The upper-level manager, the executive-level manager, is also known as the senior vice president of patient care, vice president for nursing, chief nurse executive, or chief nursing officer (CNO). Middle management reports to the vice president for nursing. According to the American Organization of Nurse Executives (1990), "A nurse executive is a registered nurse who is part of the executive management team and as such is responsible for the management of the nursing organization and the clinical practice of nursing throughout the organization."

The CNO spends the least amount of time in direct supervision. Most of the time is spent planning and making policies. He or she is responsible for establishing organizational goals and strategic plans for the patient care department (Box 9-4).

Box 9-4 UPPER-LEVEL MANAGER RESPONSIBILITIES

- Establishing organizational goals
- Establishing strategic plans for nursing
- Integrating work units to achieve the organization's mission
- Buffering the effects of the external environment on nurses within the organization

From American Organization of Nurse Executives (1992). The role and functions of the hospital nurse manager. In: *American Hospital Association advisory*. Chicago: American Hospital Association.

Key tasks that the nursing executive officer may perform include the following (adapted from Carroll, 2006, p. 33):

- *Assessment:* Understand the organization's internal environment and culture and the external environment (regulatory, technology, community, legislation) in which it functions.
- *Planning:* Forecast trends in the profession, health care, costs, reimbursement, and regulations, and develop responsive strategic plans.
- *Organization:* Based on assessment and strategic planning, bring together the appropriate mix of resources, staff, and evidence-based knowledge to assist in the meeting of strategic goals.
- *Control:* Evaluate nursing policies, programs, services, and performance to ensure that they are consistent with the organization's mission and strategic goals and the profession's standards.

Other managerial roles have evolved over the past few years. To assist the nurse manager or head nurse, the role of charge nurse (resource nurse or patient care manager) has been developed. This expanded staff nurse role grants a staff nurse managerial responsibility on a given shift. This role may be a permanent position or a rotating one. The care manager functions as a liaison between the nurse manager and the activities and staff of the off-shifts.

Key tasks that the care manager may perform include the following (adapted from Carroll, 2006, p. 33):

- Assist in shift coordination.
- Create patient assignments for the shift.
- Deal with personnel issues arising during shift (e.g., sick calls, real-time conflict management).
- Make patient care rounds during shift.

- Trouble-shoot problems that occur during shift.
- Assist staff members with making decisions and prioritizing care.
- Use resources efficiently.
- Perform staff evaluations (this will depend on the organization).
- Serve as liaison between staff of off-shift and first-line management.

COMPETENCIES OF CLIENT CARE MANAGERS

Client care managers use organizational resources and routines while providing direct client care. Use time productively; collaborate with the interdisciplinary work group. And use leadership characteristics to manage others within the nursing work group. More specifically, to manage client care, entry-level nurses perform the following tasks (Wywialowski, 2004, pp. 4-5):

- Identify organizational resources and determine when they are needed.
- Work within various nursing service delivery patterns.
- Use position descriptions to establish the scope and limitations of their own and other nursing work group member practices.
- Manage time purposefully and productively.
- Prioritize client needs and related care.
- Exhibit flexibility in providing care within available time constraints.
- Show initiative, flexibility, and creativity as leadership qualities.
- Think critically to make decisions required to solve client care problems.
- Defend your decisions.
- Collaborate with other health team members.
- Resolve conflicts within the work group.
- Delegate appropriately.

The role of the care manager differs from that of the first-line manager in that the charge nurse or care manager has more limited authority and a limited span of control. The charge nurse may or may not perform staff evaluations; this will depend on the organization. The charge nurse may have more knowledge of staff performance, especially if the position deals with the off-shifts. The typical workday of a care manager or charge nurse is presented in Box 9-5.

Box 9-5   TYPICAL CLIENT CARE MANAGEMENT ROUTINES

7:00–7:30 A.M.: Receive change-of-shift report.

7:30–8:00 A.M.: Complete preliminary assessment of assigned client needs; complete assigning client care to coworkers; administer scheduled drugs and treatments before meals or with meals.

8:00–9:30 A.M.: Administer drugs to be given after meals and per agency schedules; complete detailed assessments of acutely ill clients and provide comfort and personal hygiene measures; note changes in medical plans and other interdisciplinary diagnostic or treatment programs.

9:30–10:00 A.M.: Administer scheduled drugs and detailed assessment of stable clients; provide comfort and personal hygiene measures; implement exercise treatments.

10:00–11:30 A.M.: Obtain feedback from coworkers regarding progress and special needs; provide assistance to coworkers, and plan to receive

assistance from others for complex procedures; administer drugs before meals; involve clients in routine health education programs.

11:30 A.M.–1:00 P.M.: Take lunch break and cover for coworkers while they are on break; monitor unstable clients; assist clients with meals; administer scheduled drugs and those to be given with meals.

1:00-2:00 P.M.: Monitor client progress; provide comfort measures; promote client rest periods; administer drugs to be taken after meals and as scheduled.

2:00–2:45 P.M.: Monitor unstable clients; seek feedback from coworkers; complete care plan revisions and documentation not completed earlier; organize data for change-of-shift report; involve clients in health education programs.

2:45–3:30 P.M.: Give change-of-shift report.

From Wywialowski E: *Managing client care.* St. Louis, MO: Mosby, 2004.

SUMMARY

The role of the manager is very different from that of the nurse. While nurses need to have strong management skills to deliver patient care, there are additional skills and tasks that are needed to be a nurse manager at any level. Not every nurse will want to be a nurse manager, even through they manage patient care on a

daily basis. As a new nurse moves into a managerial role, it is important to realize that a different set of skills and knowledge is required to advance in this role. The Association of Nurse Executives has many resources for these roles, and the American Nurse Credentialing Center manages the certification examinations for nurses working in nursing administration.

CLINICAL CORNER

Mentoring for Leadership and Management
Edna Cadmus

The health care environment requires leaders in all roles to master the key principles of leadership. Managing tasks alone is not leadership. Leadership requires (1) inspiring a shared vision, (2) challenging the process, (3) enabling others to act, (4) encouraging the heart, and (5) leadership for everyone (Kouzes and Posner, 2002). Kouzes and Posner identify that "It's about the practices leaders use to transform values into actions, visions into realities, obstacles into innovations, separateness into solidarity, and risks into rewards."

In addition, the leader needs to be able to operate under evidence-based management tenets identified in the Institute of Medicine (2004) report on work environment. These five tenets are (1) balancing efficiency and patient safety, (2) promoting trust, (3) creating and managing change, (4) implementing shared decision-making around work design and flow, and (5) establishing a learning environment.

The chief nursing officer (CNO) of the organization has a prime responsibility to ensure that opportunities for education as well as coaching are available to leaders at all levels and roles in the organization. She or he must ensure that leaders are challenged to continue to

Continued

CLINICAL CORNER—cont'd

grow in a learning environment. The CNO needs to ensure that there is a shared and clear vision so that managers and staff can translate this vision into action.

Coaching leaders require a clear understanding of what level they are at, from novice to expert, and what generational characteristics direct their leadership and learning style. For example, are they Baby Boomers or Generation X-ers? This makes a difference in how they learn and want to be coached. Manion (1998) describes the process of coaching as a process of setting mutual goals, addressing needs, identifying performance and motivational factors of the individual, defining expectations, teaching and educating, observing, and providing feedback.

One way to begin this process is through the use of a 360-degree feedback tool such as the Leadership Practice Inventory tool. This helps the leader in understanding his or her strengths in leadership and where he or she may want to develop a plan with a coach to help enhance leadership abilities. Feedback should be solicited from peers inside and outside the department—those who report to the individual as well as those with whom he or she reports. Determining who would provide the most thoughtful feedback is an important step. Once feedback is received, it should be looked at by the coach and the leader as a roadmap to help strengthen skill sets. Keeping it separate from an evaluation process is important as it is less threatening to the leader. Also, the coach selected by the leader

should be someone who has limited, if any, supervision of the person.

Setting mutual and clear expectations and providing learning opportunities for the leader in areas where he or she needs development are important in goal setting. Providing timely and direct feedback cannot be overlooked.

The data from the 360-degree tool can also be aggregated for the CNO to help understand the departmental needs overall. Often, similar needs exist and can be provided through formal education or workshops. The Nursing Advisory Board is one way of providing opportunities for nurse leader development; examples include such topics as accountability, conflict resolution, creating innovation, and change.

While on-the-job opportunities and education can be provided, formal education needs to be in the equation. First-line leaders today require a skill set that is complex and well rounded. Formal education at a master's level needs to become the minimal preparation. This route provides a safe haven for learning skills that can be applied to the work setting.

References
Institute of Medicine. (2004). *Keeping patients safe*. Washington, DC: National Academies Press.
Kouzes, J., & Posner, B. (2002). *The leadership challenge*. 3rd ed. San Francisco: Jossey-Bass.
Manion, J. (1998). *From management to leadership*. Chicago: American Hospital Publishers.

EVIDENCE-BASED PRACTICE

Why Do Nurse Managers Stay? Building a Model of Engagement

Mackoff, B., & Klauer Triolo, P. (2008). Why do nurse managers stay? Building a model of engagement. Journal of Nursing Administration, 38(3), 118-124.

The short tenure of nurse managers suggest an urgent need for a new model to understand and build engagement that translates into longevity and excellence in nurse managers. Given the current and projected shortage of nurses, the short tenure of nurse managers is of prime concern. To gain a fresh perspective about this problem, the researchers of this study sought to build an actionable model of nurse manager engagement by studying 30 outstanding long-term nurse managers in six settings.

The study revealed rich data linking individual signature behaviors to nurse manager vitality and longevity. The analysis identified 10 individual signature behaviors that revealed the experiences, capabilities, and attributes of long-term individual managers.

Mission-Driven: Characterized as motivated and driven to action by a sense of meaningful mission and context, the ability to be oriented toward a purpose; the bigger picture can be seen as it relates to the day-to-day operational issues without losing sight of the values at the bedside.

Generativity: The ability to find pleasure and satisfaction in caring for and contributing to the next generation.

Ardor: Ardor is defined as warmth, animation, and excitement. This element of ardor was noted in the

EVIDENCE-BASED PRACTICE—cont'd

excitement about staff, colleagues, and leadership; dedication to patient care; and commitment to the organization.

Identification: The comments of these nurse managers suggest that achievement by identifying with the work of others is a crucible in the engagement of a nurse manager, whose former bedside patient care has been replaced with managerial tasks and goals.

Boundary Clarity: This is defined as the capacity to build strong connections with others without losing the sense of self. These managers cultivated strong, internal boundaries and created emotional insulation, restoring boundaries through disengagement and modeling and displaying appropriate boundaries.

Reflection: The ability to leverage lessons from experience, observe themselves and note the effect of their behavior on others, and scan for cues about self and others in workplace situations.

Attunement: Regard of the individual and appreciation of each person's contribution to the organization the capacity to understand diverse perspectives and to set aside assumptions to hear the whole story.

Self-Regulation: Using restraint to keep emotions in check, suspend judgment, and conserve energy.

Change Agility: Challenging the process, welcoming and initiating change, and seeking change through new learning.

Affirmative Framework: Using an optimistic explanatory style; generates positive expectations and models resilient behavior.

The researchers of this study believe that organizations can address the current leadership vacuum and minimize the nursing shortage by building on a model of engagement. We will see increased tenure of new and experienced nurses by investing in nurse managers as the key drivers of health workplace cultures.

NCLEX® EXAM QUESTIONS

1. The nurse manager on the labor and delivery unit evaluates that one of the staff nurses has leadership qualities. Which of the following is a basis for this judgment?
   1. The nurse works overtime every week.
   2. The nurse stays long after her shift is over to chart.
   3. The nurse uses a monthly forum to review current knowledge content.
   4. The nurse uses a negative approach when evaluating staff skills.

2. As a nurse, you are aware that one element that is the same when comparing the nursing process and the management process is:
   1. identification of needs
   2. identification of resources
   3. planning
   4. control

3. One main difference between an ideal leader and an organization-focused manager is that an:
   1. ideal leader maintains the status quo
   2. organization-focused manager is creative

   3. ideal leader is a risk-taker
   4. organization-focused manager is a visionary

4. Which of the following is NOT the middle-level manager's responsibility?
   1. People within the departments they supervise
   2. Liaison between upper management and first-level manager
   3. Establishment of organizational goals
   4. Activities within the departments they supervise

5. The middle-level manager:
   1. makes hospital-wide decisions
   2. supervises a number of upper-level managers
   3. is responsible for the people and activities on a 24-hours-a-day/7-days-a-week basis
   4. is responsible for his or her specific shift only

6. You are mentoring a new nurse. You know that which of the following is NOT a mentor's responsibility?
   1. Discuss means to correct chronic tardiness.
   2. Offer criticism on nursing skills.
   3. Perform a nurse's probation period review.
   4. Evaluate the nurse's exact break and lunch times.

Continued

NCLEX® EXAM QUESTIONS—cont'd

7. The four skill sets needed by good leaders are:
   1. self-awareness, self-management, social awareness, and relationship management
   2. self-awareness, self-management, social control, and relationship management
   3. self-awareness, self-control, social awareness, and relationship management
   4. self-awareness, self-management, social awareness, and relationship performance

8. Ruiz (1997) defines the "four agreements" that leaders must make with themselves. They are as follows:
   1. Be impeccable with your word, take nothing personally, make no assumptions, and always do your best, no more and no less.
   2. Be impeccable with your actions, take nothing personally, make no assumptions, and always do your best, no more and no less.
   3. Be impeccable with your word, take nothing personally, make assumptions, and always do your best, no more and no less.
   4. Be impeccable with your word, take nothing personally, make no assumptions, and be appreciative of your staff.

9. Leader competencies are a necessary aspect of a leader's role. As a leader, you are aware that the following is needed for this role:
   1. a clear vision and owned purpose
   2. a pessimistic attitude with colleagues
   3. a negative approach with families
   4. a membership with more than three committees

10. The vice president of nursing is responsible for:
   1. establishing organizational goals and strategic plans for nursing
   2. developing and maintaining daily assignments
   3. prioritizing events during disaster plan implementation
   4. overseeing the mission and vision of the organization

Answers: 1. 3   2. 3   3. 3   4. 3   5. 3   6. 1   7. 1   8. 1   9. 1   10. 1

REFERENCES

American Organization of Nurse Executives. (1990). The role and functions of the hospital nurse manager. In: *American Hospital Association advisory*. Chicago: American Hospital Association.

American Organization of Nurse Executives. (1992). The role and functions of the hospital nurse manager. In: *American Hospital Association advisory*. Chicago: American Hospital Association.

Bennis, W. (1994). *On becoming a leader*. New York: Addison-Wesley.

Carroll, P. (2006). *Nursing Leadership and Management: A Practical Guide*. Clifton Park, NY: Thomson Delmar Learning.

Ruiz, D. M. (1997). *The four agreements: a practical guide to personal freedom (a Toltec wisdom book)*. San Rafael, CA: Amber-Allen.

Sullivan, E., & Decker, P. (2001). *Effective leadership and management in nursing*, 5th ed. Upper Saddle River, NJ: Prentice Hall.

Wywialowski, E. F. (2004). *Managing client care*. 3rd ed. St. Louis: Mosby.

Information Management

Computers have made a dramatic impact on the health care environment in the past ten years. The use of computerized record systems and computerized order entry systems has been linked to improvements in patient safety and increases in hospital efficiency. These systems have also increased the potential access to information and data, making our work environments rich in information. How we react to this information is important, and the use of this information in driving improvement is a key function of organizations that are continually learning and moving toward "best practice."

This section deals with improving organizational performance, information systems, and the use of data for improvement.

CHAPTER 10

Improving Organizational Performance

Chapter Objectives

1. Identify the key focus of performance improvement.
2. Discuss trends in quality improvement.
3. List three drivers of quality.
4. Outline two models of performance improvement.
5. Identify three clinical outcome measures.
6. Identify major patient safety goals.
7. Describe four nursing outcomes specific to desired specialty.
8. Relate a clinical activity to a performance model.

Definitions

Sentinel event Unexpected occurrence involving death or serious physical or psychological injury

Risk management Organized program to prevent the incidence of preventable accidents, injuries, and errors

National Patient Safety Goals Set of nationwide goals set by The Joint Commission, to focus performance in areas of patient safety

Six Sigma Performance improvement model based on the idea of minimal defects and concerns

Root cause analysis Retrospective review of the event, to evaluate potential causes of the problem or sources of variation in the process

Lean management Performance improvement model dealing with minimization of waste in processes

Outcome Measurable result related to a strategic objective

Retrospective review Analysis of past events, usually through a chart audit

IMPROVING ORGANIZATIONAL PERFORMANCE

The year 1998 was a pivotal year in the quest for improvement in health care. In that year, the Institute of Medicine issued a report, *To Err Is Human: Building a Safer Health System*, detailing the problem of medical errors in health care. The Advisory Commission on Consumer Protection and Quality also released a report calling for a national commitment to improve quality, concluding that "there is no guarantee that any individual will receive high quality care for any particular health problem … the health care industry is plagued … with errors in health care" (Advisory Commission on Consumer Protection and Quality, 1998). It was found that these quality concerns occur typically because of ways in which care is organized. Health care organizations were challenged to ensure that services were safe, effective, patient centered, timely, efficient, and equitable.

Performance improvement (PI) has been shown to be a powerful tool to help health care organizations become safer and more efficient and patient centered. Total quality management (TQM), which is also referred to as PI or quality improvement (QI), had been used in industry since the 1950s and had been related to improvements in productivity and quality.

HISTORICAL PERSPECTIVES

In the 1950s, the Joint Commission on Accreditation of Healthcare Organizations was formed and the evaluation of care delivered in health care institutions began. During the 1960s, the American Nurses Association began to develop standards of nursing practice, which become the basis for early quality assurance (QA) programs. In the 1970s, the U.S. Congress established Professional Standards Review Organizations (PSROs) to review the quality and cost of care delivered to Medicare and Medicaid recipients. QA required audits of care. These audits measured basic compliance, emphasizing what was done "wrong," but did little to advance a philosophy of learning from performance.

Health care costs became a major issue in the 1980s, and society began to question the efficiency and effectiveness of health care (Phelps, 1997). Health care administrators turned to industry for lessons learned in managing efficiency. Industry had adopted quality management techniques in the 1950s. An early proponent was W. Edwards Deming, who worked with the Japanese automotive industry after World War II. His 14-point management philosophy is the underpinning of TQM. The 14 points follow:

1. Create constancy of purpose toward improvement of product and service, with the aim to become competitive and to stay in business, and to provide jobs.
2. Adopt the new philosophy. We are in a new economic age. Western management must awaken to the challenge, must learn their responsibilities, and take on leadership for change.
3. Cease dependence on inspection to achieve quality. Eliminate the need for inspection on a mass basis by building quality into the product in the first place.
4. End the practice of awarding business on the basis of price tag. Instead, minimize total cost.

Move towards a single supplier for any one item, on a long-term relationship of loyalty and trust.
5. Improve constantly and forever the system of production and service, to improve quality and productivity, and thus constantly decrease costs.
6. Institute training on the job.
7. Institute leadership. The aim of supervision should be to help people and machines and gadgets to do a better job. Supervision of management is in need of an overhaul, as well as supervision of production workers.
8. Drive out fear, so that everyone may work effectively for the company.
9. Break down barriers between departments. People in research, design, sales, and production must work as a team, to foresee problems of production and in use that may be encountered with the product or service.
10. Eliminate slogans, exhortations, and targets for the workforce asking for zero defects and new levels of productivity. Such exhortations only create adversarial relationships, as the bulk of the causes of low quality and low productivity belong to the system and thus lie beyond the power of the work force.
11. a. Eliminate work standards (quotas) on the factory floor. Substitute leadership.
    b. Eliminate management by objective. Eliminate management by numbers, numerical goals. Substitute leadership.
12. a. Remove barriers that rob the hourly paid worker of his right to pride in workmanship. The responsibility of supervisors must be changed from sheer numbers to quality.
    b. Remove barriers that rob people in management and engineering of their right to pride in workmanship. This means, abolishment of the annual or merit rating and management by objective.
13. Institute a vigorous program of education and self-improvement.
14. Put everybody in the company to work to accomplish the transformation. The transformation is everybody's job (Deming, 2000a, pp. 23-24).

Deming believed that an industry consists of multiple processes and decisions, which are interrelated, and developed a "system of profound knowledge" (Deming, 2000b):

- All work consists of multiple processes
- Differences in work are the result of the system of work, not individual worker performance
- New work designs are based on our understanding of how work processes relate to one another
- An understanding of what motivates people

His model for improvement was the PDCA (Plan–Do–Check–Act) cycle, which remains in widespread use today. Juran (1989) elaborated on Deming's work in TQM. He believed that quality "did not happen by accident" but was the result of a quality trilogy—planning, control, and improvement. In 1960, Crosby defined *quality* as the extent to which processes were in conformance with the requirements of the customer. He was known for believing that things should be done "right the first time" and for the philosophy of "zero defects" (Nielson et al., 2004). While these three proponents of quality improvement focused on work processes, Donabedian (1992) contributed the idea of *outcome* as part of the overall quality structure. Outcomes involve the results achieved, and they reflect the effectiveness of the process components. This outcomes focus allows institutions to measure themselves against the standards and the competition. A compendium of past and present quality terms is presented in Table 10-1.

KEY FOCUS OF PERFORMANCE IMPROVEMENT

This focus on outcomes has moved health care from a compliance model toward one of "best practice." While accrediting bodies and federal regulators set minimum standards of compliance, many hospitals are now moving toward a model of "best in class." Examples of organizations that recognize such "best practice" are American Nurses Association and its Magnet Award for Nursing and the Malcolm Baldrige National Quality Award for performance excellence. Hospitals winning the Magnet Award can be accessed at http://www.nursingworld.org/ancc/magnet/index.html. The hospitals that have been recognized by receiving the Malcolm Baldrige National Quality Award can be accessed at http://baldrige.nist.gov/Contacts_Profiles.htm.

The key focus of PI includes

- Meeting and exceeding the needs of the customer
- Building organizational learning into each work process
- Continually evaluating and improving work processes
- Assessing all customer requirements
- Constantly striving to "do it better"

It is vital to remember that all PI must be "data driven" and not based on anecdote.

DRIVERS OF QUALITY

The key focus of the quality movement is the meeting of the needs of the customer. In organizations striving for "best practice," this may mean exceeding the needs of the customer.

Obviously, the key customers of health care are the patient and family; they are at the center of all drivers of quality. Other customers of the hospital include the physicians and the community. Bronson Methodist Hospital in Kalamazoo, Michigan, has defined the patient (and family) and the community as key customers, with key requirements and market segments as given in Table 10-2.

What is important is that each set of customers has specific requirements that need to be met by the health care organization. The degree to which these key requirements are met forms a base for the patient satisfaction measures of the institution. Other customers include regulators, partners, and payers.

Quality outcomes also are a key requirement of the patient and the community. How do hospitals measure quality outcomes? There are a variety of means.

Table 10-1   PAST, PRESENT, AND EVOLVING QUALITY TERMS

Past Quality Terms	Present Quality Terms	Evolving Quality Terms
Quality control	Total quality management	Quality management
Quality assurance	Continuous quality improvement	Quality improvement
		Performance improvement
		Performance excellence

Adapted from Yoder-Wise, P. (2003). *Leading and managing in nursing* (p. 175). St. Louis: MO: Mosby.

Table 10-2   KEY CUSTOMER AND STAKEHOLDER GROUPS, REQUIREMENTS, AND MARKET SEGMENTS

Group	Requirements	Market Segment
Customer group: Patients (including families)	Quality outcomes Communication Empathy Responsiveness Efficiency	Inpatients and outpatients Geographic location (service area) Service lines Age demographics
Stakeholder group: Community	Leadership and support Access to healthcare services Health information Quality outcomes	Type of organization Geographic location

From Bronson Methodist Hospital. (2007). Baldrige application. Retrieved March 11, 2007, from http://baldrige.nist.gov/PDF_files/Bronson_Methodist_Hospital_Application_Summary.pdf.

OUTCOME MEASURES

The key to PI is the "result" of all actions taken to improve patient care. While it is important to "do what we say we do," it is more important to "do it well." So, just how well do we deliver patient care?

Patient care units have an abundance of data available to them. One common outcome used by patient care units is *patient satisfaction*. A majority of health care organizations across the United States measure patient satisfaction. Two of the common vendor satisfaction measures are Press Ganey and Gallup. These data can be segmented to list the performance of specific units/shifts. The key requirements of the patient/family at Bronson Methodist Hospital are listed in Box 10-2. They were identified as: communication, empathy, responsiveness, and efficiency.

Patient satisfaction surveys are customized to include information on the key requirements of the patients of an institution. With the use of nationwide surveys, hospitals can compare their performance with that of other local hospitals, of similar hospitals, and of best-in-class performers. See Figure 10-1 provides an example of a patient satisfaction data set.

Other data sets available to the nurse include the National Database of Nursing Quality Indicators® (NDNQI®), a program of the American Nurses Association National Center for Nursing Quality. The database collects and evaluates unit-specific nurse-sensitive data from hospitals in the United States and internationally. Participating facilities receive unit-level comparative data reports to use for QI purposes. Nursing-sensitive indicators reflect the structure,

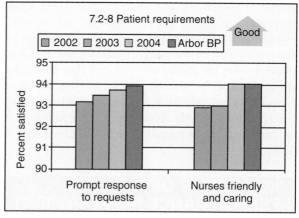

Figure 10-1 • Bronson Methodist Hospital. (2007). Baldrige application. Retrieved March 11, 2007, from http://baldrige.nist.gov/PDF_files/Bronson_Methodist_Hospital_Application_Summary.pdf.

Example of a patient satisfaction data set. This graph shows that in 2002, 93.3% of patients thought that nurses promptly responded to their needs, and that in 2004, this increased to 94%. The local best practice was 94. Arbor BP, Arbor Best Practice.

process, and outcomes of nursing care (Box 10-1) (National Center for Nursing Quality, 2007).

Nurses will need to know the outcomes that directly affect their unit. Common outcomes for all units are infection rates, patient satisfaction, and performance on The Joint Commission (TJC)'s Core Measures. The Core Measures are specific to the unit, so it is important for you to know which measure or indicator reflects your unit and your level of performance. The initial

Box 10-1 MENU OF INDICATORS CURRENTLY BEING COLLECTED

- Patient falls NQF
- Patient falls with injury NQF
  - Injury level
- Pressure ulcer rate
- Hospital-acquired pressure ulcer rate
- RN satisfaction
- Nursing hours per patient day NQF
  - Registered nurses (RN) hours per patient day
  - Licensed practical/vocational nurses (LPN/LVN) hours per patient day
  - Unlicensed assistive (UAP) hours per patient day
- Staff mix NQF
  - RN
  - LPN/LVNs
  - UAP
  - Percent agency staff
- RN education/certification
- Pediatric pain assessment, intervention, reassessment (AIR) cycle
- Pediatric peripheral intravenous infiltration
- Psychiatric physical/sexual assault

CORE measures include Heart Failure, Acute Myocardial Infarction, Pneumonia, Surgical Infection, and Pregnancy. Others measures are Pain Management and Children's Asthma Care. Participating hospitals collect data related to their performance on the specific measures, and these measures are then reported to TJC. This data set allows for nationwide comparison on performance. TJC's Core Measures are available at http://www.jointcommission.org/PerformanceMeasurement/PerformanceMeasurement/default.htm.

There is also a wide variety of other outcomes that are used by hospitals, and they include financial measures (e.g., cash on hand, market share, and length of stay), human resource measures (e.g., employee satisfaction and productivity), and ethical measures (e.g., community service and financial audits). Hospitals determine the outcomes to be used as part of the strategic planning process. Reporting of the identified outcomes often occurs via a scorecard, which gives a visual representation of current performance on the key outcomes (Figure 10-2).

The first rule of PI is that it must be data driven; therefore, based on information derived from some of the various data sets available to the institution, a "concern" or a variance in process will be identified. In reaction to this "concern," a PI project will be initiated. These projects usually follow one of the following models.

A second rule of PI is that PI activities should be based on what is important to the customers. Your energies should be concentrated on what is important to them.

MODELS OF QUALITY

FOCUS Method

F—Focus on an opportunity for improvement.
O—Organize a team involved with the process.
C—Clarify the current process.
U—Understand the causes of variation in the process.
S—Based on evidence, Select the improvement.

Plan–Do–Study–Act (PDSA) Cycle

This model is based on Deming's PDCA model that was discussed earlier.
Plan—Plan a change, with activity aimed at improvement.
Do—Carry it out.
Check/Study—Study the results: what happened? What did you learn? Did the change work?
Act—Adopt the change; rework the change.
Many organizations combine these models into a PDCA-FOCUS model (Figure 10-3).

As organizations have matured in the PI journey, a new process, Six Sigma, is being used in conjunction with PDSA. The objective of Six Sigma quality is to reduce process variation to no more 3.4 "defects" per 1 million. DMAIC is the acronym. It is a data-driven quality strategy for improving processes (Box 10-2).

EVIDENCE-BASED PRACTICE

This model describes the integration of research evidence with clinical experience to improve outcomes. The process for evidence-based practice includes (Sackett, Straus, Richardson, Rosenberg, and Hayes, 2000) the following:

- Formulation of a question from current clinical concerns

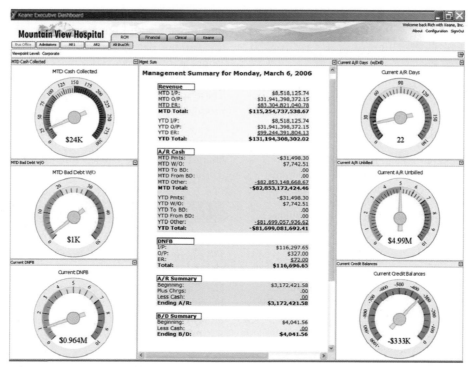

Figure 10-2 • Scorecard. Clinical Dashboard Metrics. Retrieved September 8, 2008 from http://www.dashboardzone.com/hospital-dashboard-clinical-dashboard-metrics.

Box 10-2   SIX SIGMA: DMAIC

Define the customer, their critical to quality (CTQ) issues, and the core business process involved.
- Define who customers are, what their requirements are for products and services, and what their expectations are.
- Define project boundaries the stop and start of the process.
- Define the process to be improved by mapping the process flow.

Measure the performance of the core business process involved.
- Develop a data collection plan for the process.
- Collect data from many sources to determine types of defects and metrics.
- Compare to customer survey results to determine shortfall.

Analyze the data collected and process map to determine root causes of defects and opportunities for improvement.

- Identify gaps between current performance and goal performance.
- Prioritize opportunities to improve.
- Identify sources of variation.

Improve the target process by designing creative solutions to fix and prevent problems.
- Create innovate solutions using technology and discipline.
- Develop and deploy implementation plan.

Control the improvements to keep the process on the new course.
- Prevent reverting back to the "old way."
- Require the development, documentation and implementation of an ongoing monitoring plan.
- Institutionalize the improvements through the modification of systems and structures (staffing, training, incentives).

Six Sigma is a registered trademark and service mark of Motorola, Inc.

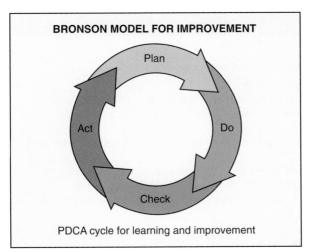

BRONSON MODEL FOR IMPROVEMENT

Plan

Act

Do

Check

PDCA cycle for learning and improvement

Figure 10-3 • PDCA model. Bronson Methodist Hospital. (2007). Baldrige application. Retrieved March 11, 2007, from http://baldrige.nist.gov/PDF_files/Bronson_Methodist_Hospital_Application_Summary.pdf.

- Access of relevant research
- Analysis of the evidence using established criteria
- Plan change in practice
- Implement change in practice
- Evaluate results

As a nurse, you will be asked to participate in process improvement teams. These teams are usually formed in reaction to a "concern" or variance in a process. These teams are usually interdisciplinary in nature and form the "O" of the PDCA-FOCUS model. You will receive team-based education as you join the team. Also, you will receive "just in time" training on the multiple data collection methods used by improvement teams. These include pareto analysis, surveys, audits, cost-benefit analysis, decision matrix, and fishbone diagram. Some teams will have a certified Six Sigma member who is responsible for data interpretation. As you mature in mature improvement, you will receive education specific to the institution's model.

LEAN CULTURE

The underlying principle of "lean" is that all processes contain waste. Womack and Jones (2003) define *lean* as a "way to do more and more with less and less—less human effort, less equipment, less time, and less space—while coming closer to providing customers with what they want" (p. 15).

One of the challenges of implementing lean in health care is that it requires people to identify waste in the work in which they are so invested. All workers want to feel their work is valuable, perhaps most especially health care workers. Recognizing that much about their daily tasks is wasteful and does not add value can be difficult for health care professionals. A nurse who is hunting for supplies is doing it to serve the needs of patients. Nurses may not see this as wasted time, and may not stop to wonder why those supplies aren't where they need them every time they need them. But if the supplies were always readily available, the time nurses spend hunting for them would instead be devoted to something more appropriate to their skills and expertise (Miller, 2005, p. 8).

RISK MANAGEMENT

Risk management can be defined as an organized program to prevent the incidence of preventable accidents, injuries, and errors (Kavaler and Spiegel, 2003). These errors, accidents, and injuries incur unintended cost to the institution, and the risk management department is charged with defining the situations that place the health care institution at risk.

The National Patient Safety Goals further emphasize the importance of the risk management function (Box 10-3). These goals were formed based on the Institute of Medicine 1998 report. This is a nationwide initiative with an overall goal of making specific improvements in patient safety of hospitals across the nation. The goals highlight problem areas and focus on systemwide solutions.

Many health care institutions have integrated the risk management and PI activities. This relates to the process management nature of the risk management function. For example, Goal 2E ("Implement a standardized approach to "hand off" communications, including an opportunity to ask and respond to questions") integrates activities of both a risk management department and PI. Lessons are being learned from the aviation and race car industries in the area of hand-offs, and processes are being designed to further enhance patient safety and reduce adverse events. The risk management department also investigates all identified accidents, injuries, errors, and adverse events. TJC requires all health care institutions to report sentinel events. A *sentinel event* is:

Box 10-3 NATIONAL PATIENT SAFETY GOALS (2008)

Goal 1	Improve the accuracy of patient identification.
1A	Use at least two patient identifiers when providing care, treatment or services.
Goal 2	Improve the effectiveness of communication among caregivers.
2A	For verbal or telephone orders or for telephonic reporting of critical test results, verify the complete order or test result by having the person receiving the information record and "read-back" the complete order or test result.
2B	Standardize a list of abbreviations, acronyms, symbols, and dose designations that are not to be used throughout the organization.
2C	Measure and assess, and if appropriate, take action to improve the timeliness of reporting, and the timeliness of receipt by the responsible licensed caregiver, of critical test results and values.
2E	Implement a standardized approach to "hand off" communications, including an opportunity to ask and respond to questions.
Goal 3	Improve the safety of using medications.
3C	Identify and, at a minimum, annually review a list of look-alike/sound-alike drugs used by the organization, and take action to prevent errors involving the interchange of these drugs.
3D	Label all medications, medication containers (for example, syringes, medicine cups, basins), or other solutions on and off the sterile field.
3E	Reduce the likelihood of patient harm associated with the use of anticoagulation therapy.
Goal 7	Reduce the risk of health care–associated infections.
7A	Comply with current World Health Organization (WHO) Hand Hygiene Guidelines or Centers for Disease Control (CDC) hand hygiene guidelines.
7B	Manage as sentinel events all identified cases of unanticipated death or major permanent loss of function associated with a health care–associated infection.
Goal 8	Accurately and completely reconcile medications across the continuum of care.
8A	There is a process for comparing the patient's current medications with those ordered for the patient while under the care of the organization.
8B	A complete list of the patient's medications is communicated to the next provider of service when a patient is referred or transferred to another setting, service, practitioner or level of care within or outside the organization. The complete list of medications is also provided to the patient on discharge from the facility.
Goal 9	Reduce the risk of patient harm resulting from falls.
9B	Implement a fall reduction program including an evaluation of the effectiveness of the program.
Goal 13	Encourage patients' active involvement in their own care as a patient safety strategy.
13A	Define and communicate the means for patients and their families to report concerns about safety and encourage them to do so.
Goal 15	The organization defines safety risks inherent in its patient population.
15A	The organization identifies patients at risk for suicide. [Applicable to psychiatric hospitals and patients being treated for emotional or behavioral disorders in general hospitals—NOT APPLICABLE TO CRITICAL ACCESS HOSPITALS]
Goal 16	Improve recognition and response to changes in a patient's condition.
16A	The organization selects a suitable method that enables health care staff members to directly request additional assistance from a specially trained individual(s) when the patient's condition appears to be worsening. [Critical Access Hospital, Hospital]

From The Joint Commission. Retrieved July 2, 2009, from http://www.jointcommission.org/PatientSafety/NationalPatientSafetyGoals/07_hap_npsgs.htm. Goals for other types of health care organizations may be accessed at http://www.jointcommission.org/PatientSafety/NationalPatientSafetyGoals/.

- An unexpected occurrence involving death or serious physical or psychological injury, or the risk thereof. Serious injury specifically includes loss of limb or function. The phrase "or the risk thereof" includes any process variation for which a recurrence would carry a significant chance of a serious adverse outcome.
- Such events are called "sentinel" because they signal the need for immediate investigation and response.
- The terms "sentinel event" and "medical error" are not synonymous; not all sentinel events occur because of an error and not all errors result in sentinel events.

When a sentinel event is identified, a root-cause analysis is performed by a team that includes those directly involved in the process. This root-cause analysis is a retrospective review of the event, to evaluate potential causes of the problem or sources of variation in the process. In a root-cause analysis of the "hand-off" procedure in the discussion of handoffs (Box 10-4), it was found that there was no systemized process for the hand-off and that multiple failures of communication occurred due to this lack of process. This process was then changed and evaluated, and the outcomes were positive.

The major outcome of PI is the creation of a learning organization (Baldrige, 2007, p. 2). This means that learning

- Is a regular part of daily work
- Is practiced at personal, unit and organizational levels
- Results in solving problems at their source ("root cause")
- Is focused on building and sharing knowledge throughout the organization
- Is driven by opportunities to effect significant, meaningful change

This is the outcome of institution-wide PI.

SUMMARY

It is important for nurses and organization administrators to continually learn from their performance. Health care organizations have a long history of collecting information on performance, but in the past 10 years, the emphasis on performance has changed as the health care environment has become more competitive. TJC requires organizations to collect information on the Core Measures and to determine how the individual hospital is performing. It is important for the nurse to know the levels of performance based on actual data. These results may be shown is dashboard form to allow the reader to make a quick determination of performance to target based on color. The use of data for PI is one means of continually learning about one's performance and making improvements based on reviews of performance. As a new nurse, it will be important to realize that, as nurses in clinical practice, the review of data provides the opportunity to improve our practice to better meet the needs of the patient.

Box 10-4   PATIENT HAND-OFFS

Patient hand-offs occur thousands of times a day in hospitals. Patients are transferred from unit to unit, brought to surgery, from surgery to postanesthetic care unit (PACU), from PACU, and transferred to a unit. Many hand-offs go off without a hitch, but devastating mistakes can happen during any of them.

"If you transfer a patient to the ICU after surgery and the ventilator isn't ready, you're really riding on the edge" of patient safety, says Allan Goldman, head of the pediatric intensive care unit at Great Ormond Street Hospital and a chief architect of the hospital's collaboration with Ferrari.

A 2005 study in *The Wall Street Journal* found that nearly 70% of all preventable hospital mishaps occurred because of communication problems, and that many of these breakdowns occur during patient hand-offs.

In 2003, the surgeons at London's Great Ormond Street Hospital noted the efficiency of the pit stops of the Ferrari race car team and concluded that patient handovers were haphazard in comparison. The physicians traveled to Italy to meet with individuals at Ferrari headquarters and began to incorporate some of the lessons learned in their own processes. For instance, in a Formula One race, the "lollipop man" (with the paddle) ushers the car in and signals the driver when it is safe to go ... it is not always clear in the hospital who is in charge.

Back in London, the physicians also sought the advice of two jumbo jet pilots and wrote a seven-page protocol for patient hand-offs. After numerous improvements and changes, "information handover omissions" fell 49% and the number of technical errors fell 42%.

(From Naik, G. Hospital races to learn lessons of Ferrari crew. *The Wall Street Journal*, November 14, 2006.)

CLINICAL CORNER

Improving Organizational Performance
Julie Sturbaum

Reducing Health Care–Acquired Infections in a Skilled Unit

In April 2008, our team began to work on reducing hospital-acquired *Clostridium difficile* infections on the skilled unit at our hospital. The first step was to identify who should participate in the work. Key leaders, including the chief nursing officer, the nurse manager on the unit, the medical director for the unit, the program manager for infection prevention and control and an influential frontline staff nurse, were recruited for the team.

Identifying Barriers to Compliance With Infection Prevention Strategies

The team examined barriers to compliance with proven infection prevention strategies such as hand hygiene, contact precautions, and cleaning patient care equipment. Once barriers were identified, changes in systems and processes underwent a trial using rapid-cycle Plan–Do–Study–Act (PDSA) improvement strategies. For example, one barrier to compliance with contact precautions was the absence of supplies like gowns, gloves, and masks at the patient's door. Our small test of change was to establish standardized times to restock the supplies outside the patient's doors. Before and after the test of change, we collected data on the number of isolation carts that were missing supplies. We found that by implementing standardized times to restock the supplies, we had fewer missing supplies. The data collected regarding presence or absence of supplies told us our test of change had been successful in removing the barrier of missing supplies. The PDSA cycle was repeated numerous times as we worked to remove barriers to compliance with proven infection prevention strategies.

Progress toward the goal of reducing *C. difficile* infections on the skilled unit was monitored using data collected on the following measures over several months:

1. Days between cases for *C. difficile* infections
2. Days between cases for methicillin-resistant *Staphylococcus aureus* (MRSA) infections
3. Percentage of environmental cleanings completed appropriately
4. Percentage of patient encounters with compliance for contact precautions
5. Percentage of patient encounters with compliance for hand hygiene
6. Percentage of patients with *C. difficile*–associated disease
7. Rate of occurrence of MRSA bloodstream infection (BSI) and hospital-acquired pneumonia (HAP) per 1000 patient-days
8. Rate of occurrence of vancomycin-resistant enterococcus (VRE) urinary tract infections (UTI) and BSI per 1000 patient-days
9. Risk priority number from the failure–modes–effects analysis

Results

The results accomplished by implementing these changes were significant for our Transitional Care Unit. Compliance with hand hygiene improved from 66% in April 2007 to 94% in April 2008, and compliance with contact precautions improved from 60% in April 2007 to 90% in April 2008.

While we did not meet our aim of achieving a 30% reduction in *C. difficile* disease on the unit, we did meet our goal of 30 days between *C. difficile* infections in March/April 2008. As of April 30, 2008, we have had no MRSA BSIs or cases of HAP for 193 days and no VRE BSIs or UTIs for 11 months. In addition, our VRE colonization incidence declined to a new low during the 12 months of this work.

The lessons we learned in breaking down barriers to compliance with infection prevention strategies have disseminated to other units in the hospital.

EVIDENCE-BASED PRACTICE

Best Practices: Understanding Nurses' Perspectives

From Novak, D., Dooley, S., & Clark, R. (2008). Best practices: understanding nurses' perspectives. Journal of Nursing Administration, 38, 448–453.

The recent rise in popularity and support for evidence-based best practice has brought to light the fact that many nursing practices are done a certain way because "that's the way we have always done it" and not because there is evidence to support it. As part of a Virginia hospital's transition to the integration of evidence into practice, the Nursing Research Council designed a study that assessed nurses' views of best practice and the organizational supports and barriers to successfully navigating practice changes with the

EVIDENCE-BASED PRACTICE—cont'd

inclusion of recommended strategies for success. It has been proved time and again that the integration of current knowledge into daily practice improves patient care by increasing the likelihood that the best clinical decisions are being made at the right time with the result being the achievement of positive patient outcomes and increased nurse autonomy. This qualitative study's aim was to gain a clearer understanding of nurses' perceptions of best practice and the personal and institutional barriers that may exist that prevent the adoption of evidence-based practice. Data were collected over a 9-month period using personal interviews, focus group discussions, and questionnaires involving nine nurses who actively participated in nursing shared governance committees and were nominated by unit directors. Following 1-hour interviews including six open-ended questions and performed by an experience study investigator, seven of the nine nurses participated in a discussion to develop ways to facilitate the use of evidence in a nurse's daily practice. Participants were then given a questionnaire to complete if they had any additional follow-up thoughts or suggestions. Five synthesizing statements

and their supporting themes and exemplars were written and used to define "best practice." The study investigators concluded the focus group by facilitating the participants' creation of the following definition: "Best practice is an ongoing process of deliberate, thoughtful teamwork that has a ripple effect. It is critically linking knowledge within the organization and externally to deliver the best care (product) at the bedside."

In conclusion, the study found that nurses with varying experience and educational preparation offered a variety of views about best practice. Overall, they were enthusiastic and shared a sense of readiness to move beyond evidence-based mandates and begin the developmental process. Participants emphasized the need for a clear understanding of how "best practice" is incorporated at the bedside and the importance of a clearly established and visible philosophy of care that embraces the priority of best practice. Specific recommendations were provided by the group and will be used to guide future organizational practice structures.

NCLEX® EXAM QUESTIONS

1. Key drivers of quality include EXCEPT but:
   1. the patient and family
   2. The Joint Commission
   3. finances
   4. insurance companies
2. Risk management includes:
   1. the management of all employees
   2. the identification of financial risk
   3. use of processes to minimize injury
   4. oversight of all PI activities
   5. 2 and 3
3. The National Patient Safety Goals:
   1. form the basis of all PI activities
   2. are a nationwide initiative
   3. are mandated by the Institute of Medicine
   4. will improve patient safety
4. The National Database of Nursing Quality Indicators:
   1. evaluates all nursing activities

   2. is measured by all nursing agencies
   3. includes unit-specific nursing measures
   4. measures nurse satisfaction
   5. 3 and 4
5. A sentinel event:
   1. is the basis of all PI
   2. must be reported to TJC
   3. evidences poor patient care
   4. is a medical error
6. An example of an outcome is:
   1. the admission process
   2. pressure ulcer rate
   3. nursing satisfaction
   4. standard of care
   5. 2 and 3
7. A root-cause analysis:
   1. focuses on risk management
   2. is a Six Sigma model
   3. determines process variation
   4. is a prospective review

Continued

8. Six Sigma is a model of quality focusing on:
   1. process development
   2. improving performance
   3. decreasing the process variation
   4. statistical analysis
9. "Lean" refers to
   1. the attempt to "make do" with the smallest amount possible
   2. a type of financial arrangement in which dollars are saved

3. getting rid of waste in all work processes
4. the streamlining of all patient processes for cost saving

10. A goal of organizational learning is to make learning:
    1. the end product of all data collection
    2. part of all activities within the organization
    3. required of all employees in clinical positions
    4. match the goals of The Joint Commission.

Answers: 1. 3 2. 5 3. 2 4. 5 5. 2 6. 5 7. 3 8. 3 9. 3 10. 2

REFERENCES

Advisory Commission of Consumer Protection and Quality in the Health Care Industry. (1998). Quality First: *Better Health Care for all Americans*. Online available at http://www.hcqualitycommission.gov/final/

Baldrige National Quality Program. (2007). *Health care criteria for performance excellence*. Gaithersberg: MD: National Institute of Standards.

Bronson Methodist Hospital. (2007). Baldrige application. Retrieved March 11, 2007, from http://baldrige.nist.gov/PDF_files/Bronson_Methodist_Hospital_Application_Summary.pdf .

Clinical Dashboard Metrics. Retrieved September 8, 2008 from http://www.dashboardzone.com/hospital-dahsboard-clinical-dashboard-metrics.

Deming, W. E. (2000a). *Out of the crisis*. Cambridge, MA: Massachusetts Institute of Technology.

Deming, W. E. (2000b). *The new economics: for industry, government, education*, 2nd ed. Cambridge, MA: MIT Press

Donabedain, A. (1992). The role of outcomes in quality assessment and assurance. *Quality Review Bulletin, 18*, 356-360.

GE's DMAIC Approach. (2007). Retrieved March 11, 2007, from http://www.ge.com/capital/vendor/dmaic.htm.

Institute of Medicine. (1998). *Crossing the quality chasm: a new health system for the 21st century*. Washington, DC: National Academies Press.

The Joint Commission. (2007). National patient safety goals. Retrieved March 11, 2007, from http://www.jointcommission.org/PatientSafety/NationalPatientSafetyGoals/07_hap_cah_npsgs.htm.

The Joint Commission. (2007). Sentinel event policies and procedures. Retrieved March 11, 2007, from http://www.jointcommission.org/SentinelEvents/PolicyandProcedures/.

Juran, J. M. (1989). *Juran on leadership for quality: an executive handbook*. New York: Free Press.

Kavaler, F., & Spiegel, A. (2003). *Risk management in health care institutions: a strategic approach*, 2nd ed. Boston: Jones & Bartlett.

Miller D.B. (ed.), (2005). *Going lean in health care*. IHI Innovation Series white paper. Cambridge, MA: Institute for Healthcare Improvement; 2005:5. Online information retrieved July 30, 2009. Available at: http://www.ihi.org/IHI/Results/WhitePapers/GoingLeaninHealthCare.htm.

Naik, G. (2006). Hospital races to learn lessons of Ferrari crew. *The Wall Street Journal*, November 14, 2006.

Nielsen, D. M., Merry, M. D., Schyve, P. M., Bisognano, M. (2004). Can the gurus' concepts cure health care? *Quality Progress*, 25-34.

National Center for Nursing Quality. (2007). Nursing quality indicators. Retrieved March 11, 2007, from http://nursingworld.org/quality/database.htm.

Phelps, C. E. (1997). *Health economics*, 2nd ed. Reading, MA: Addison-Wesley.

Sackett, D., Strauss, S., Richardson, W., Rosenberg, W., & Haynes, R. (2000). *Evidence-based medicine: how to practice and teach EBM*, 2nd ed. Edinburgh: Churchill Livingstone.

Womack, J., & Jones, D. (2003). *Lean thinking: banish waste and create wealth in your corporation*. New York: Free Press.

Yoder-Wise, P. (2003). *Leading and managing in nursing*. St. Louis: Mosby.

CHAPTER 11

Hospital Information Systems

Chapter Objectives

1. Define *electronic health records (EHRs)* and *electronic medical records (EMRs)*.
2. Relate National Patient Safety Goals to the adoption of EMRs.
3. Analyze the driving forces behind the implementation of electronic record keeping.
4. Review the components of a hospital-wide EMR.
5. Differentiate between an EMR and a hospital information system.
6. Discuss obstacles to use of the EMR.
7. Analyze the role of the nurse in the implementation and use of the EMR.
8. Differentiate between the levels of computer competencies required of new nurses versus experienced nurses.

Definitions

Electronic health record Information relating to the past or future physical/mental health, or condition of an individual that resides in electronic systems used to capture, transmit, receive, store, or manipulate data for the primary purpose of providing health-related services

Electronic medical record Information relating to the medical care received by an individual; usually institution specific residing in electronic systems that are hospital or health system based

Decision support Provision of assistance via a computer application for the purpose of assisting the nurse in decision making

Clinical information systems Used for the collection, integration, and distribution of information to the appropriate department

Nursing information system Part of a hospital system that standardizes nursing records across the system

Computerized provider order entry (CPOE) Automated systems for providers to enter patient care orders and to access decision support databases

ELECTRONIC HEALTH RECORDS

A true electronic health record (EHR) is a complete record of an individual's health-related data. The U.S. Department of Health and Human Services (DHHS) is spearheading an initiative to build a national electronic health care system that would allow patients and their caregivers to access their complete health records anytime and anywhere (DHHS, 2003).

After this announcement, both private and public organizations joined forces to develop an EHR. Included in this effort is the DHHS, the U.S. Department of Veterans Affairs (VA), the Institute of Medicine (IOM), The Robert Wood Johnson Foundation,

The Healthcare Information and Management Systems Society (HIMSS), and HL7 (Health Level 7, a health care standards developer) (HL7, 2004). A goal of this project is to have a sharing of data on a nationwide level across institutions. For example, if an individual from California entered a trauma center in New Jersey, the trauma center would be able to access the individual's record from California. While the health care system has not reached such a level of integration, the VA has a system that allows access of the medical record across the nation for all patients of the VA system.

The term *electronic health record* is loosely used to include any patient care record that is collected and stored in an electronic fashion. A majority of health care institutions are moving toward the creation of computerized medical records to be used within the organization. The patient record has a variety of uses. The first use is the documentation of patient care and a means of communication among members of the health care team. The second use is to provide legal and financial records, and the third is to provide data for research and continuous performance improvement (Young, 2000). In the era before computers, the management of patient records in health care organizations was based on manual file processing systems. In many hospitals, the medical records department remains a large filing system for all paper charts. Ask any nurse with experience, and he or she will tell you about requesting the "old chart" for a patient and receiving a truckload of paper documentation that may go back years. Additionally, one of the major complaints of individuals reading paper charts has always related to the illegible handwriting often seen in many areas of the chart.

The IOM reports (1997, 2000, 2001) dealing with the patient safety issues facing the U.S. health care system all discussed the importance of electronic patient records in the improvement of safety, quality, and efficiency of health care in the United States. In 1991, the IOM issued a report calling for the elimination of paper-based records within 10 years. Progress, however, has been slow and the goal has not been met (IOM, 2000; Overhage et al., 2002). The financial costs for the implementation of such systems are high, and in this era of cost containment, many institutions do not have the financial resources to initiate such systems. The motivation is not to have a paperless system per se but rather to make important patient information available and useable to all appropriate caregivers. Box 11-1 lists advantages and disadvantages of the EHR.

While there are many disadvantages to the EHR/computerized health record, the movement to health care institutions of an overall culture of safety has

---

Box 11-1   ADVANTAGES AND DISADVANTAGES OF THE ELECTRONIC HEALTH RECORD

Advantages of the Electronic Health Record
- Storing data in small space
- Accessible from remote sites to many people at the same time
- Information retrieval is almost instantaneous.
- Provides clinical alerts, expert systems, and reminders
- Links clinicians to protocols, care plans, critical paths, literature databases, pharmaceutical information, and other databases of health care knowledge
- Automated programs can create customized views to meet the needs of various specialties.
- Improves risk management and provides outcomes assessment
- Improves clinicians' productivity
- Provides more accurate capture of financial charges and billing efficiency
- Increases patient satisfaction

Disadvantages of the Electronic Health Record
- Startup costs for hardware, software, installation, maintenance, increased technical personnel, training, and future upgrades are considerable.
- Learning curve for a new system of documentation is steep.
- Confidentiality, privacy, and security of the information are concerns.
- New hardware is nonportable or portable and breakable.
- Issues surrounding entry of data remain.
- Technical understanding is required to maintain the system.
- Downtime is an issue.

Adapted from Young, K. (2000). *Informatics for healthcare professionals* (pp. 99-104). Philadelphia: F.A. Davis.

resulted in a strong push to implement computerized health records or hospital-wide information systems.

There are a wide variety of hospital information systems. Some systems include all patient data (e.g., physician orders, laboratory results, electronic charting, decision supports, etc.). Others may be more function specific and are limited to certain types of data such as medication order entry and documentation. Other systems provide decision support such as pharmacy drug reminders, drug interactions, and best practice guidelines. Most of the information systems are individualized to the specific health care agency or system and are not nationwide. The EHR differs from a hospital information system. A hospital information system incorporates all information used in both patient care and the management of the structures and processes that support the care delivered at a particular institution.

The primary and secondary uses of the hospital-wide information system are as follows (adapted from IOM, 1997):

Primary Uses

- Patient care delivery
- Patient care management
- Patient care support processes
- Financial and other administrative processes

Secondary Uses

- Education
- Regulation
- Research
- Public health and Homeland Security
- Policy support

The functionality of any information system within a health care agency should address the following:

- *Improve patient safety*—Each year in the United States, tens of thousands of people die as a result of preventable adverse events in health care (IOM, 2000).
- *Support the delivery of effective care*—It has been suggested that only about 55% of Americans receive recommended medical care that is consistent with evidence-based practice guidelines (McGlynn et al., 2003).
- *Facilitate the management of chronic illness*—More than half of people with chronic conditions have three or more health providers. Physicians and patients report difficulty in the coordination of

care with multiple providers (Leatherman and McCarthy, 2002; Partnership for Solutions, 2002).
- *Improve efficiency*—Efficiency is the avoidance of waste. With the staffing and financial challenges faced by many institutions, it is imperative that processes be improved.
- *Feasibility of implementation*—This takes into account the financial capability of an institution to support such a system, as well as the personnel capacity for support (Committee on Data Standards for Patient Safety, 2003).

The core functionalities for a computerized health information system are as follows:

- *Health information and data*—EHRs with defined datasets such as medical and nursing diagnoses, a medication list, allergies, demographics, clinical narratives, and laboratory test results can ensure access to current patient data by those who need it.
- *Results management*—Managing all types of results (laboratory tests, radiograph results) electronically has the distinct advantage of allowing access to the results in a more efficient timeframe than with paper-based results. The automated display of results may also lead to a decrease of redundant testing (Bates and Gawande, 2003).
- *Order entry*—Computerized provider order entry (CPOE) has been shown to decrease the number of medication errors by up to 83% (Bates and Gawande, 2003).
- *Decision support*—Several studies have shown that computerized decision support improve drug dosing, drug selection, and screening for drug interactions (Abookire et al., 2000; Schiff and Rucker, 1998).
- *Electronic communication and connectivity*—Improved communication between care partners, such as pharmacy, radiology, laboratory, and nursing departments, can enhance patient safety and quality of care (Schiff et al., 2003).
- *Patient support*—A multidimensional telehealth system has demonstrated the ability to decrease the stress for some caregivers of patients with Alzheimer's disease (Bass et al., 1998).
- *Administrative processes*—Electronic staffing systems allow nurse managers extra time to manage care instead of creating staffing schedules.
- *Reporting and health management*—Health care agencies have multiple reporting manually.

THE VIRTUAL HOSPITAL

An example of a decision support system is the Virtual Hospital. The Virtual Hospital is known as a digital library for health information. Established by the University of Iowa, this medical multimedia textbook takes full advantage of hypertext links to provide navigation between documents and figures embedded in the text. The seamlessly constructed links to off-site databases bring to the screen digitized audio and visual material. It is an impressive demonstration that allows professionals and consumers to quickly seek peer-reviewed information on a variety of adult and pediatric topics. This type of reference, accessible from anywhere in the world at any time of day, offers resources to support geographically isolated practitioners and makes teaching materials available to anyone (Virtual Hospital, 2003 [http://www.vh.org]; Kearney Nunnery, 2005).

HEALTH CARE INFORMATION MANAGEMENT SYSTEM

There are a wide variety of hospital information systems (Figure 11-1) with which the nurse will come in contact. The most common functions are detailed next.

Patient Information Retrieval

Results of laboratory and diagnostic tests are posted to computer records in many agencies. These tests are then made readily available to those who need the information.

Order Entry

Entry of physicians' orders for medications, laboratory work, diagnostic tests, and other therapies is often one of the earliest aspects of patient care that is placed on the computer. With the upgrades in technology over the past few years, some organizations are moving toward the use of hand-held computers for creation of orders, which are then downloaded to the hospital system.

Nursing Data Entry

A computerized medication administration record (MAR) often is an early aspect of the computerized chart that is recorded. This is then followed up with computerized charting and full nursing documentation.

Administrative Systems

Most hospitals have computerized financial and billing systems. The federal programs of Medicare and Medicaid have required that billing be done through computerized systems that can communicate with the

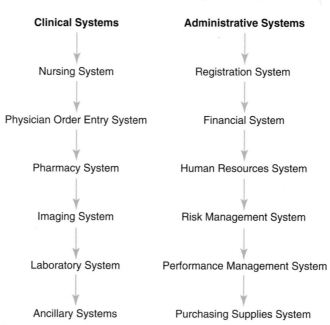

Clinical Systems

Nursing System
↓
Physician Order Entry System
↓
Pharmacy System
↓
Imaging System
↓
Laboratory System
↓
Ancillary Systems

Administrative Systems

Registration System
↓
Financial System
↓
Human Resources System
↓
Risk Management System
↓
Performance Management System
↓
Purchasing Supplies System

Figure 11-1 • Health care information management system. (From Kearney Nunnery, R. [2005]. *Advancing your career: concepts of professional nursing,* 3rd ed. Philadelphia: F. A. Davis. Used with permission.)

government agency. Some of the billing systems are integrated with the patient care delivery. One such system in common use is Pyxis SpecialtyStation, whose function is integrated throughout many functions. This comprehensive system allows a facility to track cost per patient as well as the cost of inventory. Supplies and medications are stored in the system, which usually is located on each unit. Nurses enter a code and then are able to obtain the necessary supply or medication from the locked cabinet. When each supply is taken by the nurse, the machine automatically charges the patient, reorders the supply, and maintains an inventory. Pyxis SpecialtyStation system is an advanced point-of-use system that automates the distribution, management, and control of medications and supplies. An automated perpetual inventory eliminates manual reorder processes. Par levels are set in the system to ensure products are ordered before a stock-out occurs.

There are numerous nurse management information systems with which the new nurse will become familiar. One such nursing administrative system is the Automated Nurse Staffing Office System (ANSOS). Nursing management information systems provide shift reports of personnel by type needed and assigned, staffing and productivity data by unit and area, average data on the intensity of care needed, and the cost of patient care (Rousel, 2006).

Point-of-Care Systems

Point-of-care systems may include the bedside or another point of care in the health care system. The documentation is performed wherever the patient is located. There is full accessibility of input and output patient information. One example of point-of-care systems is the PDA (personal digital assistant). These PDAs contain decision support systems, such as drug references, food–drug interaction indexes, and basic life support (BLS) or advanced cardiac life support (ACLS) guidelines. Some hand-held systems allow for documentation of patient care activities, which are then downloaded to the larger patient system via a docking deck. Many institutions with computerized charting have point-of-care systems located in areas near the patient so that the documentation can occur as the time of care. This allows the nurse to document in or near the patient room as soon as the information is collected. Information is also collected and recorded in other patient care devices, such as cardiac monitors, ventilators, and glucose monitors. Information from these systems can also be downloaded to the larger patient care system via an integrated electronic medical record (EMR).

NURSING MINIMUM DATA SET

In the move toward the development of a nationwide EHR, the need arises for a standardized nursing language that can be understood across a variety of systems. The NMDS (nursing minimum data set) represents one attempt at a standardized language (Box 11-2). There are a number of recognized standard languages in use in nursing (Table 11-1). Many of the monitoring devices used in patient care can be integrated into the clinical information system. Most cardiac monitors, glucose monitors, and ventilators have cards installed that allow for data to flow from the device to the clinical system, thus saving documentation time. The NMDS was defined to establish uniform standards for the collection of comparable essential patient data (Yoder-Wise, 2003, p. 196). The uniform minimum

---

Box 11-2 ELEMENTS OF THE NURSING MINIMUM DATA SET (NMDS)

Nursing Care Elements
1. Nursing diagnosis
2. Nursing intervention
3. Nursing outcome
4. Intensity of nursing care

Patient Demographic Elements
5. Personal identification*
6. Date of birth*
7. Sex*
8. Race and ethnicity*
9. Residency*

Service Elements
10. Unique facility or service agency number*
11. Unique health record number of the patient
12. Unique number of the principal registered nurse provider
13. Episode, admission, or encounter date*
14. Discharge or termination date*
15. Disposition of patient or client*
16. Expected payer for most of the bill

*Elements comparable to those in the uniform minimum health data set (UMHDS).
From Werley, H. H., & Lang, N. M. (1988). The consensually derived nursing minimum data set elements and definitions. In: H. H. Werley & N. M. Lang, eds. *Identification of the nursing minimum data set* (pp. 402-411). New York: Springer.

Standardized Terminology	Problems/ Diagnoses	Interventions	Goals/ Outcomes	Reference
Complete complementary alternative medicine billing and coding reference		×		Gianinni (2005)
Home health care classification	×	×	×	Saba (1990)
International classification for nursing practice	×	×	×	International Council of Nurses (1999)
North American Nursing Diagnosis Association (NANDA) taxonomy	×			NANDA (1999)
Nursing Interventions Classification		×		McCloskey and Bulechek (2000)
Nursing management minimum data set				Huber, Delaney, and Crossley (1992)
Nursing minimum data set	×	×	×	Werley and Lang (1988)
Nursing Outcomes Classification			×	Johnson, Maas, and Moorehead (2000)
Omaha system	×	×	×	Martin and Scheet (1992)
Patient care data set	×	×	×	Ozbolt, Fruchtnight, and Hayden (1994)
Perioperative nursing data set	×	×	×	Kleinbeck (2000)
SNOMED RT	×	×	×	Spackman, Campbell, and Cote (1997)

Table 11-1 AMERICAN NURSES ASSOCIATION–RECOGNIZED STANDARDIZED LANGUAGES

Modified from Yoder-Wise, P. S. (2003). *Leading and managing in nursing*. 3rd ed. St. Louis: Mosby.

health data set (UMHDS) is a minimum set of items of information with uniform multiple data users. UMHDSs have been developed for long-term care, hospital discharge, and ambulatory care (Yoder-Wise, 2003, p. 196).

INFORMATICS COMPETENCIES FOR NURSES

As a nurse, you will need to become comfortable with the technology of the workplace. You will also need to have a working knowledge of informatics. "*Nursing informatics* is a specialty that integrates nursing science, computer science, communicate data, information, and knowledge in nursing practice" (American Nurses Association [ANA], 2001, p. vii). In 1992, the ANA supported nursing informatics as a specialty for registered nurses and offered a certification examination for nursing informatics.

Nurse managers play a pivotal role in the adoption of information systems. In their leadership role, they have three levels of competency with information systems. As an *initial user* of information system, they need to have the following competencies:

1. Use computerized management systems to record administrative data (billing data, quality assurance data, workload data, etc.).
2. Use applications for structured data entry (classification systems, acuity level, etc.).
3. Understand client rights related to computerized information.
4. Recognize the utility of nurse involvement in the planning, design, choice, and implementation of information systems in the practice environment.
5. Incorporate a code of ethics in regard to client privacy and confidentiality.

As they become more familiar with the system, they enter a next level of competency, that of a *modifier*. In this role, they will have the following competencies:

1. Have an awareness of role of nursing informatics in the context of health informatics and information systems.

2. Participate in policy and procedural development related to nursing informatics.

3. Participate in system change processes and utility analysis.

4. Participate in evaluation of information systems in practice settings.

5. Analyze ergonomic integrity of work station, bedside, and portable technology apparatus in practice.

6. Participate in design of data collection tools for practice decision making and record keeping.

7. Participate in quality management initiatives related to patient and nursing data in practice.

8. Have an awareness of the impact of implementing technology to facilitate nursing practice.

9. Evaluate security effectiveness and parameters of system for protecting client information and ensuring confidentiality.

10. Participate in change to improve the use of informatics within nursing practice.

11. Encourage other nurses to develop comfort and competency in technology use in practice.

As, they assume mastery of the competencies and progress in management, they assume a role of *innovator*. The innovator:

1. Develops and participates in quality assurance programs using information systems

2. Participates in patient instructional program development

3. Participates in ergonomic design of work stations, bedside access stations, and portable apparatus equipment

4. Maintains awareness of societal and technological trends, issues, and new developments and applies these to nursing

5. Demonstrates proficient awareness of legal and ethical issues related to client data, information, and confidentiality

6. Designs and implements project management initiatives related to information technology for practice

SUMMARY

Information systems have become an integral part of the nursing workplace, and nurses and nurse managers need to embrace its use to assist them in making the workplace safer and more efficient. The EMR and hospital information systems are assisting the nurse to more efficiently gather the necessary patient information to make clinical decisions. As a nurse manager, you will need to role model comfort with the use of technology for those staff members who are uncomfortable with technology. You will also need to constantly evaluate the use of technology in your practice and the efficiency of your unit.

CLINICAL CORNER

Implementation of an Information Management System for a Cardiothoracic Unit
Jane O'Rourke

Unit 5 South is a 40-bed cardiothoracic surgical unit in a metropolitan hospital with an active emergency department. The cardiothoracic service is supported with a strong referral base. Two active physician groups perform an average of 720 cardiac surgical procedures annually.

Postanesthesia care	4 Beds
Cardiothoracic intensive care	6 Beds
Step-down	30 Beds

Each level of care operates with different staffing patterns and operational procedures to support patient care.

The service presently uses the clinical information system of the hospital for patient care management. This system has been found not to meet the needs of the cardiothoracic unit. The complexity of the operations leads to the leadership decision to purchase a different management information system for 5 South. The management and staff of 5 South were major players in the choice and implementation of the clinical information system in use on the unit for patient care. Given their project experience, 5 South staff put forth the following proposal for a management information system to assist with staffing, scheduling, budget planning, and operational tracking. The project is designed to meet a 12-month timeframe for completion.

Continued

CLINICAL CORNER—cont'd

Phase I
30 Days
	The vice president of surgical services appoints a committee for the project.
	The committee will consist of the following members:
	    Nurse manager
	    Clinical specialist
	    Cardiologist
	    Three staff nurses
	    Cardiopulmonary technician
	    Information technology manager

The scope of the project is drafted with timeframes for each phase and scope of work.

Request for proposal (RFP) is written.
The RFI will solicit the following information:
    Description
    Cost
    Hardware requirements
    Technological support
    Training
    Service agreement
    Information technology requirements
    System backup
    Incremental costs
    Incidental costs
    Payment schedule
    Timeframe for delivery
    Installation process
    List of references (e.g., demographic facilities)

Phase II
120 Days
RFPs are reviewed and plotted on a dashboard.
Site visits to be done at four top-choice vendor-recommended facilities.
Site visits are matched with our facility and must be using the software program for at least a year with outcome data retrievable.
Vendor will be selected by committee.
Financial expertise will be requested to detail the return on investment.
Proposal is finalized and submitted to executive staff for review.
If the proposal is acceptable, it will be presented to the board of directors at the next scheduled quarterly meeting.

Phase III
60 Days
Vendor of choice is notified.
Contract is received and reviewed by committee, executive staff, legal counsel, and finance.
Contract revisions are submitted.
Contract is finalized.
Contract is signed.
Implementation plan is devised through joint vendor and hospital meetings.
Member of hospital leadership staff is identified as the project manager to oversee the installation and accept accountability.

Phase IV
90 Days
Work plan is established by project manager.
Work plan is presented to executive staff for approval.
Super-users are identified and make site visits.
Education and installation are plotted.
Hardware and related equipment are ordered.
Super-users are educated.
Go-live dates are established.

CLINICAL CORNER—cont'd

Phase V 30 Days	Hardware is installed. Software is installed. Staff are educated. System goes live. Functionality is adjusted. Formal communication is disseminated to staff. Ongoing orientation and training are planned.

EVIDENCE-BASE PRACTICE

The Nursing Shortage: Can Technology Help?

Case, J., Mowry, M., Welebob, E. First Consulting Group. (June 2002). The nursing shortage: can technology help? Oakland, CA: California HealthCare Foundation.

As the nursing shortage worsens, hospitals will need to use every means possible to support nurses. There are far too many examples in the industry of unsuccessful implementations and poor uses of technology that have created more work for nurses. However, when the right technology is successfully implemented, monitored for effectiveness, and adequately maintained, technology can make a positive difference in the patient care environment. Technology can free nurses to concentrate on direct care by increasing efficiency and alleviating some of the burden on them. It can help make the care environment more rewarding and thus help improve recruitment and retention.

This report commissioned by the California Healthcare Foundation focuses on technological implementations considered by nurses to be successful.

Scheduling: "The Nightingale System." Nurses are able to enter their preferences for shifts via the Internet, administrators enter the requirements for the unit, and algorithms are run to produce a schedule that best meets the needs of everyone.

Communication: Wireless telephones that each nurse picks up at the beginning of the shift. This enhances communication with patients, physicians, and other personnel.

Patient Education: The "Phoenix Education System" is an electronic method of meeting patient educational needs. The system tracks who gets what as well as follow-up comprehension activities.

Automated Messaging: This can be incorporated into clinical documentation, order entry, and electronic medical record systems. An example is when a nurse documents a patient needs assistance walking, the service automatically sends a message to physical therapy.

Automated Nursing Documentation: Information can be presented in a way that supports adherence to standards and policies. Automated reminders such as pain assessment follow-up help ensure that needed information is gathered by requiring certain fields to be completed, such as documentation for using restraints.

Medication Management: A variety of systems and technologies can be used to support the medication management process at the point of care. They perform safety checks. There are medication-dispensing devices, smart intravenous pumps, and medication administration systems with barcode technology.

This report concluded that empowering nurses with the tools they need and reducing their frustration with paperwork can help to improve nurse retention and lessen the nursing shortage.

NCLEX® EXAM QUESTIONS

1. All of the following are uses of the patient record EXCEPT:
   1. documentation
   2. provision of data for research
   3. provision of legal and financial records
   4. an area to place incident report
2. The electronic patient health record may include:
   1. patient statistics
   2. medication order entry
   3. an incident report
   4. patient census data
3. The electronic health record differs from a hospital information system in that:
   1. a hospital information system incorporates all information used in both patient care and the management of the structures that provide the patient care
   2. a hospital information system does not incorporate all information used in both patient care and the management of the structures that provide the patient care
   3. a hospital electronic health record incorporates all information used in both patient care and the management of the structures that provide the patient care
   4. a hospital electronic health record does not incorporate all information used in both patient care and the management of the structures that provide the patient care
4. The core functionalities for an electronic health information system are:
   1. health information, data, and order entry
   2. patient census, data, and order entry
   3. patient acuities, patient census, and incident report
   4. incident reports and outcomes measures
5. A primary use for the electronic health information is:

6. A secondary use for the electronic health information is:
   1. education
   2. patient care management
   3. regulation
   4. research
6. A secondary use for the electronic health information is:
   1. education
   2. patient care delivery
   3. patient care management
   4. patient care support processes
7. The functionality of any electronic information system within a health care agency should address all of the following EXCEPT:
   1. improvement of patient safety
   2. support of the delivery of effective care
   3. facilitation of the management of chronic illness
   4. increasing patient stays
8. An example of a computerized billing system is:
   1. Dr Quality
   2. ANSOSS
   3. Pyxis
   4. none of the above
9. An example of a nursing data entry system is:
   1. Computerized Medication Administration Systems (MARs)
   2. nursing minimum data set (NMDS)
   3. Omincell
   4. incident reporting
10. The following patient assessment equipment have the capability of having cards installed that allow for data to flow from the device to the clinical system, thus saving documentation time:
    1. cardiac monitors and ventilators
    2. intravenous infusions and medications administered
    3. laboratory information and blood levels
    4. gastrostomy tube feedings and total parenteral nutrition infusion

Answers: 1. 4   2. 2   3. 1   4. 1   5. 2   6. 1   7. 4   8. 3   9. 1   10. 1

REFERENCES

Abookire, S., Teich, J., Sandige, H., Paterno, M., Martin, M., Kupperman, G., et al. (2000). Improving allergy alerting in a computerized physician order entry system. *Proceedings of the AMIA Annual Symposia*, 2-6.

American Nurses Association. (2001). *Scope and standards of nursing informatics practice.* Washington, DC: Author. Publication No. NIP21 3M 05/02.

Bass, D., McClendon, M., Brennan, P., & McCarthy, C. (1998). The buffering effect of a computer support network on caregiver strain. *Journal of Aging and Health, 1091,* 20-43.

Bates, D., & Gawande, A. (2003). Improving patient safety with information technology. *New England Journal of Medicine, 348,* 2526-2534.

Committee on Data Standards for Patient Safety. (2003). *Key capabilities of an electronic health record system: letter report.* Washington, DC: National Academy of Sciences.

Giannini, M. (2005). *The CAM and nursing coding manual.* Albany, NY: Delmar.

HL7. (2004). Health level 7 Unlocking the Power of Health information. Retrieved May 27, 2009, from http://www.hl7.org.

Huber, D. G., Delaney C., & Crossley, J. (1992). A nursing management minimum data set. *Journal of Nursing Administration, 22*(7/8), 35-40.

Institute of Medicine. (1991). *The computer based record: an essential technology for health care.* In R. Dick & E. Steen (Ed.), Washington, DC: National Academies Press.

Institute of Medicine. (1997). *The computer based record: an essential technology for health care* (revised edition). In R. Dick & E. Steen (Eds.), Washington, DC: National Academies Press.

Institute of Medicine. (2000). *To err is human: building a safer health system.* In L. Kohn, J. Corrigan, & M. Donaldson (Eds.), Washington, DC: National Academies Press.

Institute of Medicine. (2001). *Crossing the quality chasm: a new health system for the 21st century.* Washington, DC: National Academies Press.

International Council of Nurses. (1999). *International classification for nursing practice—Beta version.* Geneva, Switzerland: Author.

Johnson, M., Maas, M., & Moorhead, S. (2000). *Nursing outcomes classification* (2nd ed.). St. Louis: Mosby.

Kearney Nunnery, R. (2005). *Advancing your career: concepts of professional nursing* (3rd ed.). Philadelphia: F.A. Davis.

Kleinbeck, S. V. (2000). Dimensions of perioperative nursing for a national specialty nomenclature. *Journal of Advanced Nursing, 31*(3), 529-535.

Leatherman, S., & McCarthy, D. (2002). *Quality of health care in the United States: a chartbook.* New York: The Commonwealth Fund.

Martin, K. S., & Scheet, N. J. (1992). *The Omaha system: applications for community health nursing.* Philadelphia: W.B. Saunders.

McCloskey, J. C., & Bulechek, G. M. (eds.) (2000). *Nursing intervention classification* (3rd ed.). St. Louis: Mosby.

McGlynn, E., Asch, S., Adams, J., Keesey, J., Hicks, J., DeCristofaro, A., et al. (2003). The quality of health care delivered to adults in the United States. *New England Journal of Medicine, 348*, 2635-2645.

North American Nursing Diagnosis Association. (1999). *Nursing diagnoses: definitions and classification, 1999-2000.* Philadelphia: Author.

Overhage, J. M., Dexter, P. R., Perkins, S. M., et al. (2002). A randomized controlled trial of clinical information shared from another institution. *Annals of Emergency Medicine, 39*, 14-23.

Ozbolt, J. B., Fruchtnight, J. N., & Hayden, J. R. (1994). Toward data standards for clinical nursing information. *Journal of the American Medical Informatics Association, 1*(2), 175-185.

Partnership for Solutions, Johns Hopkins University. (2002). *Chronic conditions: making the case for ongoing care.* Baltimore: Johns Hopkins University.

Rousel, L. (2006). *Management and leadership for nurse administrators.* Boston: Jones and Bartlett.

Saba, V. K. (1990). Home health care classification (HHCC system). Retrieved Aprile 23, 2009, from http://www.sabacare.com.

Schiff, G., Klass, D., Peterson, J., Shah, G., & Bates, D. (2003). Linking laboratory and pharmacy: opportunities for reducing errors and improving care. *Archives of Internal Medicine, 163*, 893-900.

Schiff, G., & Rucker, T. (1998). Computerized prescribing: building the electronic infrastructure for better medication usage. *JAMA, 29*, 1024-1029.

Spackman, K. A., Campbell, K. E., & Cote, R. A. (1997). SNOMED: a reference terminology for health care. In D. Masys (ed.), *Proceedings of the American Medical Informatics Association Annual Symposium* (pp. 640-644). Philadelphia: Hanley & Belfus.

U.S. Department of Health and Human Services. (2003). News release: HHS launches new efforts to promote paperless health care system. Retrieved April 23, 2009, from http://www.hhs.gov/news/press/2003pres/20030701.html.

Werley, H. H., & Lang, N. M. (1988). The consensually derived nursing minimum data set elements and definitions. In: H. H. Werley & N. M. Lang (Eds). *Identification of the nursing minimum data set* (pp. 402-411). New York: Springer.

Yoder-Wise, P. (2003). *Leading and managing in nursing* (3rd ed.). St. Louis: Mosby.

Young, K. M. (2000). *Informatics for healthcare professionals.* Philadelphia: F.A. Davis.

CHAPTER 12

Monitoring Outcomes and Use of Data for Improvement

Chapter Objectives

1. Relate the principles of performance improvement to the monitoring of patient care data.
2. Discuss routine information monitored by nurse managers.
3. Identify methods of analyzing data in health care.
4. Identify outcomes for various areas of nursing responsibility.
5. Differentiate between *data* and *information*.
6. Analyze the role of the nurse manager in assisting unit staff to deal with the information provided by the data collected.

Definitions

Benchmarking Process of comparing the performance of an organization against a set standard or best practice

Data Factual information (as measurements or statistics) used as a basis for reasoning or decision making

Information Knowledge gained from the analysis of data collected

Outcomes What follows as a result or consequence of the planned care delivered to patients. It is the objective evaluation of performance. Outcomes can be related to all aspects of health care: patient care, financial, human resource based, leadership, etc.

Productivity Actual number of hours of care delivered as related to the number of hours of work

Core Measures Those measures determined to be vital to the delivery of safe patient care by The Joint Commission and measured throughout the country

FOUR DOMAINS OF NURSING DATA

Many of the chapters in this text have discussed areas of importance for the nurse and nurse manager. Many of these areas of importance will be measured on a routine basis. And the nurse needs to be knowledgeable of the levels of performance in these key areas.

What are the uses of outcome information? Many individuals, especially in some health care organizations, believe that very little is done with all of the information that is collected on a daily basis. In organizations that have adopted a philosophy of organizational learning, outcome data are taken very seriously and used to drive improvement. These organizations have knowledge of their level of current performance

Table 12-1 FOUR DOMAINS OF NURSING DATA

Domain	Outcomes Commonly Reviewed
Client care	Infection rates Core Measures (The Joint Commission) Patient satisfaction Access to care Unit-specific measures of care
Provider staffing	Staffing ratios Employee satisfaction Job stress Intent to leave Staff competency
Administration	Costs Overtime Use of agency nurses Productivity Turnover
Research	Best practice Evidence-based practice

Adapted from Huber, D. (2006). *Leadership and nursing care management.* Philadelphia, PA: Elsevier. P. 273.

Detect Needed Improvements

- Identify outcomes that need attention.
- Identify patient groups that need attention.
- Identify patient care processes and polices that need improvement.
- Identify possible improvements in patient care delivery.

Motivate and Help Staff

- Communicate current levels of performance.
- Hold regular monitoring reviews.
- Identify training needs.
- Recognize staff for "a job well done."

Plan for the Future

- Identify successful and "best practice."
- Test new programs or protocol changes.
- Help plan and budget.
- Continue to motivate staff.

External Reporting

- Inform senior leadership of performance.
- Inform current and potential patients and other stakeholders.
- Report to the accrediting agencies and the community.

on many levels. It is the nurse manager's responsibility to have a working knowledge of the unit's performance and to create an environment of continuous learning and improvement.

Nursing data fall into four domains (Table 12-1). Nurses need data to provide information about client care, provider staffing, administration of care and the organization, and knowledge-based research for evidence-based practice. Collecting specific sets of data related to each of these domains give nurses information about practice and its effectiveness.

USES OF OUTCOME INFORMATION

A tremendous amount of information is collected during a hospital stay. Much of these data are further analyzed and turned into information that assists the organization and nurse manager in evaluating levels of performance. The information can be used to drive organizational, departmental, unit-based, and individual improvements.

So, what are the uses for outcome information (adapted from The Urban Institute, 2004)?

THE CORE MEASURES

The patient care outcomes that are routinely collected vary from unit to unit and from institution to institution. There are nationwide measures, such as the National Patient Safety Goals and the Core Measures of The Joint Commission. These were discussed in Chapter 10. All institutions also collect information on infection rates. This information is required by both state and federal regulating agencies. Sometimes these measures are intertwined; one such example is the Core Measure of Pneumonia, which is also an infectious process. Infectious disease evidence shows two actions that result in lower mortality: administering antibiotics within 4 hours of admission and acting on the information obtained from blood cultures. By reviewing the levels of performance on these two "in-process" measures of caring for a patient with pneumonia (administering antibiotics within 4 hours of arrival and acting on information obtained from blood cultures), an organization may be able to improve their performance on the outcome for the care of the pneumonia patient.

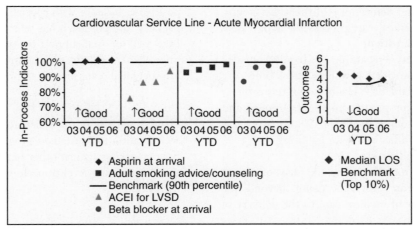

Figure 12-1 • In reviewing the chart, look at the performance of a particular hospital in the Core Measures for patient with acute myocardial infarction. North Mississippi Medical Center (2007). Retrieved September 8, 2008, from http://baldrige. nist.gov/PDF_files/NMMC_Application_Summary.pdf

In reviewing Figure 12-1, look at the performance of a particular hospital in the Core Measures for a patient with acute myocardial infarction. If you review the levels of performance for angiotensin-converting enzyme inhibitors (ACEIs) for left ventricular systolic dysfunction, you will see an improvement in performance from 2003 to 2006. You will also see improved performance for two of the other in-process measures for care of the patient with acute myocardial infarction: adult smoking advice/counseling and aspirin on arrival. Processes were created by the hospital based on performance in 2003 to make it easier to give aspirin on arrival, to give β-blockers, and to give smoking advice. This change in process led to the result of better performance in the following years. Also, it led to a lower length of stay for these patients.

Fiscal accountability by health care providers has become a theme in health care delivery systems; however, evaluation of outcomes on the basis of cost alone may minimize the importance of patient needs and the quality of the care delivered. Mechanisms related to resource identification and allocation has to be driven by internal data and information systems that consider all domains of hospital data: clinical, financial, administrative, and patient satisfaction data.

Also, many hospitals will have organization- and unit-specific dashboards that visually display current levels of performance on key indicators. For a further discussion of dashboards, go to Chapter 10.

PATIENT SATISFACTION REPORTS

One of the most common performance indicators reviewed by nurses on a routine basis is the patient satisfaction report. For this report, newly discharged patients are given a questionnaire that reflects their perception of the care received on the unit. The response to each of the questions provides data that are transformed into information that can be used by the nurse manager for improvement of care on the unit.

Data are collected routinely in a health care organization so that the organization can reflect on its performance and try to improve certain areas. The main purpose of data collection is to improve care to all individuals involved in the health care delivery. Let's use the data set for patient satisfaction as a discussion point. Most nurses on units will tell you that patient satisfaction is one of the most important performance measures in an institution. You may say to yourself that the clinical outcome should be most important measure of performance, but patient satisfaction data really provide information on a variety of areas.

Common satisfaction data results in information about:

- Accessibility—both physical access and financial access to care
- Communication skills—of the physicians, nurses, physician assistants, nurse practitioners, and others involved in direct patient care

- Personality and demeanor—of the same group
- Quality of medical-care processes—as provided directly to the patient
- Care continuity—regarding the handoffs made provider-to-provider, as well as across time
- Quality of health care facilities—in terms of having the appropriate equipment, supplies, and peripheral resources available
- Efficiency of office staff—in handling scheduling, billing, etc.

As you can see from these lists, the focus of patient satisfaction relies on providers going beyond the mechanical delivery of medical care to the delivery of a true health service.

DRIVING FORCES FOR INCREASING PATIENT SATISFACTION

The list of benefits of paying attention to patient satisfaction is long and extends to virtually every corner of the health care organization whether hospital, physician practice, home health, long-term care, and so forth. This makes sense, because the range of factors making up satisfaction is quite wide. With greater patient satisfaction comes the following benefits:

Clinical Benefits

- Greater patient trust and acceptance with treatment plans
- Increasing buy-in for treatment plans more quickly, making best use of scarce physician time
- Increasing trust, which allows caregivers to discover more factors that may affect the care needs of the patient
- Enhancing patient involvement in their own care through preventative measures, corrective measures, and so forth

Operational Benefits

- Driving efficiency into the organization by focusing on what works well with patients and eliminating what does not work well
- Cross-over trust is enhanced. For instance, a good experience in scheduling appointments can cross over into a better experience with the care provider. In addition, a good experience with the patient's primary care physician can cross over into a more

positive experience with specialists to whom the primary care physician has referred the patient.
- Increased internal support for other quality improvement efforts, such as timeliness improvement, care process improvement, etc.

Quality Accreditation Benefits

- Heightened ability to participate in quality accreditation measurement programs
- Benchmarking against other health care providers, and determining level of performance as compared with peers

Financial Benefits

- Being compensated for services by health plans and purchasers that link compensation in part to satisfaction scores
- Reduced provider staff stress and turnover
- Providing evidence of value of care to purchasers and payers

Marketing and Promotional Benefits

- Increased likelihood for being referred for services
- Increased propensity to return to the same hospital, same physician, etc.
- Improving word-of-mouth promotion of your organization
- Better comparison against competitors

Risk Management Benefits

- Reduced likelihood of malpractice litigation

Regulatory Compliance Benefits

- Positive scores as reported by the government such as when the Centers for Medicare & Medicaid Services (CMS) posts satisfaction survey results on its Hospital Compare web site.

Now that you realize the impact of patient satisfaction, it is important to review the ways that you will need to react to the information received from the surveys. Examples of the information in each of the various domains is presented in Box 12-1.

REVIEW OF PATIENT SATISFACTION OR OTHER PERFORMANCE MEASURES

A major function of outcome measurement is to raise questions. A review of the data will lead to a discussion

Box 12-1   PRESS GANEY PATIENT SATISFACTION SURVEY

Press Ganey Report

Children's specialized hospital—pediatric rehabilitation

Admissions

Speed of admissions process
Courtesy of admissions personnel

Room

Cheerfulness of room
Daily cleaning of room
Room temperature
Noise level in and around room
Television, call button, etc. working
Courtesy of housekeeping personnel

Diet and Meals

Explanations given regarding diet
Temperature of food
Quality of food
Variety of menu
Likelihood getting what you ordered

Nursing Care

Nurses' courtesy
Nurses' promptness in responding
Nurses' attitude toward call
Nurses' attention to special needs
Participate in setting personal goals
Sensitivity/responsiveness to pain
Nurses' instructions regarding home care and medications
Quality of day shift (7 A.M.–3 P.M.)
Quality of evening shift (3 P.M.–11 P.M.)
Quality of night shift (11 P.M.–7 A.M.)
How well nurses kept you informed
Availability of the nurses

Physical Therapy

Courtesy of physical therapist
Participate in setting physical patient goals
Physical therapist explained treatment and progress
Adequacy of physical therapy program
How well physical therapist helped to meet goals

Occupational Therapy

Courtesy of occupational therapist
Participate in setting occupational therapy goals
Occupational therapist explained treatment and progress
Adequacy of occupational therapy program
How well occupational therapist helped meet goals

Recreation Therapy

Courtesy and responsiveness to needs
Availability of recreational activity
Instructions/information on postdischarge activity

Psychology

Courtesy of psychologist
Psychologist concerned regarding patient's problems

Psychologist helpful regarding rehabilitation adjustment

Speech Therapy

Courtesy of speech therapist
Participate in setting speech therapy goals
Speech therapist explained treatment and progress
Adequacy of speech therapy program
How well speech therapist helped meet goals

Other Services

Volunteers

Staff who escorted you to and from room
Laboratory personnel
Respiratory therapy
Audiology
Prosthetics/orthotics service
Business office
Patient and family education programs
Telephone operators

Visitors and Family

Courtesy of people at information desk
Adequacy of visiting hours
Accommodations/comfort for visitors
Staff attitudes toward visitors
Information given to family regarding condition and treatment
Adequacy of signs in hospital

Rehabilitation physician

Physician explained rehabilitation program
Courtesy of physician
Physician's concern regarding questions and worries
Physician kept informed regarding treatment and progress
Sensitivity and responsiveness to pain
Physician informative regarding family
Physician discussed discharge plans
Availability of rehabilitation physician

Social Worker and Discharge

Courtesy of social worker
Social worker responsive to needs
Social worker assisted in discharge
Amount of notice given regarding discharge
Adequacy of equipment recommended
Training given regarding home care
Patient discharge information packet
Staff explained discharge plans
Assistance with postdischarge

Final Ratings

Staff explained what stay would be like
Overall cheerfulness of hospital
Overall cleanliness of hospital
Staff sensitivity to inconvenience
Staff had positive attitude
Staff did not push too hard

Continued

Box 12-1   PRESS GANEY PATIENT SATISFACTION SURVEY—cont'd

Care/treatment well coordinated
Staff concern for privacy
Rehabilitation program helped you meet goals
Likelihood of recommending hospital
Staff sensitivity: spiritual needs
Training given you/family for home
Overall care at hospital
Staff worked together
Pain controlled
Degree to which staff treated you with respect

Staff concerned not to frighten child
Staff efforts included you in decisions
Degree of safety and security felt
Accuracy of information received regarding service
Staff concern for questions and worries
Staff promptness; response to requests
Overall Assessment

Staff prepared you to function at home
Staff prepared you to function in community

(From Press Ganey. Used with permission.)

Box 12-2   "HOW ARE WE DOING" MEETINGS?

Who Should Participate?

Include all staff members involved in the present process or program, if appropriate. An example would be if you had an increase in the patient dissatisfaction when admitted on the evening shift, you may only need to include members of the patient care team from that shift.

When Should the Meetings Be Held?

The meetings should be held as soon as the outcome data are available. Patient satisfaction data are available on a weekly or monthly basis for many institutions. It is important to be able to react to the performance data in a timely manner. If you are reviewing patient satisfaction data that is over 6 months old, the time for action is long past! Many clinical outcome measures (Core Measures) are available on a quarterly basis. Preferably, meetings should be coordinated with the data availability schedule. The meetings should also be done regardless of the level of performance. Organizational learning can always occur, even in the best performing institutions.

How Should the Outcome Data Be Used?

Provide the latest reports to the attendees in advance, so they will know what they will need to react to.

Make sure that the data are presented in a way that is understandable to all. Do not just give them data sets ... put it in readable format. Many hospitals have in-service education on topics such as dealing with data.

What Kinds of Data Are Most Useful?

Compare recent performance to past performance or intended benchmarks or targets. Make sure that the data are reflective of the outcomes on your particular unit.

What if There Are Poor Outcomes?

Do not enter the meeting with an attitude of blame. Present the data in a matter-of-fact manner, and work with the staff to brainstorm possible ways to improve. Always keep the meeting on a positive note.

What if There Are Good Outcomes?

Congratulate the staff on a "job well done." Identify "best practices" that can be shared with the rest of the institution and begin work with the rest of the institution to share this practice. Continue to evaluate and motivate staff to high performance. Remember, complacency can lead to lackluster performance.

What Are the Next Steps?

If additional work and time are needed, create a plan to continue work.

(Adapted from The Urban Institute. (2004). *Using outcome information: making data pay off* (p. 14). Washington, DC: Author: Exhibit 7. Used with permission.)

of "How are we doing?" Most commercial patient satisfaction surveys will rate potential areas of improvement that are statistically significant—that is, those areas that will benefit most from some extra attention. Sometimes the information provided makes sense to the staff. For example, a less-than-stellar result in the patient's perception of "caring attitude by staff" may be the result of a week of higher-than-expected patient acuity accentuated by two snowstorms where staff had difficulty actually getting to work. Sometimes, though, the nurse manager may have difficulty seeking an explanation for unexpected or unusual outcomes. There are a number of ways that you can seek explanations for unexpected outcomes.

- Talk with individual staff and supervisors.
- Review patient responses to survey type questions to see if you can glean any information.
- Hold a staff meeting to review the results.
  - Staff meetings regarding performance outcomes should be routinely done, even if results are excellent or meeting targets.
- Form a focus group to identify the concern.
  - Give focus group permission to identify a potential resolution (based on data and best practice).

Do not jump to conclusions based solely on the data. Data do not tell you what caused the problem; the outcome data only identify the results. There are often processes that need to be improved. The data must be shared with the individuals involved in the process, and performance improvement meetings must be held if improvements are required.

When you are holding a staff meeting to review performance, consider the areas of discussion presented in Box 12-2.

SUMMARY

It is important for nurses to be aware of the actual level of performance based on the data. We may think that we are delivering patient-focused care, but without the data collected from the patient and family, we are really assuming the outcomes. The important results are usually determined by the organization. These results balance value for all of the key stakeholders of the organization—patients, their families, the workforce, the community, the payors, and the public.

CLINICAL CORNER

Improving Performance Based on Data— The Role of the Advance Practice Nurse
Mary Jo Assi

Acute Myocardial Infarction Door to Balloon Time

The clinical quality advance practice nurse (APN) at The Valley Hospital responsible for the acute myocardial infarction (AMI) Core Measure found that performance was not meeting goal. She then initiated weekly meetings for stakeholders to work on systems and issues to improve elements of care. A primary area of concern for immediate intervention was our door-to-balloon time (D2B) for patients with ST-segment elevated myocardial infarction (STEMI). The requirement at the time to meet the Core Measure goal was 120 minutes or less. Our average time for year-end 2005 was 152 minutes. The two areas primarily responsible for care of the STEMI patient are the emergency department (ED) and cardiac catheterization laboratory (CCL). Although both had access to specific care data, neither

was in agreement as to reasons for delay in treatment. Nursing staff and physicians from both areas believed they were doing all they could to achieve timely care for these patients. In this instance, the APN acted as an objective clinical and systems expert. She analyzed the data, identified system failures, and worked with key stakeholders from both departments to create new systems to improve care and clarify individual and department accountability. These systems included a new process for triaging patients in the ED to obtain an ECG within 5 minutes; physician agreement to streamline the on-call process to one telephone call to activate the CCL team within 5 minutes; agreement that the CCL team be on-site within 30 minutes; and immediate transport to the CCL by ED staff when the CCL team is on-site. Once new practices were instituted, the efforts of nursing staff and physicians became immediately apparent. By year-end 2006, D2B had decreased to 96 minutes. With continued focus and improvement to systems, 2007 ended with an average D2B time of 66 minutes and a further reduction through third quarter 2008 to 58 minutes.

EVIDENCE-BASED PRACTICE

Hospitals Crack Down on Deadly Infections

Modified from Francis, T. (2007). Hospitals crack down on deadly infections. The Wall Street Journal, June 26.

Hard-to-treat, drug-resistant strains of methicillin-resistant *Staphylococcus aureus* (MRSA) have become increasingly common, accounting for more than 60% of hospital staph infections. Patients with already strained immune systems are dying from these worrisome infections, and hospitals are working to prevent the spread of these infections through early identification and isolation of infected patients. While expensive, officials at Newark Beth Israel Medical Center are saying early efforts to identify patients are well worth the cost and have decreased new MRSA infections to almost zero and cut ICU patients who carry the bug from 33% to 10% in about 6 months. University of Maryland Medical Center is reporting similar results and reports that the surveillance efforts pay for themselves in prevention of costly infections. "Active surveillance" involves the screening of all patients, symptomatic and asymptomatic, when they enter the hospital. New equipment for the rapid scanning of samples is expensive but is being proved beneficial as infected patients are isolated earlier, making it less likely the bug will spread. The hospitals currently screening all patients for MRSA, approximately 28% nationwide, support their decision with an anticipated decrease in the use of vancomycin, decreased number of infections, increased patient satisfaction, decreased length of stay, and decreased infections in already weakened patients. The hospitals using the rapid scanning technology anticipate that the equipment and staff will pay for themselves in the infections they prevent.

Previously, the Centers for Disease Control and Prevention (CDC) estimated that 3.95 of every 1000 patients discharged from a hospital had been diagnosed with MRSA; more recent statistics suggest the numbers to be as high as 34 of 1000 discharged patients are infected with MRSA and at least another 12 per 1000 carry the organism without active infection. The CDC estimates that 126,000 patients are hospitalized with MRSA infections each year; 5000 of these patients will die, costing $4 billion annually in health care costs. It is seen that MRSA is no longer confined to ICUs, as it was in the beginning, and that MRSA infections are on the rise. With measures as simple as hand washing, MRSA infections in hospitals could be significantly decreased when hand washing is combined with isolation of infected patients and the use of gowns and gloves during the care of these infected patients.

NCLEX® EXAM QUESTIONS

1. What are the uses of outcome information?
   1. Detect needed improvements and motivate and assist staff.
   2. Plan daily schedule on unit and detect needed improvements.
   3. Evaluate staff for errors and discuss remediation.
   4. Provide staff support and evaluate negative behaviors.
2. Nursing data fall into four domains:
   1. client care, provider staffing, administrative, and research
   2. client care, billing, administrative, and research
   3. core values, provider staffing, administrative, and research
   4. core values, billing, administrative, and reports
3. Mechanisms related to resource identification and allocation have to be driven by internal data, and information systems that consider all domains of hospital data include:
   1. clinical, fiscal, administrative, and patient satisfaction data
   2. classification, financial, administrative, and patient satisfaction data
   3. clinical, financial, social, and patient satisfaction data
   4. clinical, financial, administrative, and patient satisfaction data.
4. The most common performance indicator reviewed by nurses on a routine basis is the patient satisfaction report. Included in this report is:
   1. the level of satisfaction of all discharged patients
   2. the nursing perception of care delivered to the patients surveyed

3. the waiting time for admission compared with peers
4. a listing of items that will result in improvements
5. The main purpose of data collected for a performance indicator is so that the organization can:
   1. reflect on its performance
   2. improve its performance
   3. compare with peers
   4. educate poor performers
6. Common satisfaction data provide results in information about all of the following EXCEPT:
   1. accessibility
   2. communication skills
   3. personality and demeanor
   4. efficiency of family member in care of patient
7. One driving force for increasing patient satisfaction is:
   1. clinical benefits
   2. community benefits
   3. classification benefits
   4. management benefits
8. Clinical benefits regarding satisfaction surveys include all of the following EXCEPT:

1. greater patient trust and acceptance with treatment plans
2. increasing buy-in for treatment plans more quickly, making best use of scarce physician time
3. increasing trust, which allows physician to discover more factors that may affect the care needs of the patient
4. evaluating patient outcomes
9. Risk management benefits regarding satisfaction surveys include:
   1. reduced incident reports
   2. reduced patient falls
   3. reduced medication errors
   4. reduced likelihood of malpractice litigation
10. Marketing and promotional benefits with respect to satisfaction surveys include all of the following EXCEPT:
    1. increased likelihood for being referred for services
    2. improving word-of-mouth promotion of your organization
    3. reduced provider staff stress and turnover
    4. better comparison against competitors

Answers: 1. 2   2. 1   3. 4   4. 4   5. 1   6. 4   7. 1   8. 3   9. 4   10. 3

REFERENCES

Huber, D. (2006). *Leadership and nursing care management*. Philadelphia, PA: Elsevier.

North Mississippi Medical Center. (2007). Retrieved September 8, 2008, from http://baldrige.nist.gov/PDF_files/NMMC_Application_Summary.pdf

Press Ganey. (2007). Patient satisfaction survey. Retrieved November 30, 2007, from www.pressganey.com.

The Urban Institute. (2004). *Using outcome information: making data pay off*. Washington, DC: Author.

Organizational Planning

It is vital to realize that while health care is seen as a compassionate calling for many, the delivery of health care is indeed a business. As a business, there are organizational requirements of budgetary planning and financial constraints. Health care in the United States is a labor- and dollar-intensive business, with the actual delivery of patient care forming the largest basis of the financial requirements. Nurses are in a major position to assist the organization in the areas of strategic planning, budgetary planning, and oversight. The nurses' unique knowledge of the day-to-day demands of patient care as well as the future needs of the community is an important variable in the strength of an organization.

This section deals with strategic planning and financial planning.

CHAPTER 13

Strategic Management and Planning

Chapter Objectives

1. Define *strategic management* and *strategic planning.*
2. Discuss the importance of the strategic planning process.
3. Identify the components of the strategic plan.
4. Compare and contrast the various types of strategic planning processes.
5. Distinguish between short- and long-term plans and objectives.
6. Identify the role of the nurse manager in the strategic planning process.

Definitions

Mission Statement defining the purpose of the organization

Vision Future-oriented statement of where the organization sees itself

Values Philosophy or behaviors determined to be vital to the organization

Environmental scan Analysis of the political, demographic, social, regulatory, and technological environments of the organization

Goals Statement of direction of the organization

Objectives Measurable statements related to the goals of the organization

Strategic context Competitive environment of the organization

Stakeholders All groups that may be affected by an organization's services, actions, and outcomes

Performance measures Quantitative tools that allow for measurement of the achievement of goals

WHAT IS STRATEGIC PLANNING?

Simply put, *strategic planning* is the process by which an organization/nursing department or unit decides where it is going over the next year or longer and how it is going to get there. Typically, the process is organization-wide and the outcome of the process that, on an organizational level, cascades down to the patient care department and the individual units and employees. The *strategic plan* is the "map" of where the organi-

zation, department, or unit is going over the next year or longer.

Strategic management is the process of setting goals and objectives for the organization/department/unit, determining the resources that are necessary to meet the goals, creating an action plan, and evaluating progress towards meeting the goals.

Strategic planning used to be the domain of the financial managers of many institutions. This philosophy has changed, and strategic planning now includes all stakeholders of the organization. Nurse managers have an important role in the strategic plan of the organization and in the implementation of action plans at the unit level that assist the organization in meeting its goals.

Managers of an organization need to focus on a series of key questions as they begin the strategic planning process (Finkler, Kovner, and Jones, 2007, p. 216):
- Why does the organization exist?
- What is the organization currently?
- What would it like to be?
- How can we make the transformation to what we want to be?
- How will we know when the transformation is done?

In answering these questions, the manager will find that the answers lead to other questions, such as, What are the strengths and challenges faced by the organization? What is its competitive status? Who are the primary stakeholders for the organization? How does the organization measure its performance? How does it learn from its performance?

ELEMENTS OF A STRATEGIC PLAN

The elements of a strategic plan include the following (Finkler et al., 2007, p. 217):
- Mission statement
- Statement of competitive challenges and strategy
- Statement of short- and long-term goals
- Statement of organizational policies
- Statement of needed resources
- Statement of key assumptions

MISSION AND VISION STATEMENTS

The first step in strategic management is the development of a mission statement for the organization. The mission statement focuses on the definition of what the organization does and aspires to do. The mission statement for some organizations is further divided into a vision, which tells the reader where the organization wants to be in the future. Many organizations also create a values statement, which includes the behaviors of importance within the organization. Some organizations include the mission, vision, and values statement in one document.

For example, the simple mission of North Mississippi Medical Center (NMMC) (2007) is:
- To continuously improve the health of the people of our region.

The corresponding vision statement of this organization is:
- To be the provider of the best patient-centered care services in America
  And the values of this organization are:
- Compassion • Accountability • Respect • Excellence • Smile (CARES)
  According to NMMC (2007):
- NMMC'S purpose is to provide compassionate health care with optimal outcomes and NMMC's Mission reflects the organization's secure roots in the communities it serves. Its ambitious Vision reflects a deeply-held commitment to excellence in every activity. The CARES Values acronym (Compassion • Accountability • Respect • Excellence • Smile) expresses NMMC's focus on exceptional customer service.

Some organizations use critical success factors as the organizing framework by which the mission, vision, and values are translated into the strategic plan. One commonly used framework is from the Studer Group, a health care consulting group that works with many health care organizations in the country. To continue with the example of NMMC:
- The Mission and Vision are translated into measurable actions through the CRITICAL SUCCESS FACTORS (CSFs): PEOPLE, SERVICE, QUALITY, FINANCIAL, GROWTH. The order of the CSFs is intentional. It starts with creating an environment that draws and nurtures the best PEOPLE to provide the best SERVICE. Great SERVICE results in happy customers and excellent QUALITY. High QUALITY and efficiency produce good FINANCIAL results and requests for more services, which results in GROWTH. All activities are organized and managed according to the CSFs, thereby creating organizational alignment and a comprehensive structure for operational excellence.

These critical success factors are also called pillars by many institutions, and in some organizations a sixth pillar, COMMUNITY, is included (Studer Group, 2008).

STATEMENT OF COMPETITIVE ENVIRONMENT AND STRATEGY

As part of the strategic planning process, it is vital for an organization to be aware of its competitive environment. This is accomplished through strategic analysis.

Sometimes, this is also called an *environmental scan*. This activity can include conducting a review of the organization's environment (e.g., a review of the political, social, economic and technical environment). Planners carefully consider various driving forces in the environment, such as increasing competition, changing demographics, and so forth. Planners also look at the various strengths, weaknesses, opportunities, and threats regarding the organization; an acronym for this activity is SWOT. As nurse managers, you will participate in the patient satisfaction initiatives of your institution. Most nurses are aware of the performance of the other units in the hospital in relation to patient satisfaction, and some are aware of the performance of the similar units in the area. An example of changing demographics and their impact on hospital planning would be a population shift to large numbers of families moving into the local area served by the institution. This information from the environmental scan might result in a facility increasing the number of services for a pediatric population. An example of technical and regulatory changes occurring is the electronic medical record, which has been strongly recommended by the Institute of Medicine as a means of decreasing hospital errors.

Other information collected for the strategic planning process comes from past performance and information collected from all stakeholders through a variety of means. These involve satisfaction surveys (patient, employees, physicians, community), focus groups with members of the community to determine issues of importance, and other means of listening to the expressed desires of the local community.

The *competitive strategy* is the organization's plan for achieving its goals. It states what services will be provided to whom. It is decided on as a direct result of the information provided by the strategic analysis and environmental scan. The organization evaluates its mission, vision, and goals in light of the information provided by the environmental scan, the identified strengths and challenges, and the demand for service. Based on this competitive strategy, the organization makes a plan that allows it to take advantage of the identified strengths and needs of the various stakeholders. The product of this process is conclusions about what the organization must do as a result of the major issues and opportunities facing the organization. These conclusions include the overall accomplishments (or *strategic goals*) the organization should achieve.

STATEMENT OF SHORT- AND LONG-TERM GOALS

According to Carter McNamara, the long- and short-term goals are the overall methods (or *strategies*) to achieve the strategic goals of the organization. An example of a short-term goal of an organization might be to improve performance on the Core Measure for Cardiac Failure, increasing from 80% to 85% compliance by the end of the year. A long-term goal might be to consistently perform at 98% to 100% at the end of 3 years. Goals should be designed and worded as much as possible to be **S**pecific, **M**easurable, **A**cceptable to those working to achieve the goals, **R**ealistic, **T**imely, **E**xtending the capabilities of those working to achieve the goals, and **R**ewarding to them, as well. (A mnemonic for these criteria is "SMARTER.")

Action Planning

Action planning is the process by which the specific goals are matched with each strategic goal. The overall organization-wide strategic goals cascade down to all departments and units and, in some cases, the individual employees. Action planning requires specifying expected outcomes with each strategic goal. These outcomes then form the basis of the performance scorecards used in most organizations. The anticipated outcomes are usually based on the competitive strategy of the organization and are often benchmarked against "best in class performers" or to where the organization wants to be in terms of performance.

Often, each objective is associated with a *tactic*, which is one of the methods needed to reach an objective. Therefore, implementing a strategy typically involves implementing a set of tactics along the way—in that sense, a tactic is still a strategy but on a smaller scale.

Action planning also includes specifying *responsibilities* and *timelines* with each objective, or who needs to do what and by when. It should also include methods to *monitor* and *evaluate* the plan, which includes knowing how the organization will know who has done what and by when.

It is common to develop an *annual plan* (sometimes called the *operational plan* or *management plan*), which includes the strategic goals, strategies, objectives, responsibilities, and timelines that should be implemented in the coming year. These are the short-term goals of the organization. The difference between short- and long-term plans and objectives relates to the time expected to accomplish them. These times vary from institution to institution, but short-term plans usually extend up to 1 year. Long-term plans vary from 3 to 5 years.

Usually, *budgets* are included in the strategic and annual plan, and with individual departmental and unit plans. Budgets specify the funds needed for the resources that are necessary to implement the annual plan. Budgets also depict how the funds will be spent. (See Chapter 14 for information on budgets.)

The strategic planning process of NMMC is diagrammed in Figure 13-1, and an example of their broad strategic plan is shown in Figure 13-2. Note that the goals are formulated according to the critical success factors identified by the organization. The performance indicators list the measures that will be used to measure progress toward achievement of the goals. The benchmarks relate the performance of the competitors or "best in class," and the targets are the short- and long-term goals.

As this organizational plan cascades down to the departments and units, it becomes more specific with action plans and timelines for measures of achievement. The action plan in Figure 13-3 includes goals that

match the overall organizational goal but are much more department specific. Also note the action steps and the outcome results.

UNIT-BASED PLANNING PROCESS

Planning typically includes several major activities or steps in the process. Different organizations often have different names for these major activities and often conduct them in different orders. Strategic planning is very individualized according to the organization.

On a unit-based level, the nurse manager will oversee the unit-based planning process. Things to accomplish include the following:

1. **Identify your purpose (mission statement)**—The mission statement for your unit should carefully mirror that of the overall organization. Remember; it is important that all levels of the organization are "on the same page." If the unit goals are different than those of the organization, there is a potential conflict.

2. **Select the goals your organization must reach if it is to accomplish your mission**—The unit and

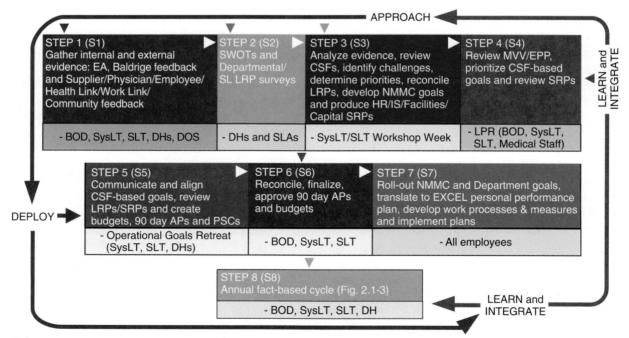

Figure 13-1 • The strategic planning process of North Mississippi Medical Center. North Mississippi Medical Center. (2006). Application for the Malcolm Baldrige Performance Excellence Award. Retrieved October 23, 2007, from http:// baldrige.nist.gov/PDF_files/NMMC_Application_Summary.pdf.

NMMC Performance Scorecard					
CSF	**Goals**	**Performance indicators**	**Benchmark**	**2006 Target**	**2011 Target**
People	Maintain a high quality workforce	Retention rate (RB) (7.4-2)	94.4%	89%	93%
Service	Improve customer service	Inpatient satisfaction (RB) (7.2-1)	90th %tile	90th %tile	95th %tile
		Outpatient satisfaction (RB) (7.2-6)	90th %tile	85th %tile	90th %tile
		ESD satisfaction (RB) (7.2-7)	90th %tile	75th %tile	80th %tile
Quality	Improve prevention and health education services				
	Improve health outcomes	Composite quality score (RB) (7.1-20)	90th %tile	90th %tile	95th %tile
Financial	Produce financial resources required to support mission and vision	BAR (RB) (7.3-10)	N/A	80	80
		Productivity by pay period (RB) (7.5-2)	5.22	5.5	5.0
		Cost per adjusted discharge (RB) (7.3-9)	$9,178	$9,900	$8,500
Growth	Expand access to health services	Inpatient total market share (GB) (7.3-15)	N/A	45%	47%
		Outpatient total market share (GB)	N/A	56%	58%
		Active medical staff members (GB) (7.6-1)	N/A	260	280

Figure 13-2 • An example of their broad strategic plan. North Mississippi Medical Center. (2006). Application for the Malcolm Baldrige Performance Excellence Award. Retrieved October 23, 2007, from http://baldrige.nist.gov/PDF_files/NMMC_Application_Summary.pdf.

Sample 90-day Action Plan • Women's and Children's Service Line (1/06-3/06)			
CSF	**Goal**	**Action steps**	**90 Day result report**
People	Maintain FT turnover rate	• Leader rounding x2 areas each day • Review rounding informateion at weekly manager meetings. • Implement 90-day AP with direct reports.	• Turnover rate at >1.6% • One 90-day AP per unit
Service	Acheive 90th percentile on inpatient satisfaction	• Nurse rounding • Bi-weekly meeting with Women/Children's patient satisfaction team	• 90th percentile or higher in patient satisfaction
Quality	Reduce practice variation in DRG 372, 373	• Physician champion identified • OM to perform CPA DRG 372-373 • PA to perform documentation analysis	• Decrease DRG 372 LOS • Assure appropriate DRG assignment
	Pediatric asthma	• Physician champion identified • Perform CPA on asthma DRG	• Decrease readmissions for pediatric asthma patients
Financial	Maintain expenses within budget	• Review OB/GYN financials with OBs • Nurse managers analyze and report OT needs to SLL	• BAR at or above 80 • Overtime below 3.0% • Expenses below budget
Growth	Develop a vision for pediatric services	• Set up meeting with LeBonheur Children's Hospital to discuss increase in pediatric subspecialties • Develop cost-benefit analysis with marketing for branding of pediatric services	• Presented draft of vision to March SLOG • Pediatric branding identified and cost-benefit reported to SLOG w/in 30 days
	Implement Women/Children's Community Advisory Board	• Recruit Advisory Board members • Develop agenda for first meeting	• First Advisory Board meeting March, 2006

Figure 13-3 • Action plan. North Mississippi Medical Center. (2006). Application for the Malcolm Baldrige Performance Excellence Award. Retrieved October 23, 2007, from http://baldrige.nist.gov/PDF_files/NMMC_Application_Summary.pdf.

personal goals of each employee must relate to accomplishment of the mission of the unit and organization.

3. **Identify specific approaches or strategies that must be implemented to reach each goal**—

Identify realistic activities that you and your staff will do to accomplish the goals.

4. **Identify specific action plans to implement each strategy**—This is where you would identify the things necessary for you and your staff to achieve

the goals. This is related to the development of the budget to assist you in the identification of resources necessary to achieve the goals.

5. **Monitor and update the plan**—As you see in the department plan, there is a 90-day monitoring of results. The careful monitoring of performance allows you and your unit to determine if your action plans are working or if they need reworking. Most strategic plans are fluid documents allowing for changes to be made as necessary.

As a nurse you will also deal with action plans that address The Joint Commission Core Measures (see Chapter 10), the National Patient Safety Goals (see Chapter 10), or particular issues of concern with your institution. Action plans for specific clinical concerns are usually managed by the performance improvement department of clinical department, but it is important that the nurse manager and staff are aware of these action plans and their role in the achievement of the overall organizational goal. An example of an action plan for a clinical goal is shown in Figure 13-4.

PURPOSES OF PLANNING

* Increases the chances of success by focusing on results and not on activities
* Forces analytical thinking and evaluation of alternatives
* Establishes a framework for decision making that is consistent with organizational strategic objectives
* Includes day-to-day and future-focused managing
* Helps to avoid crisis management and provides decision-making flexibility
* Provides a basis for managing organizational and individual performance (Rousel et al., 2006)

SUMMARY

Strategic planning is a continually evolving process in most organizations, with constant monitoring of performance to goal, achievement of strategic objectives,

---

Sample APs for Clinical Goal (Others AOS)
Goal

Overall: Improve clinical processes and outcomes
Specific: Improve tracheostomy management and outcomes

▼

Action Plans

Overall: Analyze and manage tracheostomy (perform CPA)
Specific:
* Implement structured monitoring of processes
* Analyze and improve processes with physicians and team
* Automate process improvements through order sets and protocols
* Educate staff on changes

▼

Performance Indicators

In-Process: patients receive:
* DVT and stress ulcer prophylaxis
* Ventilator weaning protocol
* Nutrition protocol
* Multidisciplinary team rounds
Outcomes: Inpatient mortality (decreased), CCU and overall LOS (decreased), cost of care (decreased)

Figure 13-4 • An example of an action plan for a clinical goal. North Mississippi Medical Center. (2006). Application for the Malcolm Baldrige Performance Excellence Award. Retrieved October 23, 2007, from http://baldrige.nist.gov/PDF_files/NMMC_Application_Summary.pdf.

---

and updating of the plan as changes occur within the environment. As a nurse manager, it is your responsibility to always be aware of the plan and your role in the plan and, as a staff nurse, to be aware of your role in assisting the organization and your unit in the achievement of the strategic goals.

CLINICAL CORNER

The Chief Nursing Officer's Role as Participant in Strategic Planning

Bonnie Michaels

Strategic planning is a process in which senior management, medical staff leadership, and hospital leadership remain focused on approved, planned initiatives and priorities set forth through the established mission, vision, and values of an organization. Typically, a plan is representative of the immediate future for the next 3 to 5 years.

I am employed as the chief nursing officer (CNO) of an organization that was previously a not-for-profit hospital, one hospital of a three-hospital system. The hospital was sold to an investor-owned for-profit entity. Within the first year of this new organization, there was clearly an identified need to formulate a new culture; design a new mission, vision, and values; and develop a new identity as a stand-alone organization. At the time of the acquisition, new departments had to be developed because the previous corporate environment consolidated support services in financial, billing, purchasing, food services, and other key support departments. All of a sudden, those in the new organization had to fend for themselves and create these needed resources as a foundation to support the clinical provision of care. Not having its own identity, the organization was thought to be the answer to everyone's needs. Expectations were high that being a stand-alone would better support the medical staff community's wants and needs and be the end-all answer for all previously identified concerns.

Strategic planning priorities, goals, objectives, and strategies to ensure the perceived strengths of the organization evolved from data analysis, physician interviews, and department manager meetings. As members of the strategic planning committee—made up of key trustees, senior management, and department heads—we started by reviewing the hospital's previous mission and strategic direction. We needed to achieve new leadership consensus so that the new organization could continue to fulfill its mission to the community. The process included the following tasks and activities:

- Strategic planning committee appointments
- Environmental data collection and analysis
- Interviews with physicians and department managers regarding the current state and future direction of this organization's clinical programs and services

- Strategic planning committee meetings and discussions and acceptance regarding:
  - Preliminary findings and conclusions
  - Development options
  - Vision, mission, and values
  - Strategic goals, objectives, and action strategies
  - Draft of a plan and executive summary for board review and approval
  - Need for facility planning and prioritizing needed plant improvements

The process made extensive use of input from trustees, medical staff, and administrators, who invested significant time analyzing data and discussing our new identity.

We also examined this hospital's demographics, payor mix, declining hospital profit margins in the state, and increasing neighboring hospital closures. We evaluated physician supply projections, looking at primary care physician need as the initial point of patient access into the health care system. Continuity of patient care requires well-trained high-quality inpatient and outpatient programs and facilities where nurses and clinicians can practice in a financially viable environment. And we projected a surplus of physician specialists and identified individual specialties for which recruitment was needed. To ensure continuity of health care in the community, primary care physicians and their close locations are particularly important as a referral base for physician specialists.

The strategic planning committee also evaluated competition of local facilities for inpatient and low-cost ambulatory care services, which included numerous physician-owned ambulatory surgery, imaging, and rehabilitation and pain management centers. We asked the question if we should be in direct competition with our physicians who owned or shared ownership of these facilities.

We evaluated our medical and nursing teaching programs and surveyed our patient catchment area and our community residents to ensure our reputation for providing high-quality patient care and the community's perception of that care. In addition, we identified issues of gaps in clinical services, the level of physician "in-network" participation, and whether there had been any erosion of referring physician loyalty and morale as a result of change in ownership. Demographic trends also reflected an aging population that are in or are close to retirement and the potential increase in chronic illnesses and the associated demand for chronic illness disease care and geriatric care.

Continued

Not always typical but important to us was employee morale. With the changes in ownership came changes in benefits and pension programs. We were fortunate that most employees elected to maintain their commitment to the new organization and community, ensuring a high level of nursing expertise that would have been a great loss to our community. We found our staff to be vested in our organization and engaged to continue to work together. They seemed to survive the unknown over the last 2 years, and middle management was identified as the talented group that was the glue that held the organization together during the rumors and due-diligence process.

We were able to develop our new mission, vision, and values with consensus building. We developed clear new standards regarding our new pillars of quality, service, integrity, people, growth, and cost. We communicate and measure these pillars in monthly reports to our board of trustees, our investors, our employees, and affiliated physicians. Communication has been enhanced because all members of the senior management team have made themselves available and visible and accessible to our physicians and staff. We are now known as an organization that is responsive to all of our constituencies and that strives to ensure a financially strong organization, with frontline staff aware that everyone can make a contribution to decreasing cost and ensuring the highest quality care. We openly measure these initiatives daily, monthly, and annually and ask for consistent feedback to ensure we are on the designated path to success. We live and breathe our strategic plan as a living document and a new culture, and as a tribute to what can be accomplished in a new thriving organization.

EVIDENCE-BASED PRACTICE

Creating a Future Worth Experiencing: Nursing Strategic Planning in an Integrated Health Care Delivery System

Drenkard, K. N. (2001). Creating a future worth experiencing: nursing strategic planning in an integrated health care delivery system. Journal of Nursing Administration, 31, *364-376. Inova Health System, Falls Church, VA, karen.drenkard@inova.com.*

It is a challenging time to be a nurse leader. Projections of a sustained nurse shortage, increasingly complex patient situations, dwindling resources, increasing technology demands, and a complicated managed care picture can change challenges into overwhelming events. A comprehensive and cohesive plan to address diverse and root causes of the problem is required.

Strategic planning is a process by which the guiding members of an organization envision its future and develop the necessary procedures and operations to achieve that future. The nurse executive team of a large nonprofit health care system undertook this process.

The steps in the strategic planning process were based on a business planning model, yet they allowed some flexibility in design. The major areas of the model include:
- Assessment of the current state
- Creation of a vision
- Gap analysis between the current state and the vision
- Plan making and priority setting using quality tools
- Engagement and meeting of nurses in the planning process
- Baseline measurements and target setting
- Refinement of the implementation plans
- Evaluation of outcomes

On completing the strategic planning process, reflection is necessary. Reflection is critical to evaluate every challenge in nursing. As part of the evaluation process, a time to review "lessons learned" is incorporated into the work plan.

Some of the lessons learned in the nursing strategic planning process include the following:
- *Get going:* There may never be a good time to start, so "Just start."
- *Keep the momentum alive:* Be confident enough as a nursing leader to "Take the lead." Momentum is important so that nurses know you are making progress.
- *Be prepared for some resistance:* Partnerships with finance, human resources, medical staff, and nursing managers all contribute to removing some resistance and creating movement toward reaching the vision.
- *Involve all stakeholders:* Inclusion of the appropriate stakeholders in the work is critical.
- *Find a way to fit it all on one page:* A concise summarization of the plan that outlines the process is necessary.

EVIDENCE-BASED PRACTICE—cont'd

- *Measure, evaluate, regroup, and update:* Flexible plans are critical, and rigor and discipline in the evaluation and measurement process are key.

A strategic plan for nursing will not necessarily eliminate difficulties of the future or make tough challenges go away. However, strategy can drive innovation, it can better integrate the parts, and it can secure synchronization from disparate players on the same team. A plan helps point the team in the same direction. We face the future more prepared by driving toward the changes in a proactive, strategic outcomes–oriented way.

NCLEX® EXAM QUESTIONS

1. The mission of an organization:
   1. sets the competitive tone
   2. states what is done by the organization
   3. measures the performance of a unit
   4. defines the philosophy of an institution
2. The vision of an organization is:
   1. a statement defining the purpose of the organization
   2. a future-oriented statement of where the organization sees itself
   3. philosophy or behaviors determined to be vital to the organization
   4. analysis of the political, demographic, and social environment of the organization
3. The purpose of an environmental scan is to assist the organization in:
   1. the setting of strategic goals
   2. measuring competitive performance
   3. developing an awareness of the social and regulatory arena
   4. determining short- and long-term business objectives
4. Strategic planning does not include:
   1. a plan to decide where the organization will go in the next year
   2. an organization-wide plan
   3. effects on patient care and patient units
   4. a community plan
5. Managers of an organization need to focus on a series of key questions as they begin the strategic planning process, including all of the following EXCEPT:
   1. Why does the organization exist?
   2. What is the organization currently?
   3. What would the organization like to be?
   4. What was included in the organizations past?
6. The mission and vision are translated into measurable actions through the critical success factors (CSFs), which include:

   1. people, service, quality, financial, and growth
   2. people, service, quality, function, and growth
   3. public, service, quality, financial, and growth
   4. people, safety, quality, financial, and growth
7. Another name for strategic analysis is a(n):
   1. economic environment
   2. environmental scan
   3. review analysis
   4. social climate
8. _____ are included in the strategic and annual plan and with individual departmental and unit plans.
   1. Resources
   2. Budgets
   3. Spreadsheets
   4. Word documents
9. Action plans for specific clinical concerns are usually managed by the performance improvement department, but it is also important that the following individuals are aware of these action plans and their role in the achievement of the overall organizational goal:
   1. nurse managers, clinical department, and staff nurses
   2. risk managers, purchasing department, and nursing assistants
   3. nurse manager, risk manager, and president
   4. nurse manager, nursing assistants, and risk manager
10. On a unit-based level, the nurse manager will oversee the unit-based planning process. Which of the following is seen as an item to be accomplished?
   1. Identify your mission statement and specific action plan to implement each strategy.
   2. Identify unit-specific policies, procedures, and protocols.
   3. Evaluate staffing needs and change as needed.
   4. Evaluate your vision and identify policies.

Answers: 1. 2   2. 2   3. 3   4. 4   5. 4   6. 1   7. 2   8. 2   9. 1   10. 1

REFERENCES

Finkler, S., Kovner, C., & Jones, C. (2007). *Financial management for nurse managers* (3rd ed.). Philadelphia: W.B. Saunders.

McNamara, C. (Authenticity Consulting, LLC). Copyright © 1997-2006. Adapted from the Field Guide to Nonprofit Strategic Planning and Facilitation. Retrieved October 23, 2007, from http://www.managementhelp.org/plan_dec/str_plan/models.htm.

North Mississippi Medical Center. (2006). Application for the Malcolm Baldrige Performance Excellence Award. Retrieved October 23, 2007, from http://baldrige.nist.gov/PDF_files/NMMC_Application_Summary.pdf.

Rousel, L., Swansburg, R., & Swansburg, R. (Eds.). (2006). *Management and leadership for nurse administrators.* Sudbury, MA: Jones & Bartlett.

Studer, Q. (2003). *Hardwiring excellence: purpose, worthwile work, making a difference.* Gulf Breeze, FL: Fire Starter Publishing.

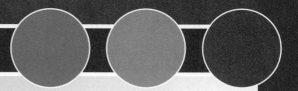

CHAPTER 14

Financial Management

Chapter Objectives

1. Define *budgeting*.
2. Differentiate between types of budgets.
3. Discuss the advantages of various budget processes.
4. Describe the key elements of budget preparation.
5. Identify the responsibilities of the nurse manager in budget preparation.
6. Discuss the responsibilities of the nurse manager in budget review.

Definitions

Budget Detailed financial plan for carrying out the activities of an organization or unit

Expenses Actual cost of activities undertaken by an organization

Revenues Income received for goods or services provided

Bottom line Income of an organization that is the result of revenue (money earned) minus expenses

Operating budget Financial plan for the day-to-day activities of the organization

Capital budget Financial plan that deals with purchases of capital assets (equipment, land, etc.)

Cash budget Financial plan that tracks cash received and spent

Cash on hand Amount of cash readily available to the organization

Direct costs Specific costs of a program; items that can be directly tied to a cost center and related to the care delivered by that cost center

Indirect costs Generalized costs (housekeeping, information technology, etc.) for support of the program and billed to the program; often called *support costs*

Variable costs Costs that vary in relation to volume and productivity

Fixed costs Costs unrelated to volume and productivity

Personnel budget Part of operating budget that deals with personnel needed to deliver care; composed of salary and benefit costs

Position control Monitoring tool used to compare actual numbers of full-time employees with the number budgeted to the control center

Budget variance Difference between actual budget and actual spending

BUDGETING PROCESS

Budget review and management represent one of the most important responsibilities of the nurse manager in this era of escalating health care costs and decreasing reimbursements. The economic stability of an organization depends on the management of the resources that are required to deliver care in a cost-effective and safe manner. Chapter 6 provided a review of the essentials of health care reimbursement.

Health care institutions are businesses, and one of the largest costs is the actual delivery of patient care. The resources required to deliver that patient care are costly and most often managed at the point of service (the unit). Nurses need to understand how to manage the cost of patient care as it relates to their clinical practice as well as to the workings of their particular unit. Also, accrediting agencies require collaborative input from staff in the development of annual budgets (The Joint Commission, 2007).

In most institutions, there is a well-defined process for the development, implementation, and evaluation of the budget. The budgeting process is a part of the overall *strategic planning process* (see Chapter 13). The organizational budget cascades down to individual departments and units. Budgets are usually developed annually for a 12-month period. The budget cycle is based on the organization's definition of the *fiscal year* (calendar [January 1–December 31] or fiscal [July 1–June 30]).

There are two major types of budgeting processes: zero-based budgeting and incremental budgeting. *Zero-based budgeting* requires the entire budget to be recreated annually starting from zero. This type of budgeting allows for the consideration of alternatives in the delivery of the service. All portions of the zero-based budget need to be justified annually. This type of budgeting also demands the proactive evaluation of the need for the services. *Incremental budgeting* is the more traditional approach, building on the previous year's budget. If there a 10% increase in funds is available, the budget may be increased by 10%. This is an easier process, but at times it allows budgets to become bloated with minimal justification of the service or at times it does not reflect the actual changes that may be anticipated for the unit.

The budgeting process can be divided into phases (Finkler and Kovner, 2001):
- Information gathering and planning
- Development of organizational and unit budgets
- Development of cash budgets, negotiation, and revision
- Evaluation

INFORMATION GATHERING AND PLANNING

In the information gathering and planning phase, the nurse manager is provided with data necessary to the development of the budget. An environmental assessment is done. This assessment provides the organization and the nurse manager with information about the changing needs of the community, changing professional requirements, economic changes that will affect the unit's function, community demographics, stakeholder needs and requirements, regulatory changes, and other items. This assessment provides the context of the needs that the unit budgets for during the next fiscal year. This environmental assessment provides the materials for the reassessment of the organization's mission, goals, and priorities. As organizational priorities are set, financial objectives are created, allocating resources to all units.

DEVELOPMENT OF ORGANIZATIONAL AND UNIT BUDGETS

Organizational and unit budgets are then created to match the financial objectives of the organization. It is important that both the financial and overall objectives of the particular unit are in concert with the organization-wide objectives and goals. The basic assumptions of the organization need to be part of the development of both organizational and unit objectives. Such assumptions may be the negotiated union contract raise for all employees, the cost of a new electronic record system, or similar items. Such assumptions are an important part of the development of the unit budget.

DEVELOPMENT OF CASH BUDGETS, NEGOTIATION, AND REVISION

The cash budget is developed after the operating and capital budgets of the unit or department are developed. It is at this stage that the unit manager's negotiating and revising skills come into play. This cash budget is usually prepared by the chief financial officer. It is the plan for the actual anticipated cash receipts and disbursements of the organization—the *cash flow*. An organization must have sufficient cash to meet its monthly obligations. Ideally, the nurse manager needs

HELPING HANDS HOSPITAL DASHBOARD RESULTS

	Q1	Q2	Q3	Annual Goal	Top 10%
QUALITY					
1. Overall patient satisfaction	88%	90%	93%	92%	95%
CORE MEASURES					
2. Acute Myocardial Infarction					
A. AMI Beta Blocker on discharge	90%	95%	98%	100%	100%
B. Smoking Cessation Advice/Counseling	98%	98%	100%	100%	100%
C. Heart Attack patients given aspirin on arrival	99%	98%	97%	100%	100%
D. Heart Attack patients given aspirin on discharge	100%	100%	100%	100%	100%
E. Heart Attack patients given thrombolytic medication within 30 min of arrival	100%	99%	100%	99%	100%
3. Surgical Care Improvement Project (SCIP)					
A. Surgery patients who received preventative antibiotic one hour before incision	94%	92%	91%	96%	98%
B. Surgery patients whose preventative antibiotic are appropriately selected	98%	92%	94%	96%	96%
FINANCIAL					
Days Cash on Hand	150	175	170	180	184
Inpatient net receivables (000s)	69,500	65,000	68,000	69,000 (per Qtr)	73,000 (per Qtr)
Average L.O.S.	4.1	3.9	4.3	3.9	3.85
Inpatient gross charges (000s)	70,000	68,000	69,500	70,050 (per Qtr)	75,000 (per Qtr)
Market Share	42%	48%	47%	49%	56%
PEOPLE					
Nursing Full Time Equivalents	400	385	396	400	400
Employee satisfaction (overall)	79%	82%	81%	88%	91%
Injury/Illness Last Time per 100 employees	5%	6%	4%	4%	2%

Interpretation   **Red** – below goal   Orange – within 2% of goal   **Green** – at goal   **Blue** – top 10% at goal

Figure 14-1 • An example of an organization-wide financial dashboard. Indiana Rural Health Association. (2008). *In patient scorecards.* Retrieved July 20, 2007, from http://www.indianaruralhealth.org/Sample%20Dashboard%20_(3_).pdf.

to be able to predict when budgeted items will be needed. Unexpected expenditures do occur and may put a strain on a cash-poor system.

EVALUATION

Evaluation of the budget occurs at both the organizational and unit levels. Many organizations have created dashboards that allow for monitoring of progress in meeting department goals. These dashboards provide a quick visual display of the unit's performance. An example of an organization-wide financial dashboard is shown in Figure 14-1. Evaluation of the budget performance is usually obtained through a process known as *variance analysis*. A positive variance (favorable) may be seen when the budgeted amount was greater than that which was actually spent. A negative variance may be seen if the budgeted amount was less than the actual spending. Variance analysis is a complex process in which the unit environment is fully investigated. A negative variance may be seen in the number of staff required during a 2-week period. However, on further investigation, it may be determined that the patient acuity was higher than anticipated, and expenses were increased in response to this increased acuity. It is the role of the nurse manager to be aware of the variances related to the unit and the reasons for the alteration in expected performance. These variance data are often used in the preparation of the next year's budget. Examples of variances seen in unit budgets are:

- Increased overtime related to greater-than-anticipated use of sick time
- Increased use of part-time personnel related to an unanticipated increase in patient acuity
- Increased expense for minor equipment due to electrical malfunction that destroyed equipment
- Increased expenses due to resignation of staff and orientation of replacement staff

Many health care organizations have flexible budgets that automatically adjust to environmental changes. A goal of most organizations is to proactively anticipate challenges through the collection of the information in an environmental assessment. An example of a proactive budget process would be the budgeting of increased staff during the influenza season.

Most organizations provide the nurse manager with fiscal reports on a routine basis (weekly, monthly, or quarterly depending on the organization). This allows each cost center manager to carefully monitor the financial activity of the unit. The budget process is a continually evolving work requiring evaluation and continual improvement.

TYPES OF BUDGETS

The overall budget is composed of a number of smaller budgets that represent specific areas of concern in the financial objective setting of an organization. The operating (expense) budget includes (1) the personnel budget, (2) costs other than for personnel, and (3) the revenue budget. Not all units prepare a revenue budget; that may be done by the finance department.

The personnel budget requires that the nurse manager forecast the anticipated workload for the year. This is done based on information gathered from the environmental assessment, review of the previous workload, and identification of the services to be provided. The calculation of staff needs is a complex procedure. First, the average daily census and occupancy rate are calculated. The total required patient care hours are calculated (Figure 14-2). Then, the number of full-time equivalents (FTEs) required to provide care is calculated based on the expected number of hours. An FTE is calculated as 2080 hours of work per year. Then, the number of full-time employees, part-time employees, and shifts needs to be calculated. Adjustments need to be made for employee benefits and nonproductive time (vacation, orientation, education, sick time, etc.) (Figure 14-3).

The next step is to prepare a daily staffing plan. This plan includes the staff mix of individuals required to provide the patient care (registered nurses, licensed practical nurses, unit clerks, patient care associates, etc.). Remember that the skill mix of staff and the

WORKLOAD CALCULATION (TOTAL REQUIRED PATIENT CARE HOURS)				
Patient Acuity Level*	Hours of Care Per Patient Day (HPPD)†	× Patient Days‡	=	Workload§
1	3.0	900		2,700
2	5.2	3,100		16,120
3	8.8	4,000		35,200
4	13.0	1,600		20,800
5	19.0	400		7,600
Total		10,000		82,420

*1, Low; 5, high.
†HPPD is the number of hours of care on average for a given acuity level.
‡1 patient per 1 day = 1 patient day.
§Total number of hours of care needed based on acuity levels and numbers of patient days.

Figure 14-2 • Workload calculation. (From Yoder-Wise, P. S. [2007]. *Leading and managing in nursing.* 4th ed. St. Louis: Mosby.)

Productive Hours Calculation

Method 1: Add all nonproductive hours/FTE and subtract from paid hours/FTE
   Example: Vacation   15 days
              Holiday   7 days
              Average sick time 4 days
              TOTAL   26 days

   26 × 8* hours = 208 nonproductive hours/FTE
   2080 − 208 = 1872 productive hours/FTE

Method 2: Multiply paid hours/FTE by percentage of productive hours/FTE
   Example: Productive hours = 90%/FTE
              (1872 productive hours of total 2080 = 90%)
              2080 × 0.90 = 1872 productive hours/FTE

Total FTE Calculation

Required Patient Care Hours ÷ Productive Hours Per FTE = Total FTEs Needed

82,420   ÷ 1872   = 44 FTEs

*Based on an 8-hour shift pattern.

Figure 14-3 • Productive hours calculation. (From Yoder-Wise, P. S. [2007]. *Leading and managing in nursing.* 4th ed. St. Louis: Mosby.)

staffing requirements are regulated. It is important that the nurse manager maintain compliance with all regulatory boards while determining the budget. Once the nurse manager has decided on the positions required to deliver care, the other labor costs can be included in the personnel budget. These other labor costs include benefits, shift differential, overtime, raises, premium pay, and so forth. Benefits are often calculated at close to an additional 30% to 40% of an individual's pay.

For costs other than personnel costs, the nurse manager will have to calculate supply and expense costs, such as supplies, education, travel to conferences, telephone, electricity, and minor equipment. Some health care institutions also require support services to be included in the budget; an example would be information technology services provided by an in-house department to a unit. These are all examples of indirect costs.

The nurse manager is dealing with only minor equipment purchases in this budget. For major items, there is a capital expenditure budget. A capital expenditure must have a life span of at least 1 year, and there is usually a dollar limit for determining if an equipment request is capital or minor. A capital expenditure usually costs more than $500 or $1000 (depending on the institution). Organizations often perform long-term planning with capital expenditures. In this manner, the organization determines priorities for such expenditures.

Each nursing unit is usually called a *cost center*. The cost center is the organizational unit for which costs can be identified and managed. While in most large health care organizations the revenue budget is prepared by the chief financial officer, the nurse manager must be aware of the revenue anticipated by the unit. Nurses working in smaller outpatient centers may be responsible for the development of the revenue budget. The calculation of the revenue budget requires knowledge of the anticipated reimbursement expected for patient care and the time of the expected reimbursement.

The majority of health care institutions orient the nurse manager to the financial aspects of the position. This also includes an orientation to the budget process of the institution and the role of the nurse manager in this process. Some health care agencies have changed the organizational structure of the unit management to include a clinical nurse manager and a business manager. The business manager may not be a nurse, but he or she works with the unit director to maintain financial efficiency in operations.

SUMMARY

The financial management of a clinical unit, as well as the entire health care institution, is the responsibility of the nurse leaders. The careful balance of health care and financial stewardship is a delicate balance that nurse leaders juggle daily. It is a learning system that all nurses work with on a daily basis.

CLINICAL CORNER

Budgetary Concerns in Implementation of an Information System on a Cardiothoracic Unit
Jane O'Rourke

The budget for the implementation of an information system on a patient care unit is operational and capital. The operational budget incorporates the costs of day-to-day activities such as staffing and disposable supplies. The capital budget includes one-time expenditures for durable items such as equipment (e.g., computer hardware). The plan for this project must include a detailed budget consisting of an operational component and capital component. The operational budget of this project outlines the staffing costs associated with the staffing hours required for the project to be functional.

Operational Budget

Trainer @ $50/hr	1 Trainer × 12 hr × 5 days	$3000
RN @ $45/hr	32 RNs × 4 hr of training	$5760
Secretary @ $20/hr	6 Secretaries × 3 hr of training	$360
Cardiorespiratory tech @ $26/hr	11 Techs × 4 hr of training	$1144
CV house physician @ $120/hr	4 Physicians × 4 hr of training	$1920
Report writer @ $27/hr	1 Report writer × 8 hr × 5 days	$1080
Informational tech @ $20/hr	5 Techs × 4 hr	$400
Total	**Training and report writing**	**$13,664**

The operational costs are primarily limited to the items related to start up. All the staff needs to be educated regarding the use of the system. Each institution has unique reports that are specific to operations. The custom-designed reports are in addition to the standardized reports that are a standard part of the software. Custom reports require detailed input from management and staff to be valuable. These reports literally take the place of manual data collection for performance improvement activities. Reports, both standard and custom, are used to support the return on the project investment.

The project evaluation is an integral part of the implementation. The evaluation summary has many components. The following questions should be answered in the project evaluation summary:

- Are the operations improved?
- What is the return on investment?
- What do the performance improvement data indicate?
- Are the staff members satisfied?
- Has the project supported the strategic plan as anticipated?

The implementation of a management information system on a clinical service demonstrates leadership consideration of both the need for change as an organization and the drive toward efficiency. The interaction and cooperation between leadership and staff are paramount to the success of any organizational change. The implementation of new projects must be congruent with the vision and strategic direction of the organization. The end goal of the change may be efficiency, but the process must be able to be financially supported as well.

EVIDENCE-BASED PRACTICE

Financial Performance of Magnet Hospitals Compared With Nonmagnet Hospitals: Is Magnet a Money Maker?

Modified from Tuazon, N. (2007). Is Magnet a money maker? Nursing Management 38(6), 24-31.

While it is touted as a nursing award, Magnet designation is important also to the health care organization as a whole and is considered the gold standard for nursing care both in the United States and abroad. Since its inception in 1995, Magnet designation has been proved to have positive outcomes on nursing quality indicators including improved patient and physician satisfaction, improved quality of patient care, and increased operating margin, but the financial impact of Magnet designation has not yet been studied. In this descriptive, nonexperimental design study, the profitability ratios between matched pairs of ANCC Magnet-designated and non-Magnet facilities in New Jersey are compared for fiscal years 2002 and 2003 including operating margin, profit margin, return on equity ratios, and return on total assets. Several classifications were compared in assigning facilities to matched pairs including classification, geographical location, tax exempt status, and bed size. The intent of the study was to assist facilities considering applying for Magnet status to determine if the significant cost associated with the Magnet application process is worth the potential rewards of designation. Significant chal-

lenges were faced in assessing the financial status of these various health care facilities that increased the complexity of the evaluation and report. The database was obtained from reports entitled *Financial Status of New Jersey Hospitals,* published by the New Jersey Hospital Association. A convenience sample of eight small, medium-size, and large Magnet hospitals was selected from the 17 potential magnet facilities, exclusions were based on several factors, and the authors recognize the limitations of the small sample size of the study. The study found that Magnet facilities, in general, outperformed the non-Magnet hospitals in all criteria with much smaller standard deviation, thus less dispersion of the group. In layman's terms, Magnet hospitals performed better financially than non-Magnet hospitals as evidenced by higher mean scores in operating margin, total margin, and return on equity.

In response to the study's findings, the author suggests that awareness of hospital leaders to the potential and actual return of Magnet recognition be increased. In addition, she suggests that the study be replicated in other states and with a larger sample size and include a longitudinal study of Magnet hospitals to compare the financial ratios prior to and after achieving Magnet designation. In support of Magnet designation, the author also recommends a study to evaluate the impact Magnet-related characteristics have on financial performances of hospitals and creative ways to fund the pursuit of Magnet designation.

NCLEX® EXAM QUESTIONS

1. As a new nurse manager, you are concerned about a negative staffing variance of the past 4 weeks. A potential reason for such a variance would be:
   1. oversupply of unlicensed personnel in the organization
   2. decreased patient acuity and staffing over the past 4 weeks
   3. staffing reduction due to voluntary furloughs
   4. higher than budgeted patient acuity and census
2. In preparation for creation of a unit budget, the nurse manager will:
   1. work with staff to set priorities
   2. develop a cash budget for the unit
   3. orient all staff to cost-conscious practices
   4. create an Excel spreadsheet to track spending

3. As a manager, you are attempting to evaluate the present status of the capital expense budget. You would look at:
   1. the cost of benefits for your staff compared with the budget
   2. the amount of money spent to date on equipment
   3. the variance reports sent to the unit on a weekly basis
   4. productivity scorecard results for staffing
4. You are attempting to determine the need for additional full-time staff. You have found that you need to cover 5200 hours of additional patient care coverage. You know that this will amount to the equivalent of:

Continued

1. 1 FTE
2. 2.5 FTEs
3. 3 FTEs
4. 5 FTEs

5. In planning for an increase in staffing, the new nurse manager must take into account:
   1. staff desires
   2. patient mix
   3. reimbursement status
   4. licensing laws

6. The majority of health care institutions:
   1. orient the nurse manager to the financial aspects of the position
   2. do not orient the nurse manager to the financial aspects of the position
   3. orient the staff nurse to the budget process of the institution
   4. do not orient the night supervisor to the financial aspects of the position

7. An example of a direct cost would be:
   1. telephone costs for entire facility
   2. copy paper for a specific unit
   3. room use for a hospital event
   4. housekeeping staff

8. An example of an indirect cost would be:
   1. housekeeping staff
   2. ink for printer on unit
   3. uniform allowance for licensed practical nurses
   4. registered nurse salary

9. The operating (expense) budget does not include:
   1. the personnel budget
   2. the costs other than personnel
   3. revenue budget
   4. off-site registered nurse continuing education seminars

10. The two major types of budgeting processes are:
    1. zero-based budgeting and incremental budgeting
    2. zero-based budgeting and alternating budgeting
    3. incremental budgeting and external budgeting
    4. incremental budgeting and personnel-based budgeting

Answers: 1. 4   2. 1   3. 2   4. 2   5. 2   6. 1   7. 2   8. 1   9. 4   10. 1

REFERENCES

Finkler, S., & Kovner, C. (2001). *Financial management for nurse managers and executives.* 2nd ed. Philadelphia: W.B. Saunders.

Indiana Rural Health Association. (2008). *In patient scorecards.* Retrieved July 20, 2007, from http://www.indianaruralhealth.org/Sample%20Dashboard%20_(3_).pdf.

The Joint Commission (2008). *Comprehensive accreditation manual for hospitals: the official handbook.* Oakbrook, IL: Author.

Tuazon, N. (2007). Financial performance of Magnet hospitals as compared to non Magnets. Is Magnet a money maker? *Nursing Management, 38*, 24, 26, 28-30.

Yoder-Wise, P. (2003). *Leading and managing in nursing.* St. Louis: Mosby.

Human Resources

This section deals with the myriad of human resource issues faced by the new nurse manager. The major challenge of a manager is moving from a patient-focused mind-set to one dealing with both patients and the interaction of the caregivers of the unit. This section addresses such topics as employment law, hiring and firing, workplace safety, legal issues, staffing and scheduling, and the evaluation of coworkers.

Much of the work of the nurse manager involves the human side of the organization—the employees. The human resource function of your job will require you to have knowledge of employment laws, union contracts, salary requirements, staff compensation, retention activities, and other areas of concern to the employees of the organization.

This unit is organized as an employee would progress through the organization.

CHAPTER 15

Management of Human Resources

Chapter Objectives

1. Discuss employment law as it relates to health care.
2. Review the recruitment process for patient care staff.
3. Identify the steps in the employment process.
4. Review the importance of a résumé in the employment process.
5. Differentiate between the various types of interviewing techniques used in health care.
6. Differentiate between various types of questions used in the employment interview.
7. Identify the role of the nurse manager in the hiring process.

Definitions

Equal Employment Opportunity Same employment opportunities must exist in an institution for all individuals regardless of race, color, national origin, religion, sex, age, or disability

Interview Formal consultation to evaluate qualifications of a potential employee

Résumé Summary of an individual's past employment, education, and honors

Recruitment Process of obtaining individuals for employment

Retention Preservation or maintenance of staff

EMPLOYEE LAW

There are a number of federal and state laws that play a major role in the employment of staff. It is very important that you have an understanding of these laws and any local or institution-specific regulations affecting the human resource function of your job. Understanding of these laws will decrease your exposure to liability in your hiring practices.

Equal Employment Opportunity Laws

Several laws have been implemented to ensure that there are equal employment opportunities for all individuals regardless of race, color, national origin, religion, sex, age, or disability. These laws are enforced by the U.S. Equal Employment Opportunity Commission (EEOC).

The federal laws prohibiting job discrimination are as follows (http://www.eeoc.gov/abouteeo/overview_laws.html):

- Title VII of the Civil Rights Act of 1964 (Title VII), which prohibits employment discrimination based on race, color, religion, sex, or national origin
- The Equal Pay Act of 1963 (EPA), which protects men and women who perform substantially equal work in the same establishment from sex-based wage discrimination
- The Age Discrimination in Employment Act of 1967 (ADEA), which protects individuals who are 40 years of age or older

- Title I and Title V of the Americans with Disabilities Act of 1990 (ADA), which prohibit employment discrimination against qualified individuals with disabilities in the private sector, and in state and local governments
- Sections 501 and 505 of the Rehabilitation Act of 1973, which prohibit discrimination against qualified individuals with disabilities who work in the federal government
- The Civil Rights Act of 1991, which, among other things, provides monetary damages in cases of intentional employment discrimination.

Included in these laws are laws that prohibit sexual harassment in the workplace (see Chapter 18). It is the responsibility of the organization to have human resource policies and procedures in place that are in compliance with the requirements of these laws (Table 15-1).

Many of these regulations relate to the hiring process, while some relate to the work environment. Those relating to the work environment (e.g., Title VII, ADA) have been discussed in other chapters.

In addition to the employment laws and regulations, many institutions are unionized. Some organizations have differing unions for different sets of employees. The nurses may be unionized under a nurses union, the environmental care employees may be represented by another union, and the licensed practical nurses may belong to a separate union. In such a multiunion environment, it is important for you to know the provisions of the union agreement(s). The union agreement(s) will affect everything from the hiring process to the delivery of patient care. If you join a unionized environment, as a new employee you will receive orientation materials to the union and its benefits and contract requirements. The new manager in a unionized environment will also receive information about all of the union rules that affect the management of the unit.

The initial contact of a potential employee starts with the actual employment process. Hospitals must provide an adequate number and appropriate types of staff consistent with the hospital's staffing and strategic plans. Integral to these efforts is the recruitment and hiring of appropriate staff.

THE EMPLOYMENT PROCESS

It is the responsibility of the organization to provide staffing adequate to deliver safe and competent care. The numbers of staff required will depend on the acuity of the patients, the requirements of the job, mandatory staffing law (if applicable), health department regulations, and hospital policies. As positions become vacant or new ones are created, the first step in the employment process is to determine the competencies required for the position. This will require a job description. Sample job descriptions are available at the following websites:

- Clinical nurse manager (http://www.anthc.org/mod/jobweb/pdf/06-236.pdf)
- Nurse manager (http://www.hr.duke.edu/jobs/descr_duhs/select.php?ID=5062)

Table 15-1   SELECTED FEDERAL LABOR LEGISLATION

Year	Legislation	Primary Purpose of the Legislation
1935	Wagner Act; National Labor Act	Unions, National Labor Relations Board established
1947	Taft-Hartley Act	Equal balance of power between unions and management
1962	Executive Order 10988	Public employees could join unions
1963	Equal Pay Act	Became illegal to pay lower wages based on gender
1964	Civil Rights Act	Protected against discrimination based on race, color, creed, national origin, etc.
1967	Age Discrimination	Act protected against discrimination based on age
1970	Occupational Safety and Health Act	Ensured healthy and safe working conditions
1974	Wagner Amendments	Allowed nonprofit organizations to unionize
1990	Americans with Disabilities Act	Barred discrimination against workers with disabilities
1991	Civil Rights Act	Addressed sexual harassment in the workplace
1993	Family and Medical Leave Act	Allowed work leaves based on family and medical needs

- Staff nurse (http://hr.duke.edu/jobs/descr_campus/select.php?ID=304)

All organizations will have a template for the job description. You need to familiarize yourself with the format in your organization. An effective job description needs to minimally include (1) title, (2) job objectives, and (3) a list of duties. As the job description is finalized, the job is "posted" according to the organization's policies. The process of "posting" is the initial stage in the nine-stage process of recruitment (Huber, 2006).

1. Position posting
2. Advertising
3. Screening
4. Interviewing
5. Selecting
6. Orienting
7. Counseling/coaching
8. Performance evaluation
9. Staff development

As a nurse manager, you will play a role in each stage of this recruitment process. Your actual role in each stage of the process will depend on the organization's hierarchal structure. As a new nurse, you need to be aware of the process to which you will be exposed in your first hire.

POSITION POSTING

Once a position becomes vacant within a hospital, the hospital posts the position internally for staff review and selection. Then the position is posted externally in the local newspapers and with staffing and recruiting agencies.

ADVERTISING

Hospitals may place ads in professional nursing journals or magazines and/or on professional organization websites. This encourages a broad range of individuals to be exposed to the position posting.

SCREENING

Hospitals use this process by reviewing applications and then determining whether the nurse meets the position criteria. Hospitals that are equal opportunity employers must meet all federal government guidelines during the screening process. Screening for nursing positions may include criminal background checks and drug and alcohol screens.

INTERVIEWING

Interviews are usually done in person, but they may also be conducted via telephone or teleconference. The interview may be one-on-one with the human resources representative and then with the nurse manager, or the interview may be conducted with multiple personnel at the same time.

SELECTING

The nurse manager or clinical director usually makes the selection for a nursing position. If the position is a management position, the nurse manager and clinical director and other members of the management team may select the candidate together.

THE INTERVIEW PROCESS

The most challenging aspect of the hiring process is to find the right person for the job. The job interview is the best way of determining the "fit" of the individual for the job and for your unit and organization. Remember, matching the job qualifications with the individual is only one aspect of the "right fit"—the personality and values of the individual also play a role in determination of the "right person for the job."

Prior to the interview process, a professional résumé is shared with individuals in the recruitment process. A résumé is a summary of professional and personal experiences—education, clinical experience, employment, skills, and interests—designed to introduce the candidate to potential employers. Often the résumé is the employer's first of impression of the candidate. As a new nurse manager, you will need to evaluate the résumé for "right fit."

For a résumé to be effective, it must be targeted to the job being applied for. A single "catch-all" résumé that a candidate expects to use in looking for various types of jobs is much less effective than several well-focused résumés that highlight pertinent experience or expertise. If, for example, a candidate planning to apply to both hospital-based and community health center–based positions might be better served by having two résumés, one focusing on hospital experience and the other focusing on the community health background. Remember, for a nurse looking for a job, the purpose of a résumé is to obtain an interview, so it must make a strong argument to the reader that you have something to offer (Vice Provost for University Life at the

University of Pennsylvania). The purpose of the resumé to the nurse manager is for evaluation of a potential candidate's education, skills, and experience related to the open position. A resumé is different from a CV (curriculum vitae) in that a resumé is a summary of your academic and work history, while a CV is a more-detailed document of work history, academic experience, publications, etc. A CV is usually used in the academic world. All nurses need to keep their resumé current; it is very frustrating to attempt to write a resumé after 5 years and try to remember everything you have accomplished! Update your resumé at least every 6 months.

RESUMÉ WRITING

Both new nurses and nurse managers and leaders need to pay attention to their resumé. Tips for resumé writing are listed in Box 15-1.

NAME AND ADDRESS SECTION

- The name and address may be centered on the page or split on each margin.
- The name should be in a slightly larger font than the rest of the resumé.
- The name should be in bold font.
- List a telephone number where you can be reached; list a home and/or a cell phone number and make sure you have an answering machine or message capability so a message can be left for you (ensure that the greeting on the answering

machine is appropriate for a potential employer to hear).
- Use an e-mail address that is professional and appropriate; avoid "cutesy" e-mail addresses such as Cutesypie@... .
- Check e-mail and telephone messages several times a day.

OBJECTIVE

Be very specific, even if you have to list more than one job title. If you cannot be specific, omit this section.

EDUCATION

- List your college name, city, and state (not street address) and the years attended.
- List the graduation date or anticipated graduation date.
- List the degree and major or program.
- Give your grade point average (GPA) (if your overall GPA is not good, give your nursing GPA [e.g., Nursing GPA 3.5]).
- Once you have graduated, you can list your degree first and then the school and date.
- If you have graduated from a college or university, you do not need to list your high school.

RELEVANT SKILLS AND EXPERIENCE OR ACCOMPLISHMENTS

Use bullet format for clinical rotations, volunteer experiences, accomplishments at other jobs if relevant, computer skills, and so on.

JOB HISTORY

- List jobs *starting with the most recent* and work back from there.
- List name of company, city, state (not street address), and years you worked (not months).
- Give your job title.
- Use bullets to state your accomplishments.
- Begin each bullet statement with an ACTION VERB. Use present tense for current job only; use past tense for all previous jobs.
- Do not use "responsible for" or "duties include"; list accomplishments in each job.
- If you have had jobs in the health care field or experience relevant to the job you are now seeking, give it more space on your resumé; jobs that are unrelated to what you are seeking can be given minimal space.

Box 15-1 TIPS FOR RESUMÉ WRITING AND PRINTING

- Resumés should be one page long, unless you have extensive experience in the position for which you are applying.
- Print on light blue, ivory, white, or beige paper (if you mail your resumé, the envelope must be the same color).
- Use Times Roman or similar font; do not use fancy fonts, underlining, or italics because they do not scan correctly.
- Margins should be 1 inch top, bottom, and sides.
- Use 12-point font if possible—no smaller than 10-point font.
- Do not use pronouns.

PROFESSIONAL AFFILIATIONS AND HONORS

- List any organizations that you were a member of as a student and/or other jobs you have had; list all honors and membership in honor societies.
- **Do not** put "References available on request" at the bottom of the résumé. References are always listed in a separate page that you can take with you to an interview.
- **Do not** list personal information (age, marital status, height, weight, etc.).

PROOFREAD! PROOFREAD! AND PROOFREAD AGAIN!

Have someone else proofread your résumé. Do not rely on computer software (Jones, 2007, p. 380). Box 15-2 provides a sample résumé for a graduate nurse.

As a nurse manager evaluating this résumé, you would realize that this new nurse has computer skills, has demonstrated leadership qualities within her nursing education, and meets the basic needs of a new staff nurse. If you were looking for a nurse with extensive experience in the cardiac setting, this candidate does not meet that need.

As a new nurse developing a first professional nursing résumé, you need to access the resources available at your school of nursing. Most schools have resources to assist you in the development of a professional CV; it is in your best interest to use these services.

EFFECTIVE COVER LETTERS

All résumés need to be accompanied by a cover letter to the institution to which you are applying. The cover letter needs to be written in a professional tone. As a new nurse, this letter will set the tone for the individual reading the cover letter. For the nurse manager, this letter will let you know if this individual is someone who may be appropriate for the position. The qualities of an effective cover letter follow (Jones, 2007, p. 383):

- Brief, neat, and without errors
- In business format
- Name and title of person to whom the letter is addressed
- Why you are interested, and what position you would like to apply for
- Appointed time for taking NCLEX-RN (for a new nurse)
- Certifications that match the posted job (for an experienced nurse)

Box 15-2 SAMPLE RÉSUMÉ FOR A GRADUATE NURSE

JANE DOE
1111 South Green Street
Anywhere, USA 00222
222-555-1212 (cell) 555-212-3333 (home)
jdoe@email.com

Job Target Long-term association with an acute care hospital acknowledged for nursing excellence
Skills
- Registered nurse highly skilled in care of the critically ill patient
- Strong ability to rapidly prioritize patient care and manage complex patient care

Education and Certifications
    University of State, Anywhere, USA
      Bachelor of Science Degree, Nursing. GPA 3.76, 2003
      Outstanding Student Award—attained for excellence in clinical area
    American Association of Critical Care Nurses— CCRN certification current to 2010
    Basic Life Support Certificate and Advanced Cardiac Life Support Certificate

Professional Experience
    Surgical Intensive Care Staff Nurse
      6/07-present
    Mercy Medical Center, Somewhere, NY
      Level II trauma center with 678 beds. 20-bed adult surgical intensive care unit
      Postcardiac, renal, and gastrointestinal surgery patient population
    Cardiac Intensive Care Staff Nurse 3/05-6/07
    Hammondton Medical Center
      Community hospital with 320 beds. 10-bed cardiac intensive care. Postcardiac intervention unit
    Staff Nurse, Telemetry 7/03-3/05
    Hammondton Medical Center
      40-bed telemetry unit
License
    State of Anywhere, USA   Registered Professional Nurse
Awards
    Staff Nurse of the Year   Hammondton Medical Center, 2006

Box 15-3 EXAMPLE OF AN EFFECTIVE COVER LETTER

May 1, 2006
Elizabeth B. Wise, PhD, RN
Director of Nurse Recruitment and Hiring
Caring Hospital USA
Joy City, LA 70777
RE: Nursing Position on Medical-Surgical Unit

Dear Dr. Wise:
I have just graduated from Caring College and would like to apply for a new graduate nurse position on Medical-Surgical Unit II at Caring Hospital. I served there as a nurse technician while attending nursing school. I plan to take the NCLEX-RN exam in early June 2009 and will be available to start work by July 1, 2009.

Having worked as a nurse technician on Medical-Surgical Unit II for 3 years, I developed positive interpersonal and professional relationships with the team. Furthermore, I am well organized, have effective time-management skills, and am enthusiastic about the prospect of returning to the unit. I am proud to have worked at Caring Hospital for 3 years in light of its high rating and Magnet status. The mission of Caring Hospital is congruent with my values.

Thank you very much for your consideration. You may reach me any time on my cell phone at (999) 709-2525. I look forward to hearing from you to schedule an interview at your convenience.

Sincerely,
Scelitta Source

From Jones, R. A. (2007). *Nursing leadership and management: theories, processes and practice.* Philadelphia, PA: F. A. Davis.

- Express appreciation for consideration and eagerness to be part of team
- How can be reached (telephone number)
- Use 9- by 12-inch envelope to send résumé and cover letter (first-class mail)
- Expect response to letter in 2 weeks
- If not, call after 3 weeks; check with Human Resources

Box 15-3 provides an example of an effective cover letter.

THE INTERVIEW

Credentials are often reviewed before or during the interview. These credentials usually consist of the following:

- Copy of the complete résumé
- Copies of nursing license or a copy of notice of passing board scores
- Two copies of a complete, typed list of all references and previous managers (one copy for the human resources department and one for the hiring manager). Be sure to include the references' complete names and titles and current addresses and telephone numbers.
- Permission for a criminal background check. Be sure to have a list of your addresses from the previous 5 to 7 years.
- Permission for a drug and alcohol screen
- For a new nurse, a copy of recent cumulative grade report to show that you are a graduation candidate and that you are not at risk for failing the licensing exam.

In many institutions, the initial interview is with the nurse recruiter. During this interview, the employment process is reviewed, the salary and benefits are reviewed in a cursory manner, and the potential employee is evaluated as to what position in the organization might be appropriate. The individual is then interviewed by the nurse manager of the particular area of interest. Some nurse managers will also include staff in the interviewing process. This is a reflection of the culture of the organization.

It is important that you have prepared for the interview and do not try to "wing it." This is important for both the job candidate and the nurse manager. As the candidate, before the interview you will need to make a self-assessment of your abilities, your strong points, and your challenges. Remember, you need to be able to put your best foot forward, and your self-awareness will greatly assist you in this endeavor. As the nurse manager, this is when the candidate is assessing your abilities and judging whether she or he would like to work with you.

STYLES OF INTERVIEWING

As you move forward to the interview process, you will need to have an idea of what you will ask or be asked. There are various styles of interviewing for the nurse manager, but you need to remember that the goal of the interview is to determine the capabilities of the individual and to determine if this individual would be an asset to the unit.

The more traditional styles of interviewing ask questions that elicit standard questions from the prospective employee. Samples of such questions would be:

- How would you describe yourself?
- What specific goals have you established for your career?
- What will it take to attain your goals, and what steps have you taken toward attaining them?
- Please describe the ideal job for you.
- How would you describe yourself in terms of your ability to work as a member of a team?
- What short-term goals and objectives have you established for yourself?
- How would you evaluate your ability to deal with conflict?
- Describe what you have accomplished toward reaching a recent goal for yourself.
- Can you describe your long-range goals and objectives?
- What plans do you have for continued study? An advanced degree?
- Can you describe your long-range goals and objectives?

Many institutions are moving toward a behavior-based interviewing technique. This technique allows the manager to more critically evaluate a person's capabilities based on the following questions:

- Describe a situation in which you were able to use persuasion to successfully convince someone to see things your way.
- Describe a time when you were faced with a stressful situation that demonstrated your coping skills.
- Give me a specific example of a time when you used good judgment and logic in solving a problem.
- Give me an example of a time when you set a goal and were able to meet or achieve it.
- Give me a specific example of a time when you had to conform to a policy with which you did not agree.
- Tell me about a time when you had to go above and beyond the call of duty in order to get a job done.
- Tell me about a time when you had too many things to do and you were required to prioritize your tasks.
- Give me an example of a time when you had to make a split-second decision.
- What is your typical way of dealing with conflict? Give me an example.
- Tell me about a time you were able to successfully deal with another person even when that individual may not have personally liked you (or vice versa).

- Tell me about a difficult decision you have made in the last year.
- Give me an example of a time when something you tried to accomplish and failed.
- Give me an example of when you showed initiative and took the lead.
- Tell me about a recent situation in which you had to deal with a very upset customer or coworker.

These questions can also be customized to deal with specific patient situations.

LAWFUL AND UNLAWFUL INQUIRIES

As the manager, there are also some rules of things to avoid in the interviewing process.

- Do not make promises that you cannot keep.
- **Do not ask about anything that the law prohibits you from considering in making your decision.** For example, do not ask about an applicant's race or religion, because you are not allowed to consider these factors in making your decision. Table 15-2 provides some ideas on how to get relevant information while staying within the bounds of the law. And do not panic if an applicant raises a delicate subject—such as disability or national origin—without any prompting from you. You cannot raise such subjects, but the applicant can.
- **Respect the applicant's privacy.** Although federal law does not require you to do so, many state laws and rules of etiquette do.

It is also a good strategy to ask the candidate if she or he has any questions of you, the interviewer. The interview is a time for both the candidate and interviewer to find the answers to any potential questions they have regarding the candidate and the organization. Box 15-4 provides guidelines for the interview process for the nurse manager.

RECRUITMENT STRATEGIES

The final stage in the recruitment process—the selection and acceptance of the candidate—often relies on many of the various recruitment activities of the organization. Many of these strategies reflect compensation, benefits, or work alternatives that are important to the nurses whom the organization is trying to recruit. Some recruitment strategies are listed in Box 15-5.

If you are the individual being interviewed, you need to know in advance which of these recruitment strate-

Table 15-2   INTERVIEW QUESTIONS THAT MAY AND MAY NOT BE ASKED

Subject	Lawful Inquiry/Areas You Can Inquire About	Unlawful Inquiry/Areas You Cannot Inquire About
Age	Are you 18 years of age or older? (to determine if the applicant is legally old enough to perform the job) If applicant is over age 21 (if job-related, e.g., bartender)	How old are you? Date of birth Date of high school graduation Age
Citizenship; national origin or ancestry	Are you legally authorized to work in the United States on a full-time basis? Ability to speak/write English fluently (if job related) Other languages spoken (if job related)	Are you a native-born citizen of the United States? Where are you from? Ethnic association of a surname Birthplace of applicant or applicant's parents Nationality; lineage, national origin Nationality of applicant's spouse Whether applicant is citizen of another country Applicant's native tongue/English proficiency
Disability	These [provide applicant with list of job functions] are the essential functions of the job. How would you perform them?	Do you have any physical disabilities that would prevent you from doing this job? If applicant has a disability Nature or severity of a disability Whether applicant has ever filed a workers' compensation claim Recent or past surgeries and dates Past medical problems
Drug and alcohol use	Do you currently use illegal drugs?	Have you ever been addicted to drugs?
Sex and family arrangements	If applicant has relatives already employed by the organization	Sex of applicant Number of children Marital status Spouse's occupation Childcare arrangements Health care coverage through spouse
Race	No questions acceptable	Applicant's race or color of skin Photograph to be affixed to application form
Religion	No questions acceptable	Maiden name (of married woman) Religious affiliation/availability for weekend work Religious holidays observed
Other	Convictions, if job-related Academic, vocational, or professional schooling Training received in the military Membership in any trade or professional association Job references	Number and kinds of arrests Height or weight, except if a bona fide occupational qualification Veteran status, discharge status, branch of service Contact in case of an emergency (at application or interview stage)

Modified from Development Dimensions International, Inc. (2003). *Legal considerations in selection; U.S. version.* Bridgeville, PA: Author.

gies are important to you. If you are the nurse manager, you need to be aware of the recruitment strategies that are made available to members of your unit. Some questions that may be asked include:
- What is the nurse-to-patient ratio?
- Is there support staff on the unit to assist nurses?

- In what ways are nurses held accountable for high qualities of practice?
- How much input do nurses have regarding systems, equipment, and the care environment?
- What professional development opportunities are available to nurses?

Box 15-4 IMPORTANT GUIDELINES FOR THE INTERVIEW PROCESS

- Prepare questions in advance on an interview guide.
- Take accurate and complete notes, without writing on the résumé or application.
- Save interview notes of all the candidates interviewed, in case of potential legal challenges.
- Use behavioral interviewing techniques in addition to skills assessments. When feasible, include an additional person in the interview process.
- Confirm that Human Resources will conduct thorough reference and background checking.
- Collaborate with Human Resources before extending an offer, promising compensation, and scheduling orientation planning.
- Human Resources will prepare an offer letter of employment for the Chief Nursing Officer's (CNO's) signature.

From Yoder-Wise, P. S., & Kowalski, K. E. (2006). *Beyond leading and managing: nursing administration for the future* (p. 319). St. Louis: Elsevier.

Box 15-5 RECRUITMENT/RETENTION STRATEGIES

- Flexible hours
- Competitive salaries
- Bonus pay
- Relocation pay
- Fixed shifts
- Weekend option program
- Part-time pay with bonus hours
- Flexible benefits packages
- Scholarships for BSN or graduate studies
- Tuition benefit plan
- Educational loan repayment
- RN specialty internships
- Professional development opportunities
- Career opportunities
- Specialty certification reimbursement
- Low nurse-to-patient ratios (workload staffing)
- Shared governance/leadership models
- Care delivery model that promotes professional care at the bedside
- Clinical ladder/career ladder
- Free parking
- Magnet recognition
- Culture of safety: zero tolerance for incivility
- Research/evidence-based practice
- NCLEX review course
- Qualified managerial support
- Clinical support; staff educators, clinical nurse specialists
- Workforce diversity
- Interdisciplinary collaboration opportunities

From Huber, D. (2006). *Leadership and nursing care management* (p. 633). Philadelphia, PA: Elsevier.

- Tell me about your culture of patient safety in this institution.
- Can you tell me how the nurses at this institution strive for excellence?
- Tell me about your commitment to the educational advancement of your nurses.

As a new nurse, it is important for you to determine the qualities of a work environment that are important to you before the interview. As a nurse manager, it is important to realize which qualities of the work environment are important to members of your staff. While pay is an important issue, it is generally not an acceptable first question to ask of an interviewer.

Many of these strategies play an important role in the satisfaction of the nurses and serve to assist with the retention of nurses. With the nursing shortage, the competition for qualified staff members is at an all-time high, and the environment created with the emphasis on some of these strategies plays a vital role in the recruitment and retention of staff.

Salary compensation is always an issue for individuals. Salaries vary according to locale, type of institution, and the professional credentials and past experience of the staff member. Salary information is often posted as part of recruitment packages.

Once the employee is hired, it is the responsibility of the organization to provide orientation, performance evaluation, training, and professional development and a professional work environment. These topics will be covered in the next chapters.

SUMMARY

Gaining employment in a health care organization is not guaranteed on graduation from a school of nursing. It is important that the recruitment process allows the nurse manager to hire individuals who will prove to be a "good fit" for that particular work environment. It is through the evaluation of the résumé and interviewing process that the candidate and nurse manager have the opportunity to evaluate the "fit" of the individual and the unit.

CLINICAL CORNER

What I Look for in a Potential Hire
Joan Orseck

After 20 years of recruitment, so much is a gut instinct that, from start to finish, this applicant is the one! However, there are certain things that will point me to this applicant and end up with a hire.

That applicant would have begun the process either with an e-mail along with a cover letter and résumé or by direct mail. The cover letter or introduction would make me want to look at the résumé and, if both have a professional tone and the experience I am looking for, I would call to make an appointment. That telephone call is very important—I can tell from the applicant's communication whether I wish to proceed. There are many times when this will end for me the process ... if one cannot communicate well on the telephone, then that person will not communicate well in any situation. I look for grammar, tone, and, yes, attitude in the applicant's voice. I wish more applicants understood the importance of this first impression.

The applicant will come to the interview after having taken a "look in the mirror." First impressions are everything. Ask any recruiter—it is hard to change one's mind after that first face-to-face meeting with the applicant. The less skin shown, the better; there should be no heavy makeup; and jewelry should be kept at a minimum. The applicant will be on time and, if there is a problem, will call to let the recruiter know.

A well-prepared applicant will come with questions and will have done homework on the hospital. It shows if the individual has gone that extra mile and has a true interest in getting the job. Behavioral interviewing is conducted to see how past situations have been handled, and the results will give the recruiter good insight into how the applicant will handle herself or himself in the future. Body language is watched closely, and I look for facial expressions ... do they match what the applicant is saying? When talking about why they have chosen nursing or telling a story about a patient experience, does the applicant's face light up? I value this highly—I want the nurse who shows compassion and commitment for this profession. We can teach someone clinical aspects if the individual is truly willing to learn, but I am a great believer that one cannot change the person. I look for personality traits because this applicant will not only be taking care of our patients but will also be an ambassador for the hospital. No one ever leaves my office without my feeling that I would want them taking care of me or a family member.

This applicant will follow up with a thank-you letter, which will tell me why he or she wants to work for us. This shows professionalism and courtesy, and both are extremely noteworthy.

EVIDENCE-BASED PRACTICE

Factors Affecting Job Satisfaction in the Registered Nurse
Kettle, J. L. (2002, Fall). Factors affecting job satisfaction in the registered nurse. *Retrieved November 20, 2008, from University of Arizona College of Nursing: http://www.juns.nursing.arizona. edu/articles/Fall%202002/Kettle.htm.*

Job satisfaction in staff nurses should be of great concern to any organization. Nurses hold the majority of positions in most health care settings, and replacement of licensed personnel is costly and time consuming. A literature search yielded the following findings as causes of job satisfaction in nursing.

One study found that nurses felt "devalued" in their job and resentful of "the perceived placing of profits over patients." Many respondents voiced concern over the idea that patient care lacked, due to organizational changes in staffing and assignment. Extrinsic work values such as job security, salary, fringe benefits, and work schedules were also considered to be important in job satisfaction. Restrictions in scheduling and limited availability of time off promote frustration and dissatisfaction.

Issues of productivity and nonproductivity have been investigated. Staff nurse views have been studied and researchers found that productivity was based on two categories, quantity and quality of work. Nonproductivity was discussed in relation to two major categories as well, organizational factors and personal factors. Organization was dependent on feelings of "being overloaded," reaction to difficult patients, and lack of teamwork. Personal problems and lack of physical or mental readiness to work also contributed to nonproductivity.

Turnover was another area that was examined. It was found that the more job stress, the lower was the cohesion, the lower was the work satisfaction, and the higher was the anticipated turnover rate. Conversely, the higher the work satisfaction, the higher was the group cohesion and the lower was the anticipated turnover.

EVIDENCE-BASED PRACTICE—cont'd

Last, the more stable the schedule, there was less work stress and lower anticipated turnover. The higher the group cohesion, the higher was the work satisfaction.

Burnout is defined as "a syndrome of emotional exhaustion and cynicism that occurs frequently among individuals who do 'people work' of some kind." There was an attempt to find a correlation between personality hardiness and the syndrome of burnout. No correlation was found. However, the authors made suggestions regarding prevention of burnout such as improved environment, additional personal time, compensation for certification requirements, age analysis, and stress management. Burnout is a significant contributor to job dissatisfaction and needs to be addressed.

Researchers have also found that lack of internal empowerment leads to job tension and frustration. Opportunity for growth and movement as well as access to challenge and an increase in knowledge and skill was found to be key in motivation toward empowerment.

In conclusion, there are many factors that contribute to dissatisfaction in the workplace. Many variables within each factor make achieving satisfaction for every individual a very difficult task. Recognition of frustrations, such as turnover, lack of internal empowerment, burnout, and elimination of external sources of stress, can decrease dissatisfaction in the health care setting.

NCLEX® EXAM QUESTIONS

1. A professional résumé consists of:
   1. your professional experience, your personal interests, and your life history
   2. your professional experience, your personal interests, your educational experience, your professional experience, your family, and your life history
   3. your personal interests, your professional interests, and your family
2. When you are listing your previous places of employment on your résumé, you would list them in the following manner:
   1. present place of employment first and proceed backward
   2. first job position followed by second, third, and fourth
   3. start in the middle and proceed to present position
   4. start in the middle and proceed to last position
3. During your first job interview, which of the following questions are acceptable?
   1. What is the nurse-to-patient ratio? Is there support staff on the unit? In what ways are nurses held accountable for high qualities of practice?
   2. Is there support staff on the unit to assist nurses? What is the director of nursing's salary? In what ways are nurses held accountable for high qualities of practice? What is the salary of the night shift nurses?

   3. What is the director of nursing's salary? Is there support staff on the unit?
4. During the interview process regarding sex and family arrangements, the interviewer may not ask:
   1. sex of applicant and marital status
   2. sex of applicant and number of family employed at institution
   3. number of children and if applicant has relatives already employed by the organization
   4. marital status and how many people live in household
5. Which of the following are employment laws in the United States?
   1. Title I and Title V of the Americans with Disabilities Act of 1990, Civil Rights Act of 1991, Sections 501 and 505 of the Rehabilitation Act of 1973
   2. Title II and Title V of the Americans with Disabilities Act of 1991, Civil Rights Act of 1991, Sections 504 and 505 of the Rehabilitation Act of 1974.
   3. Title I and title IV of the Americans with Disabilities Act of 1990, Civil Rights Act of 1992, Sections 504 and 505 of the Rehabilitation Act of 1973.
   4. Title III and title IV of the Americans with Disabilities Act of 1974, Civil Rights Act of 1989, Sections 501 and 595 of the Rehabilitation Act of 1973.

Continued

6. When listing your education on your résumé, you should include:
   1. graduation date or anticipated graduation date
   2. graduation date, degree, major, and grade point average
   3. graduation date, highest grades, and program
   4. grade point average, major, and any repeated classes

7. Which of the following are appropriate recruitment/retention strategies?
   1. Tuition benefit plan and promise of unit change in 6 months
   2. Educational loan repayment and promise of raise in 3 months
   3. Promise of change of unit in 3 months and promise of change in salary in 6 months
   4. Registered nurse specialty internships and educational loan repayment

8. A cover letter to be sent with your résumé should include:
   1. school graduated from and projected start date
   2. projected start date and medical illnesses
   3. medical illnesses and school graduated from
   4. honors received and psychological illnesses

9. It is the organization's responsibility to:
   1. provide adequate staffing
   2. provide competent care
   3. evaluate each unit's patient acuity
   4. all of the above

10. The numbers of staff required on each unit depends on:
   1. the acuity of the patients and the requirements of the job
   2. mandatory staffing law and health department regulations
   3. Both 1 and 2 are correct.
   4. Neither 1 nor 2 is correct.

Answers: 1. 2   2. 1   3. 1   4. 1   5. 1   6. 2   7. 3   8. 1   9. 4   10. 3

REFERENCES

Development Dimensions International, Inc. (2003). *Legal considerations in selection; U.S. version*. Bridgeville, PA: Author.

Huber, D. (2006). *Leadership and nursing care management*. Philadelphia: Elsevier.

Jones, R. A. (2007). *Nursing leadership and management: theories, processes and practice*. Philadelphia: F. A. Davis.

Vice Provost for University Life at the University of Pennsylvania. (2008). http://www.vpul.upenn.edu/careerservices/nursing/resume.html#sample_resume.

Yoder-Wise, P. S., & Kowalski, K. E. (2006). *Beyond leading and managing: nursing administration for the future*. St. Louis: Elsevier.

CHAPTER 16

Providing Competent Staff

Chapter Objectives

1. Discuss hospital-wide and unit-based new employee orientation.
2. Analyze the role of preceptor in nurse orientation.
3. Compare and contrast the roles of the nurse, preceptor, and human resources in orientation.
4. Analyze the progression of nursing clinical competence.
5. Review the annual mandatory competencies for patient care staff.
6. Compare and contrast the roles of manager and staff in performance appraisal.
7. Identify the steps and progression of the staff registered nurse in the clinical ladder program.
8. Discuss activities used by the nurse manager to support promotion of staff members.

Definitions

Orientation Process in which initial job training and information are provided to staff

Mandatories Name given to those educational sessions and competencies that are required by accrediting agencies

Competencies Areas in which employees are to be determined to be qualified to perform

Clinical ladder Process whereby the employee is developed for progression within a position category

Organizational learning Development of new knowledge and skills within an organization. Such learning is achieved through research, development, evaluation, and improvement cycles

Performance appraisal Process in use in an organization by which the employee is routinely evaluated according to performance standards

Performance appraisal system Process or tool used by an organization to evaluate employee performance and to set developmental goals

Preceptor Experienced individual who assists new employees in acquiring the necessary knowledge and skills to function effectively in a new environment

BENNER FIVE STAGES

As the new nurse enters the workforce, it is important to realize that this is just the beginning of the professional journey. Benner (1984) posits that the nurse moves through five stages of clinical competence: novice, advanced beginner, competent, proficient, and expert nurse.

These different levels reflect changes in three general aspects of skilled performance:

1. One is a movement from reliance on abstract principles to the use of past concrete experience as paradigms.
2. The second is a change in the learner's perception of the demand situation, in which the situation is seen less and less as a

compilation of equally relevant bits and more and more as a complete whole in which only certain parts are relevant.

3. The third is a passage from detached observation to involved performer. The performer no longer stands outside the situation but is now truly engaged in the situation.

As you read this content, think of your own areas of experience in nursing. Decide where you think you fit.

STAGE 1: NOVICE

Beginners have had no experience of the situations in which they are expected to perform. Novices are taught rules to help them perform. The rules are context free and independent of specific cases; hence, the rules tend to be applied universally. The rule-governed behavior typical of the novice is extremely limited and inflexible. As such, novices have no "life experience" in the application of rules.

"Just tell me what I need to do and I'll do it."

STAGE 2: ADVANCED BEGINNER

Advanced beginners are those who can demonstrate marginally acceptable performance, those who have coped with enough real situations to note, or to have pointed out to them by a mentor, the recurring meaningful situational components. These components require prior experience in actual situations for recognition. Principles to guide actions begin to be formulated. The principles are based on experience.

STAGE 3: COMPETENT

Competence, typified by the nurse who has been on the job in the same or similar situations for 2 or 3 years, develops when the nurse begins to see his or her actions in terms of long-range goals or plans of which he or she is consciously aware. For the competent nurse, a plan establishes a perspective, and the plan is based on considerable conscious, abstract, analytic contemplation of the problem. The conscious, deliberate planning that is characteristic of this skill level helps achieve efficiency and organization. The competent nurse lacks the speed and flexibility of the proficient nurse but does have a feeling of mastery and the ability to cope with and manage the many contingencies of clinical nursing. The competent person does not yet have enough experience to recognize a situation in terms of an overall picture or in terms of which aspects are most salient, most important.

STAGE 4: PROFICIENT

The proficient performer perceives situations as wholes rather than in terms of chopped-up parts or aspects, and performance is guided by maxims. Proficient nurses understand a situation as a whole because they perceive its meaning in terms of long-term goals. The proficient nurse learns from experience what typical events to expect in a given situation and how plans need to be modified in response to these events. The proficient nurse can now recognize when the expected normal picture does not materialize. This holistic understanding improves the proficient nurse's decision making; it becomes less labored because the nurse now has a perspective on which of the many existing attributes and aspects in the present situation are the important ones. The proficient nurse uses maxims as guides which reflect what would appear to the competent or novice performer as unintelligible nuances of the situation; they can mean one thing at one time and quite another thing later. Once one has a deep understanding of the situation overall, however, the maxim provides direction as to what must be taken into account. Maxims reflect nuances of the situation.

STAGE 5: THE EXPERT

The expert performer no longer relies on an analytic principle (rule, guideline, maxim) to connect her or his understanding of the situation to an appropriate action. The expert nurse, with an enormous background of experience, now has an intuitive grasp of each situation and zeroes in on the accurate region of the problem without wasteful consideration of a large range of unfruitful, alternative diagnoses and solutions. The expert operates from a deep understanding of the total situation. The chess master, for instance, when asked why he or she made a particularly masterful move, will just say, "Because it felt right; it looked good." The performer is no longer aware of features and rules; his or her performance becomes fluid and flexible and highly proficient. This is not to say that the expert never uses analytic tools. Highly skilled analytic ability is necessary for those situations with which the nurse has had no previous experience. Analytic tools are also necessary for those times when the expert gets a wrong grasp of the situation and then finds that events and behaviors are not occurring as expected. When alternative perspectives are not available to the clinician, the only way out of a wrong grasp of the problem is

Box 16-1   FIVE STAGES OF TRANSITION FROM NOVICE TO COMPETENT PRACTITIONER

Stage I

The nurse is overwhelmed by the number of potentially relevant details that pertain to a patient's care.

Stage II

The new nurse may suffer exhaustion while trying to manage their patients within the confines of the unit guidelines and protocols.

Stage III

Successfully embracing policy and protocol enables feelings of confidence and serves as a critical marker of readiness.

Stage IV

A period of transition in the preceptee-preceptor relationship. The preceptor serves as a resource, frequently retreating from the forefront of patient care.

Stage V

The "comfort zone" of a preceptor is withdrawn as orientation is successfully completed.

From Reddish, M., & Kaplan, L. (2007). When are new graduates competent in the critical care unit? *Critical Care Quarterly 30*(3): 199–205.

by using analytic problem solving (Benner, 1984, pp. 13–34).

Box 16-1 summarizes the five stages of transition from novice to competent practitioner.

It is important to realize that you do progress in professional competence as you work. Self-assessment to your current level of performance is an important function in nursing. Much of your progression will also greatly depend on the work environment. The organization provides the environment for the clinical progression of all staff, both for organizational needs and for the personal development of the nurse. Such professional work environments are evidenced in the various health care organizations that have achieved Magnet status (ANCC, 2008).

STAFF COMPETENCY

The Joint Commission states that a hospital must provide the right number of competent staff to meet the needs of the patients (2007). Competent staff is a staff that is qualified and able to perform the work according to professional standards. Staffing is discussed in Chapter 19. To meet the goal of providing adequate competent staff, the hospital must carry out the following processes and activities:

- The hospital provides for competent staff either through traditional employer-employee arrangements or through contractual arrangements with other entities or persons.
- Orienting, training, and educating staff
- The hospital provides ongoing in-service and other education and training to increase staff knowledge of specific work-related issues.
- Assessing, maintaining, and improving staff competence
- Ongoing, periodic competence assessment evaluates staff members' continuing abilities to perform throughout their association with the organization.
- Promoting self-development and learning. Staff is encouraged to pursue ongoing professional development goals and provide feedback about the work environment (The Joint Commission, 2007, p. 319).

The initial step in deciding staff competency in most health care organizations occurs in employee orientation.

NEW EMPLOYEE ORIENTATION

Orientation is a process in which initial job training and information are provided to staff.

Staff orientation promotes safe and effective job performance. Some elements of orientation need to occur before staff provide care, treatment, and services. Other elements of orientation can occur when staff is providing care, treatment, and services (The Joint Commission, 2007, p. 330). All employees, regardless of level of competence, are required to attend orientation. Basic to new employee orientation is education on the organization-specific function, policies, and expectations, such as mission, vision, values, stakeholder expectations, performance improvement, basic skill evaluation, and mandatory policy review. Hospital orientations can range from 3 weeks to 6 months depending on the organization and responsibilities of the nurse.

For new graduates, the orientation is often expanded to allow for mentoring to the new role. The time frame for new nurse socialization to the role, or the process of developing clinical judgment in practice, has been suggested to be as follows (Ferguson, Day, Anderson, and Rohatnsky, 2007):

- Orientation (0–20 days)
- Learning practice norms (orientation 4–6 months)
- Developing confidence (6–12 months)
- Consolidating relationships (12–18 months)
- Seeking challenges (18–24 months)

This does not mean that the formal orientation is 2 years, but the length of time for a new nurse to become fully socialized to the profession and organization.

Once an employee accepts a new position, the orientation process is outlined. The length of orientation varies from hospital to hospital and for differing groups of employees. Some hospitals differentiate between experienced staff and novice staff. This is also the time that a new employee has completed the health physical and has met all of the medical criteria for employment, such as hepatitis B immunization and immunity status, tuberculosis testing, etc.

MANDATORY CONTENT

The first part of orientation is usually organization specific. There is usually a hospital-wide orientation, which may include speakers such as the human resources representative, the infection control coordinator, the safety officer, the employee health coordinator, and the process improvement coordinator. This organization-specific orientation usually includes those educational topics that are considered mandatory by the accreditation agencies. These mandatory topics are usually reviewed on an annual basis in most health care institutions. This mandatory review allows for the determination of employee competency in knowledge in these content areas (Box 16-2).

Box 16-2   NEW EMPLOYEE ORIENTATION: MANDATORY CONTENT

- Mission and governance
- Customer contact requirements
- Code of conduct
- Fire safety
- Age-specific patient content
- Infection control
- Process improvement
- Corporate compliance
- HIPAA
- Benefits

UNIT-BASED CONTENT

There then is a unit-based or nursing-based orientation. Unit-based orientations are designed by the unit educator and nurse manager to orient the new nurse to the unit, its policies, patient needs, procedures, and protocols. For example, a nurse in a cardiac unit will receive education on electrocardiogram interpretation, cardiac drugs, cardiac arrest protocols, etc. A nurse in the labor room will receive education on fetal monitoring, neonatal resuscitation, etc. Patient care assignments will be made to match the learning of orientation. A description of the growth from novice to competent practitioner is detailed in Figure 16-1.

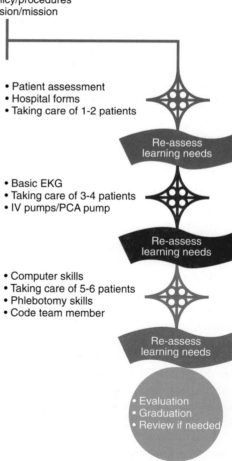

- Start orientation
- Review policy/procedures
- Hospital vision/mission

- Patient assessment
- Hospital forms
- Taking care of 1-2 patients

Re-assess learning needs

- Basic EKG
- Taking care of 3-4 patients
- IV pumps/PCA pump

Re-assess learning needs

- Computer skills
- Taking care of 5-6 patients
- Phlebotomy skills
- Code team member

Re-assess learning needs

- Evaluation
- Graduation
- Review if needed

Figure 16-1 • A sample training roadmap. Lee, V., & Harris, T. (2007). Mentoring new nursing graduates. Retrieved October 12, 2007, from http://www.minoritynurse.com/features/other/080207d.html.

PRECEPTOR MODEL

There are numerous models of nursing orientations, but most use preceptors to work with and evaluate the new employee during the orientation phase. New nurses are traditionally oriented to the professional role by "experienced" registered nurses who are knowledgeable of the "ways of nursing" in the organization. A *preceptor* can be defined as an experienced staff member who possesses excellent clinical skills and facilitates learning through caring, respect, compassion, understanding, nurturing, role modeling, and the excellent use of interpersonal communication (Speers, Strzyzewski, and Ziolkowski, 2004). There are varied methods of choosing preceptors and pairing them with orientees. In hospitals with clinical ladders, experienced nurses are required to serve as preceptors as part of their normal responsibilities. In other institutions, preceptors are chosen based on their competencies, while in other institutions, nurses are chosen based on availability. This last method often results in multiple preceptors for one orientee. This can result in frustration for the orientee, who may be receiving multiple messages from multiple preceptors (Hardy & Smith, 2001). Research demonstrates that proper pairing is key to the success of the preceptor program (Hardy & Smith, 2001). Proper pairing occurs with preceptors who are selected into the role based on competencies in both clinical nursing and the ability to facilitate learning (Speers et al., 2004).

This model can be used to assist new employees and to reward experienced staff nurses. This model provides a means for orienting and socializing the new nurse as well as providing a mechanism to recognize exceptionally competent staff nurses (Sullivan & Decker, 2005). Box 16-3 lists various functions of the preceptor.

While preceptors are used to assist with the orientation of new nurses to the organization and unit, there are also rewards for the preceptor. The experienced nurses often feel more enthusiasm and feel more involved with the new staff, while the orientees express a sense of belonging to the unit (Hardy & Smith, 2001). New graduate nurses require time to move from the role of student to expert clinician. Preceptors are an essential part of that transition (Neuman et al., 2004).

There are other roles involved in this orientation (Box 16-4).

Box 16-3   PRECEPTOR FUNCTIONS

- Assist new nurse to acquire knowledge and skills
- Tailor program specifically to needs
- Orient to unit
- Socialize within group
- Orient to unit functions
- Teach unfamiliar procedures
- Assists in development of skills
- Act as resource person
- Familiarize with policies and procedures
- Act as counselor
- Act as role model
- Time management coach
- Delegate tasks
- Assist with priority setting

CONTINUED EMPLOYEE DEVELOPMENT

Accrediting agencies require that staff competence to perform job responsibilities must be assessed, demonstrated, and maintained by the human resources department in conjunction with the education department and the nurse manager (The Joint Commission, 2007). Competency in the required organizational and unit "mandatories" must be annually evaluated. The current licensure of the individual must be maintained on record. Some states require contact hours for professional license renewal. Many health care organizations provide these contact hours through their internal education or through employee benefits, which include educational advancement.

As the employee moves from novice to expert, the organization supports the individual in achieving the required competencies and additional learning required for growth. The basis for the assessment of the individual's needs and abilities is determined through the performance appraisal process. This process allows for the evaluation of the employee against stated standards. It also allows the employee to set annual goals for future development. The aggregation of these individual learning goals then becomes part of the annual education and human resource plan of the organization.

Box 16-4 ROLES INVOLVED IN ORIENTATION

Role of Nurse Manager
- Provide leadership in the culture of the nursing unit
- Provide supportive evaluation feedback to new nurses and experienced nurses
- Demonstrate valuing of mentoring activities
- Provide workloads that are reasonable and safe (with monitoring)
- Provide full-time employment on a single nursing unit
- Provide educational experiences
- Provide collaborative team experiences where possible

Nurse Managers Retention Strategies
- Assist new nurses to manage stress
- Increase levels of responsibility slowly
- Maintain a level of challenge through provision of additional responsibilities
- Acknowledge continuing education needs
- Provide encouragement and support in their transition
- Maintain an appropriate staff mix wherein they can practice safely

Human Resource Role
- Provide adequate orientation programs

- Ongoing support to address higher levels of learning
- Approve leaves for absences or educational study
- Support educational opportunities
- Coordinate new nurse employment on single units
- Initiate formal evaluative processes for performance appraisal
- Support a learning organization approach
- Provide resources and learning opportunities
- Acknowledge the contributions of mentors

Creative Engagement and Retention Strategies
- Support and encourage certification programs
- Facilitate service for education agreements
- Support clinical leadership
- Invest in the employee
- Provide extended learning experiences to enhance practice
- Provide adequate staff for safe patient care
- Provide oversight of new nurses by experienced nurses
- Encourage institutional commitment to mentorship
- Support "respectful workplace" initiatives

From Ferguson, L., Day, R., Anderson, C., & Rohatinsky, N. (2007). The process for mentoring new nurses into professional practice. Conference presentation at the National Healthcare Leadership Conference, 2007. Retrieved October 12, 2007, from http://www.healthcareleadershipconference.ca/assets/PDFs/Presentation%20PDFs/June%2012/Pier%209/The%20Process%20of%20Mentoring%20New%20Nurses%20into%20Professional%20Practice.pdf.

PERFORMANCE APPRAISAL PROCESS

In the beginning, performance appraisal began as a method to justify salary increases for employees. Today, the performance appraisal is used to determine rewards but also to further assist the employee in setting performance goals for the year. Staff career progression begins with goal setting at the annual performance appraisal process.

It is important that the nurse and the nurse manager know the bases on which the individual is being rated. If you are the nurse being evaluated, ask for a copy of the tool being used. If the evaluation is based on the job description, make sure that both the nurse and manager have a copy. Most nursing departments develop departmentwide or unit-specific goals, and all nurses, regardless of their position, are expected to contribute to these goals. Other organizations expect nurses to accomplish individual goals. It is important

to know how you are evaluating or being evaluated. Behaviors appropriate during the evaluation process are listed in Box 16-5.

As a nurse being evaluated:
- Know what you are being rated on.
- Before the review, carefully think about the period since your last review.
- Review the previous year's goals.
- Keep track of your performance and accomplishments along the way.
- Use examples to illustrate how you met the standard.
- Remain positive; acknowledge errors and show how you learned from them.
- Receive criticism well.
- Clarify expectations.
- Accept praise.

There are three main phases of the performance appraisal process:
1. Planning for the Interview

Box 16-5   LIST OF RECOMMENDED SUPERVISOR AND STAFF NURSE BEHAVIORS FOR PERFORMANCE APPRAISAL

Manager Behaviors

Records routinely scheduled, observations of the nurse's performance relative to position, professional standards, and job description competencies in a variety of situations.

Validates interpretation of nurse's performance.

Offers counsel and support as required, citing position and professional standard expectations.

Plans a date and time collaboratively with the nurse.

Communicates to nurse what will be needed for evaluation meeting.

Confirms the interview in writing.

Reviews nurse's past evaluation record.

Completes the written evaluation.

Staff Nurse Behaviors

Utilizes position and professional standard expectations daily.

Documents specific patient outcomes that reflect planned nursing interventions.

Asks for clarification of expectations when there is doubt, citing position responsibilities and professional standards.

Summarizes accomplishments during the evaluation period.

Prepares a list of activities that advance career to the next level.

Collaborates with the supervisor relative to date, time, and expected preparation for the evaluation interview.

Modified from Grohar-Murray, M. E., & DiCroce, H. R. (2003). *Leadership and management in nursing* (p. 223), 3rd ed. Upper Saddle River, NJ: Prentice Hall.

2. Participating in the appraisal Interview
3. Using evaluation results

PLANNING FOR THE INTERVIEW

Preparing for the evaluation is important to the nurse. In preparing, one should always list strengths and weakness, accomplishment of last year's goals, and future goals.

The nurse manager must also be prepared with proper documentation for this interview with specific examples of performance. There must be a correlation between the evaluation and the job description and goals of the institution.

PARTICIPATING IN THE APPRAISAL INTERVIEW

This is the time for discussion specific to the employee only. The first topic of discussion is the individual's accomplishments and successes. This begins the interview on a positive note. The process should be carried out in a professional and sequential manner. If the employee is being recommended for improvement in certain areas, these specific areas must be addressed at the interview and the employee is granted a certain amount of time to improve on the lacking skills or performance. If disciplinary action is warranted due to inferior performance, the nurse manager should have readily available to the employee means to correct the performance, such as counseling or reeducation.

Box 16-6   SUPERVISOR AND STAFF NURSE RESPONSIBILITIES

Supervisor Responsibilities

Conducts the interview.

States judgments about the nurse's performance.

Provides justification for salary.

Encourages new goals.

Agrees upon future goals.

Staff Nurse Responsibilities

Shares documented evidence of significant professional outcomes.

Clarifies performance.

States future goals.

States actions to meet goals.

Modified from Grohar-Murray, M. E., & DiCroce, H. R. (2003). *Leadership and management in nursing* (p. 227), 3rd ed. Upper Saddle River, NJ: Prentice Hall.

USING EVALUATION RESULTS

Health care organizations have in place a method for goal attainment and outcome management. This plan may include items such as if employee goals were met and, if not, what the plan is to assist the employee in meeting these goals in a timely manner. There may be a process improvement plan in place for evaluation of this process. Also, the employee is asked to set goals for the upcoming year along with outcome measures. These goals and outcome measures will form a portion of the next performance appraisal. The responsibilities of the supervisor and the staff nurses during the performance appraisal are listed in Box 16-6.

As the goals of all employees are set and the organizations sets the strategic challenges and objectives for the next year, education and human resource plans are developed. Ongoing education, including in-services, training, and other activities, is mandated by The Joint Commission (2007) to include at a minimum the following:

- Occurs when job responsibilities or duties change
- Increases knowledge or work-related issues
- Is appropriate to the needs of the population(s) served and to comply with law and regulation
- Emphasizes specific job-related aspects of safety and infection prevention and control
- Incorporates methods of team training, when appropriate
- When and how to report adverse events
- Is offered in response to learning needs identified through performance improvement findings and other data analysis (i.e., data from staff surveys, performance evaluations, or other needs assessments)
- Is documented

The above list only refers to the education that is mandated. Health care organizations develop a myriad of educational programs to further support the professional growth of employees and the mission of the organization.

As nurses progress from novice to expert, many health care facilities have a system that allows for promotion of nurses along clinical ladders. Education and benefits for progression in clinical competence form the basis for such ladders.

CLINICAL LADDERS

Clinical ladders are programs that reward nurses for their advancement in nursing. It permits horizontal advancement, allowing excellent clinicians to remain in their role at the bedside. Nurses advance through a determined number of levels within a position category based on predetermined criteria. When a level is reached, there are additional advantages for the nurse. When the highest level for a particular position has been reached, advancement requires additional education in nursing.

Clinical ladders were developed in organizations in reaction to Benner's concept of *Novice to Expert* (1984). They were developed as a means to promote an individual's growth as a professional nurse on the path to expert status. Using organizationally established criteria in conjunction with an interview, health care organizations decide on the merits of individual clinical advancement. The process for Professional Clinical Career Ladder progression is usually both clinically and academically based.

Rockingham Memorial Hospital (RMH) supports an environment that promotes professionalism and excellence in nursing care. The following are some areas of clinical practice and professional excellence that are recognized in this clinical ladder program:

- Professional nursing service
- Clinical nursing competence
- Leadership skills
- Continuing education
- Evidence-based practice in nursing
- Nursing career plans
- Volunteer nursing/health service outside of hospital
- Customer service and hospital-wide initiatives for excellence
- National certification in nursing specialty area
- Shared governance participation on hospital or unit committees
- Health education for staff patients, and others

Objectives

- Promote, recognize, and reward excellence in clinical practice and professionalism of RMH nursing staff
- Promote exceptional bedside nursing patient care and clinical performance by participation in the areas of leadership, continuing education, and through evidence-based practice participation
- Provide clear delineation of nursing competence levels
- Utilize nurses who have been educationally prepared for a variety of levels of practice
- Encourage excellence in practice to ensure quality care of patients.
- Champion recruitment and retention of qualified registered nurses
- Commitment to customer service and RMH excellence standards
- Promote participation in volunteer community and health nursing service

Automatic Advancement Levels I and II:

- **Clinical Nurse I**—Clinical ladder entry level for a new graduate bedside registered nurse. After successful completion of department orientation, a nurse will automatically advance to a Clinical Nurse I.

- **Description**—A new bedside registered nurse developing nursing skills, expanding knowledge, and assuming job responsibilities.
- **Clinical Nurse II**—After completion of a year of employment, and receiving a satisfactory PACE Evaluation, a bedside registered nurse will automatically advance to Clinical Nurse II level. A newly hired, experienced registered nurse (with at least 1 year of recent nursing experience) will be placed at a Clinical Nurse II level. After successful completion of department orientation and first successful PACE evaluation, may advance to higher clinical ladder levels following all program requirements. All RN's will remain at Clinical Nurse II level if they do not choose to advance to higher levels.
- **Description**—An experienced bedside registered nurse capable of independent patient care. Actively developing more advanced nursing skills and knowledge through education and involvement in nursing activities beyond basic job requirements and responsibilities.

Automatic Advancement Levels III, IV, and V:

- **Clinical Nurse III**—Requires annual portfolio submission and complying with all clinical ladder program requirements. Advancement to this level requires self-paced and self-motivated participation.
- **Description**—A bedside registered nurse highly skilled in patient care. Provides leadership and mentorship abilities. Active involvement in continuing education and in nursing activities beyond the basic job requirements and responsibilities.
- **Clinical Nurse IV**—Requires annual portfolio submission and complying with all clinical ladder program requirements. Advancement to this level requires highly self-paced and self-motivated participation.
- **Description**—A bedside registered nurse who has a broad base of advanced nursing experience. Recognized for professional nursing leadership and knowledge. Leadership extends to education

and development of others. Involvement in multiple nursing activities beyond basic job requirements and responsibilities. Acquiring research skills by participating in evaluation of clinical outcomes to improve nursing through evidence-based practice.

- **Clinical Nurse V**—Requires annual portfolio submission and complying with all clinical ladder program requirements. Advancement to this highest level on the clinical ladders requires extraordinary and exceptional self-paced and self-motivated participation.*Must be nationally certified in nursing specialty**
- **Description**—A bedside registered nurse who has exceptional advanced nursing experience. Recognized for expert professional nursing leadership and knowledge. Leadership is recognized at a role-model level. Involvement in multiple nursing activities beyond the basic job requirements and responsibilities. Active and ongoing professional involvement in improving nursing through evidenced-based practice, such as research activities, writing a published nursing article, etc. All submitted evidence-based practice submissions and research materials must be presented in a professional format with extensive information such as charts, graphs, studies, stats, outcomes, etc.

(Clinical Ladders developed by Rockingham Memorial Hospital; retrieved September 2, 2009, from http://www.rmhonline.org/rmh_human_resources/pages/RMH_clinical_ladders.html)

SUMMARY

Health care organizations are responsible for the level of competency of all employees. Competency assessment starts with the initial orientation for all employees and continues throughout the term of employment. Nurses progress on a continuum of competency from novice to expert during their careers according to the work of Benner (1984). This continuum forms the basis for many career development opportunities available to the nurse. These opportunities are related to job function during the performance appraisal process.

CLINICAL CORNER

Shared Governance and Staff Education

Rosemarie D. Rosales

East Orange General Hospital is committed to keeping its nurses motivated to lifelong learning. Our shared governance model, which started in 2005, forms the basis for our professional growth. The Professional Practice Council was the first council to get off the ground in 2005. The chair and co-chair were staff nurses, and the facilitators of the council were directors. This council was responsible for approval of policies for patient care and standards of nursing practice. It was given the charge of coordinating the festivities of the Nurses' Week Celebration in 2006. The nurses' week-long event was planned and executed by the council and its members. It was able to raise the funds for nurses to support some of their special projects. This council was also instrumental in the introduction of the clinical ladder program with approximately 30 nurses receiving awards at different levels. In 2006, staff nurses were encouraged to pursue educational advancement. Our chief nursing officer (CNO) was instrumental in getting this started with a partnership with a local college. From this single partnership, we have expanded the options available to our nurses from on-site registered nurse to bachelor of science in nursing programs to affiliations with a doctor of nursing practice program.

Our shared governance expanded with the formation of the Performance Improvement (PI)/Educational Council in 2006. The chair and co-chair of this council were initially directors, and after a few months, the members elected the chairs and co-chairs. The staff nurses of both councils became engaged and felt empowered as members of these councils. In June of this same year, these two councils coordinated the festivities of the unlicensed personnel week. It was another huge success, and they were very proud of their accomplishments. The PI/Education Council was placed in charge of the PI activities and the educational initiatives of the Patient Care Services Division. The council started weekly practice alerts to spark educational endeavors for the staff. Because of the increasing activities of the council, the decision was made to separate the council into the PI Council and the Education Council. The PI Council continued to review the PI activities, and the Education Council assisted in the educational initiatives of the division. Issues identified in the PI Council paved the way for the creation of a committee to review deviations in practice or issues.

The Peer Review Committee is composed of staff nurses, and they review quality referral cases. Recommendations are made to correct the identified process or system issues. Our leadership is very transparent in its commitment to providing safe, high-quality care to our patients and customers.

The commitment of our CNO to education was evident when he increased the number of clinical educators to four full-time equivalents, with one of them being on the night shift. All the clinical educators are master's prepared. This is the commitment our institution has in providing excellent education to our staff nurses. We were one of the first in the state to provide a clinical educator on the night shift. The leadership of the Patient Care Services Division believes that a night shift educator will help the orientees and new staff as they transition to their role as new nurses.

To assist our nurses in complying with the 30 continuing education units (CEUs) required to renew licenses, we introduced e-learning with our yearly subscription to CE Direct from Nursing Spectrum. We enrolled 100 full-time staff nurses, and we gave priority to those whose licenses will expire in 2008. The staff nurses were very pleased with this endeavor. They have been using CE Direct, and we awarded more than 1000 CEUs every year.

We also nurtured our staff nurses in providing them with opportunities for promotion. We developed them to become clinical coordinators and assisted them in their transition to specialty units such as telemetry and critical care. This helped in the retention of our nurses and in recruitment for our specialty areas. In 2007, we promoted some of our qualified nursing assistants to patient care technicians (PCTs) by providing them with the PCT training. To date, we have at least five PCTs in every clinical unit. We also extended the training of our staff members who are willing to become unit secretaries.

Leadership in our institution believes in promotion from within for our qualified staff. Last year, we promoted a clinical educator to a nurse manager, two clinical coordinators to an assistant director and a nurse manager, and, most recently, a clinical documentation specialist to manager for guest relations. All these endeavors have contributed to increasing the staff morale and have proved that the institution is committed to employee satisfaction.

EVIDENCE-BASED PRACTICE

An Evidence-Based Protocol for Nurse Retention

Gess, E., Manojlovich, M., & Warner, S. (October 2008). An evidence-based protocol for nurse retention. Journal of Nursing Administration, 38, *441–447.*

The ongoing nursing shortage that is being faced by the United States and worldwide will have a detrimental effect not only on nurses and health care economies but more importantly on the safety and well-being of patients. In a cyclical fashion, the nursing shortage leads to nursing dissatisfaction that leads to nursing turnover that leads to a nursing shortage, making replacing those nurses more complicated and costing health care billions of dollars a year. Nursing turnover is estimated to cost 4 to 5 times more than the health care industry estimates and most of these costs are indirect, as a result of predeparture decrease in productivity, position vacancy expenses, and orientation costs of new hires until they reach a productive level. In response to this, an evidence-based protocol for nurse retention has been designed based on current literature by experienced nurse managers for use by frontline managers in assisting in retaining critical nursing staff. Recognizing that nurse managers are critical in the retention of nurses and the minimal support available to assist this group in retaining nurses, the authors developed a focused protocol and interventions that can be viewed as a cost-effective way to address the high rates of nursing turnover which can be tailored to individual units of hospitals. While organizational commitment to nursing has been identified repeatedly in the literature as being critical to nurse retention, little useful material or protocols have been provided to ensure that the bedside nurse feels and understands an institution's commitment to each individual, thus increasing their satisfaction and decreasing their chance of leaving their position. In this protocol, autonomy, recognition, and communication have been identified as measurable ways to increase organizational commitment on the nurse manager level and were selected because they positively influence job satisfaction, organizational commitment, and retention.

The protocol begins with a self-assessment of the organization to identify current practices. Next, the authors instruct the nurse manager on the methods for calculating the rate of nursing turnover on her individual unit using a Nursing Turnover Measurement Form. Next, the Anticipated Turnover Scale is explained and suggested for use with staff to allow for a better feel for the stability and anticipated staffing changes on the unit. Together, these tools will be used to identify areas of weakness where increasing organizational commitment will be beneficial in decreasing staff turnover. With the information collected during this baseline assessment, the direction of attention is determined and the authors provide suggestions for ways to initiate change and increase satisfaction with autonomy, recognition, and communication. The impact the nursing shortage will have on health care demands that the critical issues of nurse retention and turnover be evaluated and addressed in ways that provide recognition to our most valuable assets through better communication and supported autonomy.

NCLEX® EXAM QUESTIONS

1. In an institution that encourages clinical ladder programs, the number of ladder positions is usually:
   1. four
   2. three
   3. five
   4. six
2. Competencies are usually completed by every employee at the institution:
   1. annually
   2. biannually
   3. every 6 months
   4. none of the above
3. Which of the following is(are) the main phase(s) of the performance appraisal process?
   1. planning for the interview
   2. participating in the evaluation interview
   3. using evaluation results
   4. all of the above
4. All of the following are the supervisor's responsibilities during an interview EXCEPT:
   1. conducting the interview
   2. stating judgments about the nurse's performance relative to position and standard expectations beginning with positive accomplishments

Continued

NCLEX® EXAM QUESTIONS—cont'd

3. providing justification for rewards or disciplinary action based on criteria
4. stating goals for the immediate future

5. Which of the following is(are) justification(s) for career development?
   1. to provide equal employment opportunity
   2. to improve use of personnel
   3. to improve quality of work life
   4. all of the above

6. Which of the following is NOT the role of a preceptor?
   1. counselor
   2. supervisor
   3. role model
   4. resource person

7. In the process of developing clinical judgment in practice, the orientation usually is within:
   1. 0–20 days
   2. 4–6 days
   3. 4–6 months
   4. 6–12 months

8. In the process of developing clinical judgment in practice, the development of confidence is usually within:
   1. 0–20 days
   2. 4–6 days
   3. 4–6 months
   4. 6–12 months

9. There are _____ stages of transition from novice to competent practitioner.
   1. three
   2. four
   3. five
   4. six

10. Benner stated that a nurse moves through _____ stages of clinical competence.
    1. four
    2. five
    3. six
    4. seven

Answers: 1. 1   2. 1   3. 4   4. 4   5. 4   6. 2   7. 1   8. 4   9. 3   10. 2

REFERENCES

American Nurses Credentialling Center (ANCC). (2008). The Magnet Recognition Program. Retrieved November 8, 2008, from http://www.nursecredentialing.org/Magnet.aspx.

Benner, P. (1984). *From novice to expert: Excellence and power in clinical nursing practice.* Menlo Park, CA: Addison-Wesley.

Ferguson, L., Day, R., Anderson, C., & Rohatnsky, N. (2007). The process for mentoring new nurses into professional practice. Conference presentation at the National Healthcare Leadership Conference, 2007. Retrieved October 12, 2007, from http://www.healthcareleadershipconference.ca/assets/PDFs/Presentation%20PDFs/June%2012/Pier%209/The%20Process%20of%20Mentoring%20New%20Nurses%20into%20Professional%20Practice.pdf.

Grohar-Murray, M. E., & DiCroce, H. R. (2003). *Leadership and management in nursing,* 3rd ed. Upper Saddle River, NJ: Prentice Hall.

Hardy, R., & Smith, R. (2001). Enhancing staff development with a structured preceptor program. *Journal of Nursing Care Quality, 15,* 9-17.

The Joint Commission. (2007). *Hospital accreditation standards.* Oakbrook Terrace, IL: Author.

Lee, V., & Harris, T. (2007). Mentoring new nursing graduates. Retrieved October 12, 2007, from http://www.minoritynurse.com/features/other/080207d.html.

Neuman, J., Brady-Schluttner, K., McKay, A., Roslien, J., Tweedell, D., & James, K. (2004). Centralizing a registered nurse preceptor program at the institutional level. *Journal for Nurses in Staff Development, 20,* 17-24.

Reddish, M., & Kaplan, L. (2007). When are new graduates competent in the critical care unit? *Critical Care Quarterly, 30*(3), 199-205.

Speers, A., Strzyzewski, N., & Ziololkowski, L. (2004). Preceptor preparation: an investment in the future. *Journal for Nurses in Staff Development, 20,* 127-133.

Sullivan, E. J., & Decker, F. J. (2005). *Effective leadership and managemnet in nursing,* 5th ed. Upper Saddle River, NJ: Prentice-Hall.

CHAPTER 17

Personal and Workplace Safety

Chapter Objectives

1. Differentiate between workplace safety and patient safety.
2. Explain why violence in the workplace is of particular concern for nurses.
3. Differentiate between abuse and assault.
4. Compare and contrast lateral and vertical violence.
5. Identify legal issues concerning workplace violence.
6. Identify issues of importance for safety in the workplace.
7. Discuss potential safety hazards in the workplace.
8. Review measures to protect the employee.
9. Identify interventions designed to deal with workplace violence.
10. Identify signs and symptoms of impaired practice.
11. Discuss the role of the nurse and nurse manager is dealing with impaired colleagues.
12. Explain the role of the employee assistance program.

Definitions

Employee assistance program (EAP) Confidential, short-term counseling service for employees with personal problems that affect their work performance

Horizontal violence Coworker act of assault, verbal abuse, threats, battery, manslaughter, or homicide

Muggings Aggravated assaults, usually conducted by surprise and with intent to rob

Physical assaults Attacks ranging from slapping and beating to rape, homicide, and the use of weapons such as firearms, bombs, or knives

Sexual harassment Unwelcomed sexual advances, request for sexual favors, or other verbal or physical conduct of a sexual nature when this conduct explicitly or implicitly affects an individual's employment, unreasonably interferes with an individual's work performance, or creates an intimidating, hostile, or offensive work environment

Impaired practice Professional working while under the influence of a mind-altering chemical such as alcohol or drugs

Threats Expressions of intent to cause harm, including verbal threats, threatening body language, and written threats

Vertical violence Actual or threatened act of assault, verbal abuse, threats, battery, manslaughter, or homicide from an employee to a manager

Workplace safety Prevention of employee workplace injuries, incidents, and personal injury while at work

Workplace violence Any violent act, including physical assaults and threats of assault, directed toward persons at work or on duty

WORKPLACE VIOLENCE

In a national survey of registered nurses conducted by American Nurses Association (ANA) in 2001, 88% of working nurses reported that health and safety concerns influence their decisions to continue working in the field of nursing as well as the kind of nursing work they choose to perform. Hospitals are perceived as places of safe haven, but in reality they are potential breeding grounds for many types of incidents, ranging from disruptive staff, patients, and families to chemical and infection exposure. Nurses have a right to a safe workplace. In fact, a safe workplace is necessary for the provision of patient care (ANA, 2007). Hazardous material exposure was covered in Chapter 7. This chapter deals with issues of concern for the nurse dealing with potentially explosive workplace situations.

Workplace violence ranges from offensive or threatening language to homicide. The National Institute for Occupational Safety and Health (NIOSH) defines *workplace violence* as violent acts (including physical assaults and threats of assaults) directed toward persons at work or on duty. Workplace violence can be divided into four categories: violence by strangers, clients (patients), coworkers, and personal relations (AACN, 2004). It has been reported that 82% of nurses surveyed had been assaulted during their careers and that many assaults go unreported (Erickson & Willams-Evans, 2000; ICN, 2001).

More than 5 million U.S. hospital workers from many occupations perform a wide variety of duties. They are exposed to many safety and health hazards, including violence. Recent data indicate that hospital workers are at high risk for experiencing violence in the workplace. According to estimates of the Bureau of Labor Statistics (BLS), 2637 nonfatal assaults on hospital workers occurred in 1999—a rate of 8.3 assaults per 10,000 workers. This rate is much higher than the rate of nonfatal assaults for all private-sector industries, which is 2 per 10,000 workers.

Employee assaults may be from patients, families, and coworkers. Assault can range from minor to major assaults. Outbursts of violence can affect the employee with disability, psychological trauma, or death. Several risk factors may lead to violence in the health care setting (Tomey, 2006):
- People under the influence of alcohol or drugs
- Working understaffed
- Long waiting times
- Overcrowded waiting rooms
- Working alone
- Unlimited public access
- Poorly lit corridors, rooms, parking lots
- Contact with public
- Exchange of money
- Working in community-based settings
- Hospitalized prisoners
- Isolated work with patients during exams and treatments

Hospitals are microcosms of society and, as such, are socialized to violence.

Workplace violence is a multifaceted event with the potential to increase in frequency and scope (Ehrmann & Zuzelo, 2007). As a nurse and manager, you need to have a basic understanding of the risk for workplace violence to intervene in effective, efficient, and meaningful ways. You have already earned about potentially violent patients and how to handle them, but you need to be able to transfer some of this knowledge to the potentially violent employee. Boxes 17-1 and 17-2 provide warning signs of physical violence.

While there is no universal strategy to prevent workplace violence, all hospitals have developed security plans to protect the employee from an unsafe workplace. The risk factors vary from hospital to hospital and from unit to unit. You have learned many ways of assessing individuals for altered levels of dealing with stress as well as intervening in such situations. These are important to remember.

Maintain behavior that helps diffuse anger.
- Present calm, caring attitude.
- Do not match the threats.
- Do not give orders.

Box 17-1   WARNING SIGNS OF VIOLENCE

- Attendance problems
- Carelessness at work
- History of physical violence
- Performance problems
- Personality changes
- Poor hygiene
- Substance abuse
- Social isolation

From Tomey, A. M. (2004). *Guide to nursing management and leadership* (p. 162), 7th ed. St. Louis: Mosby.

Box 17-2 SIGNS OF IMPENDING PHYSICAL VIOLENCE

- Clenched jaws or fists
- Increased movement
- Increased respirations
- Pacing
- Shouting threats
- Staring or pointing
- Use of profanity

From Gates, D. M., & Kroeger, F. (2003). Violence against nurses: the silent epidemic. *ISNA Bulletin, 29*, 25-29; National Institute for Occupational Safety and Health (NIOSH). (April 2002). Occupational violence. Retrieved March 20, 2008, from http://www.cdc.gov/niosh/topics/violence/. DHHS (NIOSH) publication No. 2002-101.

- Acknowledge the person's feelings (e.g., "I know you are frustrated").
- Avoid any behavior that may be interpreted as aggressive (e.g., moving rapidly, getting too close, touching, or speaking loudly).
  Be alert.
- Evaluate each situation for potential violence when you enter a room or begin to relate to a staff member, patient, or visitor.
- Be vigilant throughout the encounter.
- Do not isolate yourself with a potentially violent person.
- Always keep an open path for exiting—do not let the potentially violent person stand between you and the door.
  Take these steps if you cannot defuse the situation quickly.
- Remove yourself from the situation.
- Call security for help.
- Report any violent incidents to your management.
  When you are dealing with potential staff violence or patient and family violence, it is important to maintain the safety of the patient care situation. If possible, remove the potentially violent individual from the patient care area.

CONFLICT MANAGEMENT

In managing the conflict, you will need to determine the cause of the conflict. First, determine the basis of the conflict. Is there difficulty between two shifts (intergroup) or two individuals (interpersonal)? Often, there is conflict between shifts that spill over to stressful situations. Some of these conflicts may relate to perceptions of work left undone by one shift or other work-related concerns. Second, you will need to analyze the source of the conflict. Conflict management techniques stress the importance of open and honest communication and assertive dialogue. It is important that during conflict situations the nurse manager views the total situation and uses positive communication. Conflict resolution techniques are described in a variety of ways by a variety of authors (Tomey, 2004; Yoder-Wise & Kowalski, 2006). The following is a list of strategies for conflict resolution, the third step of conflict management (Huber, 2006, p. 528):

- *Avoiding*—If you avoid the problem, you can trick yourself into believing that there is no problem.
- *Withholding or withdrawing*—In this situation, parties remove themselves from participation in a solution; this does not resolve a conflict.
- *Reassuring*—Parties do not withdraw but try to make everyone feel good. In this situation, reassuring strategies are used to diffuse strong conflicts; this may be a way of hindering open communication.
- *Accommodating*—This is often used in vertical conflict when there is a power differential. It may also be used when one individual has a vested interest in a solution that may be relatively unimportant to the other individual.
- *Competing*—This is an assertive strategy in which one individual's needs are satisfied at another's expense.
- *Compromising*—This strategy is used when both individuals play a part in the decision. It is a basis of conflict management.
- *Confronting*—Individuals will speak for themselves in a way that the other individual hears the concern.
- *Collaborating*—Parties work together to find a mutually beneficial solution.
- *Bargaining and negotiating*—This involves both parties in a back-and-forth discussion to reach a level of agreement.
- *Problem-solving*—The goal is to find a workable solution for all parties.

Box 17-3 provides a model for managing conflict.

Box 17-3 MODEL FOR MANAGING CONFLICT

Determine the basis of the conflict.
- Intrapersonal
- Interpersonal
- Group
- Intergoup
- Organizational

Analyze the sources of the conflict.
- Cultural differences
- Different facts
- Separate pieces of information
- Different perceptions of the event
- Defining the problem differently
- Divergent views of power and authority
- Role conflicts
- Number of organizational levels
- Degree of association
- Parties dependent on others
- Competition for scarce resources
- Ambiguous jurisdictions
- Need for consensus
- Communication barriers
- Separation in time and space
- Accumulation of unresolved conflict

Consider alternative approaches to conflict management.
- Avoiding
- Accommodating
- Compromising
- Collaborating
- Competing

Choose the most appropriate approach.
Implement the conflict management strategy.
Evaluate the results.

From Tomey, A. M. (2004). *Guide to nursing management and leadership* (p. 144), 7th ed. St. Louis: Mosby.

Box 17-4 HORIZONTAL VIOLENCE IN THE WORKPLACE

- Nonverbal behaviors such as the raising of eyebrows or making faces in response to comments by the victim
- Verbal remarks that could be characterized as being snide or abrupt responses to questions raised by the victim
- Activities that undermine the victim's ability to perform professionally, including either refusing or not being available to give assistance
- The withholding of information about a practice or patient that will undermine a victim's ability to perform professionally
- Acts of sabotage that deliberately set up victims for negative situations in their work environment
- Group in-fighting and establishment of cliques designed to exclude some staff members
- Failure to resolve conflicts directly with the individual involved, choosing instead to complain to others about an individual's behavior
- Failure to respect the privacy of others
- Broken confidences

From Longo, J., & Sherman, R. (2007). Leveling horizontal violence. *Nursing Management, 38,* 35.

HORIZONTAL VIOLENCE IN THE WORKPLACE

Many of the issues that interfere with workplace safety arise from the interactions that routinely occur between staff members. In times of stress, there is often miscommunication among colleagues. Most of these conflicts can be resolved with open communication. There is, however, a growing concern among health employees about horizontal violence between staff members. *Horizontal violence* is an act of aggression toward another colleague (Box 17-4). It may range from verbal or emotional abuse or extend to physical abuse. Subtle acts of horizontal abuse may include belittling a fellow staff member, withholding information, or freezing a colleague out of group activities. As a nurse, the challenge will be to identify behaviors that could be considered horizontally violent. Some of this behavior occurs between physicians and nurses. Two thirds of nurses say that they have experienced such abuse at the hands of physicians (Cook, 2001; Rosenstein, 2002).

Horizontal conflict is based on differences between colleagues. *Vertical conflict* relates to differences between managers and staff associates. These differences are often related to inadequate communication, opposing interests, and lack of shared attitudes. If staff members continue with horizontally violent behavior, the outcome is low morale and stress (Rosenstein, 2002). As a new nurse leader, it will be your responsibility to stop such behavior. The following steps are recommended to stop the cycle (Longo, 2007, p. 36):
- Analyze the culture of your work unit: observe for verbal and nonverbal cues in the behavior of your staff.
- Name the problem when you see it and use the term "horizontal violence."

- Raise the issue at staff meetings and educate your staff about horizontal violence to help break the silence.
- Allow staff members to tell their stories if horizontal violence is part of the culture of the unit.
- Ensure there is a process for dealing with this issue if it occurs in your unit and be responsive when issues are brought to your attention.
- Engage in self-awareness activities and reflective practice to ensure that your leadership style does not support horizontal violence.
- Provide your nursing staff members with training about conflict management skills and empower them to defend themselves against bullying behavior.

SEXUAL HARASSMENT

Some instances of abuse may be forms of sexual harassment. Sexual harassment can result from collegial interpersonal conflict. *Sexual harassment* is a form of sex discrimination that violates Title VII of the Civil Rights Act of 1964. It is defined as unwelcomed sexual advances, request for sexual favors, or other verbal or physical conduct of a sexual nature when this conduct explicitly or implicitly affects an individual's employment, unreasonably interferes with an individual's work performance, or creates an intimidating, hostile, or offensive work environment (The U.S. Equal Employment Opportunity Commission, 2009).

All employment agencies are required to have sexual harassment policies and reporting procedures. This will be part of your new hire and mandatory annual education. When exposed to an incident of sexual harassment, it is important to remember that it needs to be confronted immediately. Confront the harasser with a statement such as, "I want you to know that I do not want you telling me sexual jokes." If the behavior continues, inform your immediate supervisor.

While incidences of interpersonal conflict are inevitable in any workplace, it is the responsibility of both staff and leadership to recognize concerns and then intervene appropriately if the workplace is to be conducive to a satisfying and professional workplace.

As a nurse and nurse manager, you must do the following (AACN, 2004, p. 2):
- Actively develop a culture where violence is not tolerated, incidents are promptly addressed and

managed, and comprehensive support for coworkers who experience violence is provided.
- Advocate for enforceable violence management policies in the workplace and hold others accountable for their behavior.
- Participate in educational training on violence awareness and prevention.
- Mentor colleagues on how to respond when incidents occur.

VIOLENCE: OCCUPATIONAL HAZARDS IN HOSPITALS

As a nurse manager, you may be involved in the development of a comprehensive violence prevention program. No universal strategy exists to prevent violence. The risk factors vary from hospital to hospital and from unit to unit. The goal of the violence prevention program is to identify risk factors in specific work scenarios and to develop strategies for reducing them (NIOSH, 2002).

Occupational Safety and Health Administration (OSHA) has identified eight essential components for a violence prevention plan:
1. Management commitment
2. Employee involvement
3. Work site analysis
4. Prevention of hazards
5. Training and education
6. Prompt recognition, control, and monitoring
7. Record keeping
8. Evaluation

This follows a model that is similar for the work of the hospital-wide safety committee (see Chapter 7).

The safety committee has the responsibility of developing and implementing the environmental controls within a hospital setting. This committee is also responsible to document that physical rounds are made in the facility and outside of the facility to maintain the hospital's environmental and administrative controls for violence prevention (Box 17-5).

All hospitals are required to have a new employee/ volunteer/student orientation program as well as an annual employee/volunteer program that must be clearly documented. The human resources department of the hospital is required to maintain these records. The state board of health and/or The Joint Commission usually requests these documents on an inspection or a

Box 17-5 HOSPITAL'S ENVIRONMENTAL AND ADMINISTRATIVE CONTROLS FOR VIOLENCE PREVENTION

Environmental Controls

- Install emergency alarms
- Install monitoring systems (cameras)
- Install metal detectors
- Provide security escorts to parking lots/decks
- Provide adequate waiting areas to prevent overcrowding
- Provide staff members with secure, lockable bathrooms
- Provide adequate lighting
- Replace lights immediately if defective
- Provide video for high-risk areas

Administrative Controls

- Establish liaison with local police and fire departments.
- Report incidents of violence.
- Require employees to report assaults and/or threats.
- Provide a trained response team.
- Distribute visitor passes.
- Maintain proper reports of incidents.
- Develop and implement hospitalwide safety plan (see Chapter 7).
- Enforce all safety and security policies and procedures (see Chapter 7).
- Distribute staff identification badges (enforce use of same).

Box 17-6 EMPLOYEE EDUCATION

- Workplace violence prevention policy and procedure
- Early recognition of escalating behavior
- Early reaction response plan of violent behavior
- Cultural and ethnic diversity awareness plan
- Location and activation of emergency alarms
- Awareness of emergency exits
- Awareness of employee roles in the event of workplace violence

survey. Required employee education is documented in Box 17-6.

Precise record keeping is required in the event of an incident. The hospital will have either a policy and procedure for a written incident report or a computer-based program. Whether your hospital uses the written form or the computer-based program, the exact date, time, and occurrence must be properly documented. The follow-up of the event is also clearly documented for future reference. The documents are used for impending court cases, review of types of employee and/or visitor injuries, needlestick injuries, or bodily harm.

WORKPLACE VIOLENCE CHECKLIST

As a new nurse contemplating working within a facility, the checklist in Box 17-7 can serve as an assessment of the personal safety of the facility.

IMPAIRED EMPLOYEES

Sometimes issues of staff conflict are symptomatic of other personal issues that may be impairing a staff member. Such issues may be stress at home, financial difficulties, or actual impairment from drugs and/or alcohol. While all staff members will have personal issues that affect the workplace at various times, it is important for you to know when these personal issues interfere with workplace and/or patient safety.

In December 1998, the ANA estimated that 7% of nurses in the United States are impaired by alcohol or drugs. Some of this addictive behavior is accentuated by the constant availability of mind-altering drugs, while some nurses come to the workplace with addictive difficulties.

Boxes 17-8 and 17-9 provide signs and physical symptoms of alcohol or drug dependency.

Marquis and Huston (2006, p. 663) discuss the profile of the impaired nurse and group characteristics into three primary areas: personality/behavior changes, job performance changes, and time and attendance changes.

COMMON PERSONALITY/BEHAVIOR CHANGES OF THE CHEMICALLY IMPAIRED EMPLOYEE

- Increased irritability with patients and colleagues; often followed by extreme calm
- Social isolation, eats alone, avoids unit social functions
- Extreme and rapid mood swings

Box 17-7   WORKPLACE VIOLENCE CHECKLIST

This checklist helps identify present or potential workplace violence problems. Employers also may be aware of other serious hazards not listed here.

Periodic inspections for security hazards include identifying and evaluating potential workplace security hazards and changes in employee work practices which may lead to compromising security. Please use the following checklist to identify and evaluate workplace security hazards. **TRUE** notations indicate a potential risk for serious security hazards:

___**T**___**F** This industry frequently confronts violent behavior and assaults of staff.

___**T**___**F** Violence has occurred on the premises or in conducting business.

___**T**___**F** Customers, clients, or coworkers assault, threaten, yell, push, or verbally abuse employees or use racial or sexual remarks.

___**T**___**F** Employees are NOT required to report incidents or threats of violence, regardless of injury or severity, to employer.

___**T**___**F** Employees have NOT been trained by the employer to recognize and handle threatening, aggressive, or violent behavior.

___**T**___**F** Violence is accepted as "part of the job" by some managers, supervisors, and/or employees.

___**T**___**F** Access and freedom of movement within the workplace are NOT restricted to those persons who have a legitimate reason for being there.

___**T**___**F** The workplace security system is inadequate (e.g., door locks malfunction, windows are not secure, and there are no physical barriers or containment systems).

___**T**___**F** Employees or staff members have been assaulted, threatened, or verbally abused by clients and patients.

___**T**___**F** Medical and counseling services have NOT been offered to employees who have been assaulted.

___**T**___**F** Alarm systems such as panic alarm buttons, silent alarms, or personal electronic alarm systems are NOT being used for prompt security assistance.

___**T**___**F** There is no regular training provided on correct response to alarm sounding.

___**T**___**F** Alarm systems are NOT tested on a monthly basis to ensure correct function.

___**T**___**F** Security guards are NOT employed at the workplace.

___**T**___**F** Closed circuit cameras and mirrors are NOT used to monitor dangerous areas.

___**T**___**F** Metal detectors are NOT available or NOT used in the facility.

___**T**___**F** Employees have NOT been trained to recognize and control hostile and escalating aggressive behaviors and to manage assaultive behavior.

___**T**___**F** Employees CANNOT adjust work schedules to use the "buddy system" for visits to clients in areas where they feel threatened.

___**T**___**F** Cellular phones or other communication devices are NOT made available to field staff to enable them to request aid.

___**T**___**F** Vehicles are NOT maintained on a regular basis to ensure reliability and safety.

___**T**___**F** Employees work in areas where assistance is NOT readily available.

From Occupational Safety and Health Administration (OSHA). (2003). *Guidelines for preventing workplace violence for health care and social service workers* (rev. 2003). Washington, DC: OSHA, U.S. Department of Labor. Retrieved December 9, 2004, from www.osha.gov/SLTC/etools/hospital/hazards/workplaceviolence/checklist.html; Huber, D. L. (2006). *Leadership and nursing care management* (p. 681), 3rd ed. Philadelphia: Elsevier.

- Euphoric recall of events or elaborate excuses for behaviors
- Unusually strong interest in narcotics or the narcotic cabinet
- Sudden, dramatic change in personal grooming or any other area
- Forgetfulness ranging from simple short-term memory loss to blackouts
- Change in physical appearance, which may include weight loss, flushed face, red or bleary eyes, unsteady gait, slurred speech, tremors, restlessness, diaphoresis, bruises and cigarette burns, jaundice, and ascites
- Extreme defensiveness regarding medication errors

Box 17-8 SIGNS OF ALCOHOL OR DRUG DEPENDENCY

- Family history or alcoholism or drug abuse
- Frequent change of work site (same or other institution)
- Prior medical history requiring pain control
- Conscientious worker with recent decrease in performance
- Decreased attention to personal appearance
- Frequent complaints of marital and family problems
- Reports of illness, minor accidents, and emergencies

- Complaints from coworkers
- Mood swings, depression, suicide attempts
- Strong interest in patients' pain control
- Frequent trips to the bathroom
- Increasing isolation (night shift request; eating alone)
- Elaborate excuses for tardiness
- Difficulty in meeting schedules and deadlines
- Inadequate explanation for missing work

From Sullivan, E., Bissel, L., & Williams, E. (1988). *Chemical dependency in nursing: the deadly diversion.* Menlo Park, CA: Addison-Wesley Nursing.

Box 17-9 PHYSICAL SYMPTOMS OF ALCOHOL OR DRUG DEPENDENCY

- Shakiness, tremors of hands, jitteriness
- Slurred speech
- Watery eyes, dilated or constricted pupils
- Diaphoresis
- Unsteady gait

- Runny nose
- Nausea, vomiting, diarrhea
- Weight loss or gain
- Blackouts (memory losses while conscious)
- Wears long-sleeved clothing continuously

From Sullivan, E., Bissel, L., & Williams, E. (1988). *Chemical dependency in nursing: the deadly diversion.* Menlo Park, CA: Addison-Wesley Nursing.

COMMON JOB PERFORMANCE CHANGES OF THE CHEMICALLY IMPAIRED EMPLOYEE

- Difficulty meeting schedules and deadlines
- Illogical or sloppy charting
- High frequency of medication errors or errors in judgment affecting patient care
- Frequently volunteers to be medication nurse
- Has a high number of assigned patients who complain that their pain medication is ineffective in relieving their pain
- Consistently meeting work performance requirements at minimal levels or doing the minimum amount of work necessary
- Judgment errors
- Sleeping or dozing on duty
- Complaints from other staff members about the quality and quantity of the employee's work

COMMON TIME AND ATTENDANCE CHANGES OF THE CHEMICALLY IMPAIRED EMPLOYEE

- Increasingly absent from work without adequate explanation or notification; most frequent absence on a Monday or Friday

- Long lunch hours
- Excessive use of sick leave or requests for sick leave after days off
- Frequent calling in to request compensatory time
- Arriving at work early or staying late for no apparent reason
- Consistent lateness
- Frequent disappearances from the unit without explanation

It is your responsibility as a nurse and nurse manager to report any issues of coworker behaviors. You should be alert to any signs and symptoms (see Box 17-4) of a coworker under the influence and be aware of methods of reporting. You should report the health care worker to your immediate supervisor. It is the supervisor's responsibility to take further action. In keeping with the institution's policies and procedures, the Human Resources Department should be alerted to assist the supervisor or nurse manager with confronting the employee. Reporting laws and consequences vary in each state. Clear documentation regarding the employee must be kept. Documentation should include tardiness, absenteeism, patient or coworker complaints, records of controlled substances on the unit, and physical signs and symptoms both observed and reported. (See

Box 17-10 EXAMPLES OF NEW JERSEY BOARD OF NURSING LEVEL I MANDATORY REPORTING

- Suspected drug diversion
- Misappropriation
- Theft
- Physical and verbal abuse
- Sexual abuse or exploitation
- Intoxication on duty
- Failing to account for wastage of controlled medication

employee assistance program discussion later in this chapter.)

Health care workers who abuse drugs or alcohol place both the patient and their fellow staff at considerable risk. It is important for you to know your responsibilities when dealing with an impaired nurse. The safety of the patient is paramount. Many state boards of nursing have adopted mandatory reporting of suspected impairment. Look to the rules and regulations in your state to determine your responsibility.

An example is the New Jersey Board of Nursing Level I mandatory reporting, which always requires the following to be reported (Box 17-10):

- Conduct that clearly violates expected standards of care and may result in various degrees of harm
- Conduct that demonstrates a pattern of poor judgment or skill

AMERICAN NURSES ASSOCIATION CODE OF ETHICS

The ANA Code of Ethics for nurses does not distinguish the cause from the effect.

In a situation where a nurse suspects another practitioner may be impaired, the nurse's duty is to take action designed both to protect patients and to assure that the impaired individual receives assistance in regaining optimal function. This advocacy role does not stop once the impairment is identified. Nurses in all roles should advocate for colleagues whose job performance may be impaired to assure that they receive appropriate assistance, treatment and access to fair institutional and legal processes. This includes supporting the return to practice of the individual who

has sought assistance and is ready to resume professional duties (ANA, 2002).

Many boards of nursing have set up advocacy programs for impaired nurses to provide them with the assistance necessary to overcome the addiction. Information about these programs are available on state board websites.

But what do you do immediately when you suspect a coworker is coming to work impaired? You call your immediate supervisor. Different hospitals have differing procedures on handling such situations, and it is important to follow the procedure. *What you do not do is nothing.* Many state boards of nursing have investigatory units that will assist the agency in uncovering suspected drug diversion or unsafe practice. In these situations, the health care agency refers the complaint to the state board, which then investigates and determines final action. In such a situation, if the complaint is found to be valid, the state board will have the nurse surrender her license to practice. She is then referred to assistance and is monitored by the state board. Reinstatement of the license can occur depending on the rules and regulations of the state board. Nurses can also voluntarily surrender their license if they think that they are in need of assistance.

In the late 1970s, the ANA began efforts to secure assistance for chemically and mentally impaired nurses (Haack & Yocum, 2002). The assistance is in the form of diversion programs, intervention, or peer assistance programs. It is a voluntary, confidential program for registered nurses whose practice may be impaired due to chemical dependency or mental illness.

EMPLOYEE ASSISTANCE PROGRAMS

All of the issues dealt with in this chapter may be assisted with the use of employee assistance programs (EAPs). The majority of health care employers across the United States have created EAPs. An EAP is a confidential, short-term counseling service for employees with personal problems that affect their work performance. EAPs grew out of industrial alcoholism programs of the 1940s. EAPs should be part of a larger company plan to promote wellness that involves written policies, supervisor and employee training, and an approved drug testing program (Canadian Centre for Occupational Health and Safety, 2007).

These programs allow employees to confidentially deal with concerns that may be causing problems in their personal or professional life. As a nurse manager you may refer staff members to this program. An example of an employee issue would be continual patterns of lateness and/or attendance. More serious issues may be for a drug or alcohol abuse problem. A referral can also be a self-referral. EAPs always protect the employee's privacy and assist employees in getting the help that they need without fear of a break of confidentiality. Family members may also use the EAP in some institutions. Exact steps for the referral process should be in the hospital's policy and procedure manual.

EAP services provide counseling to employees and their families in an attempt to help the employee and his or her family return to a functional unit. EAPs may provide assistance in dealing with the following issues:

- Personal issues
- Job stress
- Relationship issues
- Eldercare, childcare, parenting issues
- Harassment
- Substance abuse
- Separation and loss
- Balancing work and family

- Financial or legal
- Family violence

Some EAP providers are also able to offer other services including retirement or layoff assistance and wellness/health promotion and fitness (e.g., weight control, nutrition, exercise, or smoking). Others may offer advice on long-term illnesses, disability issues, counseling for crisis situations (e.g., death at work), or advice specifically for managers/supervisors in dealing with difficult situations (Canadian Centre for Occupational health and Safety, 2007).

SUMMARY

As shown from the information presented in this chapter, health care agencies are stressful places with potentials for unexpected behavior and perhaps violence. A safe personal workplace is the responsibility of all employees and senior leadership. As a nurse, you need to be aware of the risks of your work environment and the interventions necessary for your protection. As a nurse manager, you need to proactively work with both administration and employees to provide a safe workplace for your employees and patients. EAPs provide support for employees experiencing stress. You need to protect both yourself and the patient and be aware of the safety policies of your institution, OSHA, and the state board of nursing.

CLINICAL CORNER

Lateral Violence: Can She Take It and Can She Make It?

Karen M. Stanley

New graduate nurses are among the most vulnerable to becoming a victim of lateral violence. Some experienced nurses seem to believe it is their "duty" to make sure the new grad has what it takes to make it in their unit. Successful assimilation of the new grad into the nursing staff is a key responsibility of the preceptor, charge nurse, and nurse manager, as illustrated by the following vignette.

A new graduate nurse is in the second week of her orientation in the surgical intensive care unit (ICU) of an academic teaching hospital. Because this new grad had successfully worked as a tech on the unit while in nursing school, the nurse manager hired her, knowing that some of the nurses

oppose hiring any new grads. The preceptor assigned to orient this new graduate is an experienced ICU nurse and an excellent teacher who is committed to seeing that this new nurse succeeds. However, she has been assigned to teach a basic life support course during the morning today, and the charge nurse has been asked to act as preceptor to the new grad. This charge nurse's opinion that new grads do not belong in the ICU setting is well known, but on this busy day there is no other preceptor available. During the interdisciplinary rounds on a very complex patient assigned to the new grad, the charge nurse grills her about aspects of the patient's medical condition that even experienced nurses may not know. Although embarrassed for the new grad, none of the nurses, physicians, or other team members speak up to help the new grad. Two of the charge nurse's closest friends are heard in the background laughing and saying, "Get her!"

CLINICAL CORNER—cont'd

This is an example of sabotage where the new graduate is set up to fail and to look bad in front of the team. It is also an example of the negative behaviors that often drive new graduates out of a unit—and sometimes out of nursing altogether.

How can this negative situation be reversed for the vulnerable new grad?

1. *Individual intervention* by the preceptor to provide support and encouragement as well as education to the new graduate to repair the damage done to her self-confidence; this includes suggestions of what the new grad can say if a similar situation occurs
2. *Private discussion* between preceptor and charge nurse confronting the negative charge nurse's behavior

3. *Group meeting* with nurse manager, all preceptors, and all charge nurses to develop a plan for teaching new grads and other new staff in a way that is supportive rather than unfair "testing"
4. *Educational offering* about lateral violence in nursing that teaches all staff how to manage episodes of lateral violence and includes them in developing an action plan to eliminate lateral violence from their unit
5. *Intervention with staff* that illustrates how lateral violence behaviors among staff members compromises the care and safety of patients

EVIDENCE-BASED PRACTICE

Hospital Safety Climate and Its Relationship With Safe Work Practices and Workplace Exposure Incidents

Gershon, R. R., Karkashian, C. D., Grosch, J. W., et al. (2000). Hospital safety climate and its relationship with safe work practices and workplace exposure incidents. American Journal of Infection Control 28(3), 211-221.

Research has identified a wide range of hazards in the hospital work environment. In addition to biological, physical, and chemical, there are also psychosocial hazards. The best known of these is job stress. This includes rotating shifts, heavy workloads, lack of autonomy/control, and poor supervision. All are linked to ill health and increased risk of workplace injury. Another psychosocial factor is organizational culture and climate, which is created by leadership style and institutional goals. An important example of organizational culture is "safety climate."

Safety climate refers to the "summary of perceptions that employees share about the safety of their work environment." Employees' safety-related perceptions are based on several factors, including management decision making, organizational safety norms, and expectations and safety practices, policies, and procedures. These factors all communicate an organization's commitment to safety. Organizations with strong safety climates consistently report fewer workplace injuries than do ones with weak safety climates. This is not only because the workplace has well-developed effective safety programs but also because the very existence of these programs sends "cues" to employees regarding management's commitment to safety. Evidence shows that a safe environment in turn further affects behavior because of the influence workers have on one another.

Early research in industry identified several key aspects of safety climate, including management's involvement in safety programs, high status and rank for safety officers, strong safety training, orderly plant operations, good housekeeping, and an emphasis on recognition of the importance of safety climate to productivity. The importance of safety climate in health care setting has just recently become a focus.

As the health care environment increasingly emphasizes reengineering, restructuring, and improved productivity, the safety climate grows in importance. Studies done to measure hospital safety indicate that safety climate is correlated with employees' compliance with safe work practices and with workplace exposure incidents. This new hospital safety climate scale can be a valuable assessment tool for hospitals and part of their overall risk management program, which is especially important given the seriousness of potential outcomes. Administrations that are supportive of strong safety will not only improve compliance with safe work practices but also benefit from the far-reaching implications inherent in the safety climate message.

NCLEX® EXAM QUESTIONS

1. You are placed in a situation where a coworker, on seeing a patient in a revealing nightgown, says to you, "What I wouldn't give to see you in such a nightgown." An appropriate response on your part would be:
   1. "Thanks a lot for that comment."
   2. "What do you mean by that?"
   3. "That is an inappropriate comment."
   4. inform your immediate supervisor

2. You are the nurse giving report to the oncoming shift when you notice that an incoming nurse has alcohol on her breath. On asking her if she had a drink, she responds, "Yes, I had a small one before coming to work, but I am perfectly fine." What is the FIRST thing that you should do?
   1. Stop report and ask her to leave the building.
   2. Continue with report and ask to speak with the nurse after report.
   3. Have a coworker call the nursing supervisor.
   4. Excuse yourself from report and call the nursing supervisor.

3. You are counting the narcotics with the oncoming nurse and find a discrepancy in the count of the Tylenol with Codeine. This is not the first time this has occurred on your shift. You have a suspicion as to which nurse is "taking" the medication but are not 100% sure. What is the FIRST thing you should do?
   1. Confront the suspected nurse.
   2. Call the nursing supervisor immediately.
   3. Do nothing until it happens again.
   4. Wait to see if it occurs again and then report.

4. Violence in the workplace is of particular concern for nurses because:
   1. nurses work in a facility that is open to the public 24/7, families are stressed due to hospitalization of loved one, and nurses are sometimes required to care for convicts
   2. nurses work in a facility that is open to the public 24/7, families are at the bedside, and nurses are sometimes required to care for convicts
   3. nurses work in a facility that is considered a large facility, families are stressed due to hospitalization of loved one, and nurses are sometimes required to care for convicts
   4. nurses work in a facility that is open to the public 24/7, families are stressed due to hospitalization of loved one, and nurses are sometimes required to care for combative patients

5. Potential safety hazards in the workplace for nurses may include the:
   1. parent of a child who wishes to spend the night at the bedside
   2. convict with 24-hour police watch at the patient door
   3. teenage patient who has a lot of visitors
   4. shortage of nurses on the night shift

6. As a newly hired registered nurse, you will receive a new employee orientation that will include:
   1. obtaining consents for surgery
   2. safe use of hospital equipment
   3. local fire department policies
   4. local police department procedures

7. If you are working as a new nurse on the 7 P.M. to 7 A.M. shift and a patient's family member arrives after visiting hours and is clearly under the influence of drugs and/or alcohol, the FIRST thing you would do is:
   1. call for backup assistance from your colleague
   2. call 911 and inform them of the issue
   3. approach the visitor directly and say visiting hours are over
   4. call security and the nursing supervisor immediately

8. As a registered nurse, you are aware that there are many stressors for the new nurse today. You feel as if you need to speak with someone about this. What are your options?
   1. Go to see a psychiatrist when your benefits start in 3 months.
   2. Request information on your hospital's employee assistance program.
   3. Tell a coworker how stressed you are.
   4. Speak to a family member about your concerns.

9. An example of horizontal violence is:
   1. verbal remarks about a patient
   2. activities that undermine the victim's ability to perform professionally
   3. giving information about a practice or patient
   4. talking and laughing with other colleagues

10. Your colleague has threatened to slash your car tires if you do not switch days off with her. What is the FIRST thing you should do?
    1. Do nothing and hope she will not do it
    2. Tell her if she does, you will report her
    3. Tell her if she does it to you, you will do it to her
    4. None of the above are proper reactions

Answers: 1.3   2.4   3.2   4.1   5.2   6.2   7.4   8.2   9.2   10.4

REFERENCES

American Association of Critical Care Nurses. (2004). *Position statement: workplace violence prevention*. Aliso Viejo, CA: Author.

American Nurses Association, Department of Government Affairs. (2007). *Health care worker safety*. Retrieved March 20, 2008, from http://www.anapoliticalpower.org.

American Nurses Association. (2002). Provision 3.6 of ANA professions response to problems of addictions and psychiatric disorders in nursing. Resolution 2002. Retrieved July 20, 2007, from http://www.nursingworld.org/MainMenuCategories/ThePracticeofProfessionalNursing/workplace/ImpairedNurse/Response.aspx.

Canadian Centre for Occupational health and Safety. Employee assistance programs (EAP). Retrieved July 27, 2007, from http://www.ccohs.ca/oshanswers/hsprograms/eap.html.

Cook, J., Green, M., & Topp, R. (2001). Exploring the impact of physician verbal abuse on perioperative nurses. *AORN Journal, 74*, 317-320, 322-327, 329-331.

Ehrmann, G., & Zuzelo, P. R. (2007). *Conference abstracts: 2007*. Presented at the NACNS National Conference, February 28–March 3, 2007, Phoenix, AZ.

Erikson, L., & Williams-Evans, S. (2000). Attitudes of emergency nurses regarding patient assaults. *Journal of Emergency Nursing, 26*, 210-215.

Gates, D. M., & Kroeger, F. (2003). Violence against nurses: the silent epidemic. *ISNA Bulletin, 29*, 25-29.

Haack, M. R., & Yocum, C. J. (2002). State policies and nurses with substance abuse disorders. *Journal of Nursing Scholarship, 34*, 89-94.

Huber, D. L. (2006). *Leadership and nursing care management*, 3rd ed. Philadelphia, PA: Elsevier.

International Council of Nurses (ICN). (2001). *Anti-violence tool kit*. Geneva, Switzerland: Author.

Longo, J. (2007). Horizontal violence among nursing students. *Archives of Psychiatric Nursing, 21*, 177-178.

Longo, J., & Sherman, R. (2007). Leveling horizontal violence. *Nursing Management, 38*, 34-37, 50-51.

Marquis, B., & Huston, C. (2006). *Leadership roles and management functions in nursing: theory and application*, 5th ed. Philadelphia: Lippincott Williams & Wilkins.

National Institute for Occupational Safety and Health (NIOSH). (April 2002). Occupational violence. Retrieved March 20, 2008, from http://www.cdc.gov/niosh/docs/2002-101/. DHHS (NIOSH) publication No. 2002-2101.

National Institute for Occupational Safety and Health (NIOSH). (April 2002). Workplace violence. Retrieved May 11, 2009, from http://www.cdc.gov/niosh/docs/2002-101/. DHHS (NIOSH) publication No. 2002-2101.

Occupational Safety and Health Administration (OSHA), U.S. Department of Labor. (2003). *Guidelines for preventing workplace violence for health care and social service workers*. Washington, DC: Author. OSHA publication 3148 (rev. 2003).

Rosenstein, A. (2002). Nurse-physician relationships: impact on nurse satisfaction and retention. *American Journal of Nursing, 102*, 26-34.

Sullivan, E., Bissel, L., & Williams, E. (1988). *Chemical dependency in nursing: the deadly diversion*. Menlo Park, CA: Addison-Wesley Nursing.

The U.S. Equal Employment Opportunity Commission. (2009). *Sexual harassment*. Retrieved May 11, 2009, from http://www.eeoc.gov/types/sexual_harassment.html.

Tomey, A. M. (2004). *Guide to nursing management and leadership*, 7th ed. St. Louis: Mosby.

Yoder-Wise, P. S., & Kowalski, K. E. (2006). *Beyond leading and managing: nursing administration for the future*. St. Louis: Elsevier.

CHAPTER 18

Legal Issues in Health Care

Chapter Objectives

1. Differentiate between negligence and malpractice.
2. Explain why the nurse is at risk for legal issues.
3. Identify issues of importance for patient charting.
4. Discuss potential risk factors in health care setting.
5. Identify issues of importance in the Nurse Practice Act.
6. Explain why nurses must be aware of each state's Nurse Practice Act.

Definitions

Personal liability Responsibility and accountability of individuals for their own actions or inactions

Corporate liability Responsibility of an organization for its own wrongful conduct

Policies and procedures Written standardized protocol that is authorized by the health care organization

Risk management activities Clinical and administrative activities that organizations undertake to identify, evaluate, and reduce the risk of injury to patients, staff, and visitors and the risk of loss to the organization itself

Informed consent Consent for treatment given by a patient after three requirements are met: the patient has the capacity to consent, consent is voluntary, and the patient receives information regarding treatment in a manner that is understandable

Patient Self-Determination Act Federal law requiring every heath care facility receiving Medicare or Medicaid to provide written information to adult patients concerning their right to make health care decisions

Advance directive Document that allows the competent patient to make choices regarding health care before it is needed

Living will Advance directive that indicates what an individual dictates regarding treatment or lifesaving measures in the future

Durable power of attorney for heath care decisions Document that permits an individual to give a surrogate or proxy the authority to make decisions for that person in the event that he or she becomes incompetent

The Omnibus Budget Reconciliation Act (OBRA) of 1987 One provision of this act provides patients the right to be free from any physical or chemical restraint imposed for the purpose of discipline or convenience and not required to treat medical symptoms

Restraint Direct application of physical force to a patient, with or without the patient's permission, to restrict his or her freedom of movement. The physical force may be human, mechanical devices, or a combination thereof

Tort Private or civil wrong or injury, including action of bad faith breach of contract, for

which the court will provide a remedy in the form of an action for damages

STATE BOARD OF NURSING

As a nurse you are well aware that you are held accountable for all of your actions both as an individual nurse and as the nurse managing the care of others. It is important, therefore, to have an understanding of legal issues and their impact on the profession. The first contact that you will have will be the state licensing authority and the laws of that authority. The first thing you will do after graduation is pass the NCLEX examination. Upon passing this milestone, you will receive your license to practice professional nursing. This license is given by the individual state where you are practicing and the license is governed by the statutory regulations of that particular state.

State boards of nursing in each state define those actions and duties of a nurse that are allowable by the profession guided by the state's practice act and common law. Nurse Practice Acts affect all areas of nursing practice. Nurse Practice Acts set educational standards, examination requirements, and licensing requirements and regulate the nursing profession in each particular state. State boards of nursing exist to foster public protection, to ensure consumer protection from fraud and abuse, and to respond to changes in the health care practice environment. The National Council of State Boards of Nursing (NCSBN) serves as a central clearinghouse, ensuring that individual state actions are enforced in all states in which an individual nurse may hold licensure.

Because each state has its own practice act and regulations, all nurses need to know the provisions of the practice act of the state in which they are licensed. This is especially important in the areas of diagnosis and treatment that differ from state to state. The addresses and web addresses of the various state boards are listed in Chapter 21.

If you are a nurse licensed in one state while practicing telenursing or giving telephone triage in another state, it is imperative that you know the nursing regulations of the state in which your care is being delivered. With the advent of multistate licensures, nurses licensed in one state may legally practice in some other states without obtaining additional licensure. The state in

which you practice is the state under whose regulations you are accountable. Not all states have multistate licenses, so again it is imperative that you know about the practice requirements of your state.

MULTISTATE LICENSE

The process for creating a nurse multistate licensure (compact) began in 1996 at the NCSBN Delegate Assembly when delegates voted to investigate different mutual recognition models and report the findings.

- At the 1997 Delegate Assembly, delegates unanimously agreed to endorse a mutual recognition model of nursing regulation.
- Strategies for implementation were also developed in 1997. In that same year, the Nurse Licensure Compact Administrators (NLCA) was established to manage compact implementation and to develop compact rules.
- In 1998, the NCSBN Board of Directors approved a policy goal relating to mutual recognition, which included the goal to "remove regulatory barriers to increase access to safe nursing care."
- The RN and LPN/VN Compact began January 1, 2000, when it was passed into law by the first participating states: Maryland, Texas, Utah, and Wisconsin.

Since 1998, the compact has included registered nurses (RNs) and licensed practical or vocational nurses (LPN/VNs) (Nurse Licensure Compact Administrators, 2008).

The states that participate in the Compact have agreed to work toward general uniformity in the laws that regulate nursing. Each state, however, retains complete authority in nurse licensing (Table 18-1).

How does this work for an individual nurse seeking nursing licensure? Each nurse has a state of legal residency, which he or she already declares each year to the Internal Revenue Service. This is the primary state in which the nurse resides; typically where the nurse pays federal taxes, lives most of the year, and has a driver's license. The nurse maintains an active nursing license in that state. If the state is part of the multistate Compact, the

Table 18-1	NURSE LICENSURE COMPACT (NLC) STATES

Compact States	Implementation Date
Arizona	7/1/2002
Arkansas	7/1/2000
Colorado	10/1/2007
Delaware	7/1/2000
Idaho	7/1/2001
Iowa	7/1/2000
Kentucky	6/1/2007
Maine	7/1/2001
Maryland	7/1/1999
Mississippi	7/1/2001
Nebraska	1/1/2001
New Hampshire	1/1/2006
New Mexico	1/1/2004
North Carolina	7/1/2000
North Dakota	1/1/2004
Rhode Island	7/1/2008
South Carolina	2/1/2006
South Dakota	1/1/2001
Tennessee	7/1/2003
Texas	1/1/2000
Utah	1/1/2000
Virginia	1/1/2005
Wisconsin	1/1/2000

If you have questions regarding NLC licensure, please contact your state board of nursing in your primary state of residence for specific requirements.

**States Pending NLC Implementation
(these dates *could* be subject to change)**

Pending Compact States	Status
Missouri	Pending

From Nurse Licensure Compact Administrators. (2008). Participating states in the NLC. Used with permission.

nurse is issued an active Compact license by that state and may not have a license in another Compact state (although she or he may have an inactive license in other states). The active license will be labeled "Multistate" or "Compact" to make identification of Compact status user-friendly, until all states join the Compact.

The nurse with a Compact license has met the requirements for a nursing license in the resident state. The nurse with a Compact license may practice in any Compact state using his or her Compact license. If a complaint and disciplinary action arise, it is processed in the state where the nursing care was rendered.

What about nurses in a Compact state who want to practice in a non-Compact state? Those nurses must apply for and receive a license before practicing in any state that has not joined the Compact.

A nurse who moves to another Compact state has a grace period to apply for a new nursing license, as well as for a new driver's license. During that period, the nurse can both drive and start a new nursing job without any delays.

What about nurses who are not residents of one of the Compact states? These nurses cannot get a Compact nursing license. If they desire to practice in a Compact state, they must apply for and receive a "single-state" license in each Compact state, as well as each non-Compact state, before practicing nursing there. Like auto drivers of yore, they must be licensed in every state where they use a license (care for patients) (Nurse Licensure Compact Administrators).

DISCIPLINARY ACTION BY THE STATE BOARD OF NURSING

As a nurse manager, you are also responsible for the monitoring of the practice of employees under your supervision and ensuring that they remain current with their licensure. A list of all individuals who hold nursing licenses, registered nurses and licensed practical nurses, is maintained by the vice president of nursing. The nurse must show the original state license to the vice president of nursing or his or her designee when the new nursing license has been issued. Many state boards of nursing now have online licensee directories that give you the status of an individual's license.

The nurse and the nurse leader are responsible for protecting the license of nurses in the organization. Disciplinary actions by the state board of nursing will occur if a complaint about a nurse's action triggers an investigation. Potential situations that may trigger an investigation include:

- Impaired nursing practice (see Chapter 17)
- Negligence
- Incompetence
- Abuse

- Fraud
- Practicing beyond the scope of the license

CORPORATE LIABILITY

Corporate liability is the responsibility of an organization for its own wrongful conduct. The health care facility must maintain an environment conducive to quality patient care. Corporate liability includes (1) the duty to hire, supervise, and maintain qualified, competent, and adequate staff; (2) the duty to provide, inspect, repair, and maintain reasonably adequate equipment; and (3) the duty to maintain safety in the physical environment (Sullivan, 2001, p. 72) (see Chapter 7).

MALPRACTICE

In the delivery of patient care, there is always a potential for malpractice and negligence. *Malpractice* refers to "any misconduct or lack of skill in carrying out professional responsibilities" (Sullivan & Decker, 2001, p. 75). It is also defined as failure of a professional person to act as other prudent professionals with the same knowledge and education would act under similar circumstances.

This is one of the reasons nurses need to maintain personal malpractice insurance. The employing organization maintains blanket malpractice coverage for all employees, but it is highly recommended that individuals purchase their own personal nursing liability insurance. Most commonly, nurses are subject to legal liability arising from malpractice and negligence. Nursing negligence malpractice occurs when the nurse's actions do not meet the standard of care, when the nurse's actions are unreasonable, or when the nurse fails to act and causes harm. Harm related to nursing clinical practice commonly arises from negligent acts and omissions (unintentional torts) and a variety of intentional acts (intentional torts) such as invasion of privacy, assault and battery, or false imprisonment (Aiken, 2004). See Box 18-1 for reasons that nurses should have personal malpractice insurance.

TORT LAW

A tort is a "private or civil wrong or injury, including action of bad faith breach of contract, for which the

---

Box 18-1 REASONS THAT NURSES SHOULD HAVE PERSONAL MALPRACTICE INSURANCE

1. In the event of litigation, the facility, not the nurse, makes any decisions about settlement or defense, so the nurse's best interests may not be represented.
2. If the court determines that the nurse acted outside the scope of employment, he or she is unprotected.
3. If the nurse does, in fact, practice outside the facility's job description (professional committees, outside speaking, educational work), the facility coverage does not apply.
4. Facilities have the right to seek reimbursement from the nurse for claims paid as a result of negligence.
5. Personal assets may in some cases be attached to satisfy a judgment, or wages may be garnished.
6. Health care facility insurance is frequently a claims-made policy. This type of policy will cover the nurse only while he or she is employed by the facility, not years later when the claim is in court.
7. The cost of insurance is relatively small in relation to the peace of mind the insurance provides.

From Rowland, H., & Rowland, B. (1997). *Nursing administration handbook*, 4th ed., (p. 192) Gaithersburg, MD: An Aspen Publication, Aspen Publishers, Inc.

---

court will provide a remedy in the form of an action for damages" (*Black's Law Dictionary*, 1996, cited in Martin & Cain, 2003).

A tort can be any of the following (Carroll, 2006, p. 279):

1. Denial of person's legal rights
2. Failure to comply with public duty
3. Failure to perform private duty that harms another person

A tort can be unintentional, such as malpractice or neglect, or intentional, such as assault and battery or invasion of privacy (Fiesta, 1999). For malpractice to exist, the following elements must be present (Carroll, 2006, p. 280):

1. **A duty exists:** This is automatic when a patient is in a health care facility.

2. **A breach of duty occurs:** The nurse did something that should not have been done or did not do something that should have been done.
3. **Causation:** The nurse's action directly led to a patient injury.
4. **Injury:** Harm comes to the patient.
5. **Damages:** Compensate the patient for injury.

NEGLIGENCE

Negligence refers to the failure of an individual not to perform an act (omission) or to perform an act (commission) that a "reasonable, prudent person would or would not perform in a similar set of circumstances" (Sullivan and Decker, 2001, p. 75). *Negligence* is also defined as the failure to exercise the proper degree of care required by the circumstance.

Common negligence allegations in nursing include the following:
- Medication errors
- Patient falls
- Use of restraints
- Equipment injuries
- Failure to take appropriate nursing action
- Failure to follow hospital procedure
- Failure to supervise treatment

An institution's policies and procedures describe the performance expected of nurses. Deviation from this expected performance can result in a liability for negligence or malpractice. A nurse failing to adhere to institutional policy runs the risk of the employer denying the nurse defense in a lawsuit.

CHARTING

Most malpractice/negligence lawsuits may take place years after the actual event. When a nurse is named in a lawsuit, it is likely that the memory of the event will have greatly diminished. The documentation in the patient care record may be the most reliable source of information. Therefore, a nurse's charting ability serves a double purpose of reminding of the care delivered to that particular patient. Documentation on an electronic medical record has become standardized in many facilities. It is important to remember the rules of nursing documentation (Box 18-2).

Review Table 18-2 to determine FLAT charting (*f*actual, *l*egible, *a*ccurate, *t*imely). Which charting example relates to the standard of care for pain and

Box 18-2   FLAT CHARTING

1. **F**actual—What you see, not what you think happened
2. **L**egible—No erasures, corrections should be made with a single line drawn through the error and initialed
3. **A**ccurate and complete—For example, color of tracheostomy secretions
4. **T**imely—Completed as soon after the occurrence as possible

From Kelly-Heidenthal, P., & Marthaler, M. T. (2005). *Delegation of nursing care* (p. 145). Clifton Park, NY: Thomson Delmar Learning.

Table 18-2   EXAMPLES OF CHARTING

Charting That Says Nothing!	Appropriate Charting	Charting That Says Way Too Much and Really Says Little!
Complaining of pain. Medicated × 3 with analgesic. Relief noted, family visiting and talking about diagnosis. Appears comfortable.	2pm. Patient complaining of pain (6 rating) at surgical site. Splinting site and expressing discomfort moving about in bed. Surgical site intact with no signs of redness or swelling. Medicated with Tylenol #3. 2 tablets given by mouth. 2:45pm. Verbalized a pain rating of 2, states that he feels much more comfortable. Easily ambulating with family in hallway. No dizziness or difficulties with gait noted.	2pm Complaining of "intense pain" rating it at "the worst I've had to date at least a 6." Family milling about and appearing to make patient much more agitated. Patient holding side and moaning. Last pain medication was 6 hours ago. Medicated at 2:15 with 2 tablets of Tylenol #3. Family stated that it was "about time" he had a pain med. Within about 20 minutes, patient appeared calmer with no agitation noted.

which chart would give you the appropriate information if you were called to court 5 years after giving this pain med?

STANDARD OF CARE PAIN MANAGEMENT

Box 18-3 shows a standard of care for pain management. This standard of care would form the basis for the expectation of care delivered to all patients within an institution. Deviation from this care can be defined as *malpractice*. As stated earlier, the following clinical problems most commonly lead to malpractice/negligence lawsuits: restraints, medication errors, patient falls, privacy violations, and other adverse events. Therefore, it is important for the nurse and nurse manager to practice according to established policy and procedure.

Box 18-3   A STANDARD OF CARE FOR PAIN MANAGEMENT

Preoperative Phase

Assessment

1. Vital signs including pain and comfort goals (e.g., 0-to-10 scale)
2. Medical history (e.g., neurologic status; cardiac and respiratory instability; allergy to medication, food, and objects; use of herbs; motion sickness; sickle cell; fibromyalgia; use of caffeine/substance abuse; fear; and anxiety)
3. Pain history (e.g., preexisting pain, acute, chronic, pain level, pattern, quality, type of source, intensity, location, duration/time, course, pain effect, and effects on personal life)
4. Pain behaviors/expressions or history (e.g., grimacing, frowning, crying, restlessness, tension, and discomfort behaviors (e.g., shivering, nausea, and vomiting). Note that physical appearance may not necessarily indicate pain/discomfort or its absence.
5. Analgesic history (type [i.e., opioid, nonopioid, and adjuvant analgesics], dose, frequency, effectiveness, adverse effects, other medications that may influence choice of analgesics [e.g., anticoagulant, antihypertensive, muscle relaxants])
6. Patient's preferences (e.g., for pain relief/comfort measures, expectations, concerns, aggravating and alleviating factors, and clarification of misconceptions)
7. Pain/comfort acceptable levels (e.g., patient and family [as indicated] agree to plan of treatment/ interventions postoperatively)
8. Comfort history (i.e., physiological, sociocultural, psychospiritual, and environmental [e.g., spiritual beliefs/symbols, warming measures, music, comfort objects, privacy, positioning, factors related to nausea/vomiting])
9. Educational needs (i.e., consider age or level of education, cognitive and language appropriateness, and barriers to learning)
10. Cultural language preference, identification of personal beliefs, and resulting restrictions
11. Pertinent laboratory results (e.g., prolonged prothrombin time [PT], partial thromboplastin time [PTT], and abnormal international normalized ratio [INR] and platelet count to determine risk for epidural hematoma in patients with epidural catheter)

Interventions

1. Identify patient, validate physician's order and procedure (i.e., correct name of drug, dose, amount, route, and time, and validate type of surgery and correct surgical site as applicable).
2. Discuss pain and comfort assessment (i.e., presence, location, quality, intensity, age, language, condition, and cognitively appropriate pain rating scale [e.g., 0-to-10 numerical scale or FACES scale] and comfort scale). Assessment method must be the same for consistency.
3. Discuss with patient and family (as indicated) information about reporting pain intensity using numerical or FACES rating scales and available pain relief and comfort measures (include discussion of patient's preference for pain and comfort measures; implement comfort measures [i.e., physiological, sociocultural, spiritual, environmental support as indicated by patient]).
4. Discuss and dispel misconceptions about pain and pain management.
5. Encourage patient to take a preventive approach to pain and discomfort by asking for relief measures before pain and discomfort are severe or out of control.
6. Educate purpose of intravenous or epidural patient-controlled analgesia (PCA) as indicated; educate about use of nonpharmacologic methods (e.g., cold therapy, relaxation breathing, music).
7. Discuss potential outcomes of pain and discomfort treatment approaches.

Box 18-3   A STANDARD OF CARE FOR PAIN MANAGEMENT—cont'd

8. Establish pain relief/comfort goals with the patient (e.g., a pain rating of less than 4 [scale of 0 to 10]) to make it easy to cough, deep breathe, and turn); premedicate patients for sedation, pain relief, comfort (e.g., non-opioid, opioid, antiemetics as ordered); consider needs of chronic pain patients.
9. Arrange interpreter throughout the continuum of care as indicated.
10. Utilize interventions for sensory-impaired patients (e.g., device to amplify sound, sign language, and interpreters).
11. Report abnormal findings including laboratory values (prolonged PT/PTT and abnormal INR and platelet count among epidural patients).
12. Arrange for parents to be present for children.

Expected Outcomes

1. Patient states understanding of care plan and priority of individualized needs.
2. Patient states understanding of pain intensity scale, comfort scale, and pain relief/comfort goals.
3. Patient establishes realistic and achievable pain relief/comfort goals (e.g., a pain rating of less than 4 [scale 0 to 10]) to make it easier to cough, deep breathe, and turn upon discharge.
4. Patient states understanding or demonstrates correct use of PCA equipment as indicated.
5. Patient verbalizes understanding of importance of using other nonpharmacologic methods of alleviating pain and discomfort (e.g., cold therapy, relaxation breathing, music).

From Nursing National Guideline Clearinghouse. (2008). Retrieved October 21, 2008, from http://www.guideline.gov/summary/summary.aspx?doc_id=5526&nbr=003757&string=Nursing National Guideline Clearinghouse.

INCIDENT REPORTS

The filing of an incident reports forms the basis of organizationwide reporting from a risk management perspective. The purpose of an incident report is to provide a factual account of an incident or an adverse event to ensure that all facts surrounding the incident are reported. The incident reporting system provides the risk manager an opportunity to investigate all serious situations. Aggregated data from incident reports are used by management to improve health care processes within the organization and for the early identification of emerging risk (see Chapter 12). Refer to your agency for the process for incident reporting. In general, incident report forms should be completed by:

1. Staff member involved in the occurrence
2. Staff member who discovered the incident
3. Staff member to whom the incident was reported

Incident reports should be completed as soon after the occurrence as possible. Accurately record all details of the incident and objectively describe the description of the incident and actions taken in response to the incident. It is important not to provide subjective information stating what should or could have been done to avoid the incident. If a document includes this information, the nurse can be asked in court why he or she did not take those actions to avoid the incident. The report also needs to include patient assessment and monitoring after the incident (Carroll, 2006).

Nurses can also be mentioned as party in medical malpractice. In such situations, a nurse's liability is determined by the state's nurse practice act and the institution's policies and procedures. Above and beyond personal liability for personal clinical practice, nurses also have accountability and liability for their acts of delegation and supervision. As a primary care coordinator, the nurse manages the environment of care delivery ensuring staff competence and reporting incompetent practice are key responsibilities (see discussion of impaired practice in Chapter 17). The nurse manager can also be held accountable for the negligence of a contract employee (agency nurse) even though he or she is not an employee of a particular institution. This is why it is important that the nurse manager is aware of skills, competencies, and knowledge of all staff working with her or him. Nurse managers also need to be aware of legal issues in the area of human resources (see Chapter 15). The nurse will need to be aware of hiring standards, performance review standards, management of employees with problems, compliance with union contract, and terminations.

HEALTH CARE INFORMATION

Invasion of privacy and confidentiality is a tort violation. The Health Insurance Portability and Accountability Act (HIPAA) was enacted in 1996 to give people control over their personal information. It also made organizations that create or receive personal information accountable for protecting it. Information disclosed by patients is confidential and should be available only to authorized personnel. Nurses must obtain permission to release information to family members and close friends as well as to others. This makes it difficult when nurses attempt to release information over the telephone. The nurse must identify the caller as an appropriate receiver of such information. Also, photographs, research information, or videos of the patient may not be used without specific signed releases. Computerized information also needs to be protected. Nurses' charting on a hallway computer must not leave information visible on the computer screen to individuals in the hallway.

INFORMED CONSENT

Nurses will often be called on to witness patient consent. There are three elements of informed consent (Nathanson, 1996, cited in Rowland & Rowland, 1997, p. 188):

1. **Information and knowledge**
   For any patient to make a valid decision regarding a treatment, they must have adequate information to consider. Health care providers are responsible for informing patients of the diagnosis, prognosis, available alternatives to treatment recommended, risks and benefits of treatment options, and the risks of not accepting treatment. This information must be presented to a patient in understandable terms. Both The Joint Commission and the American Hospital Association require that hospitals meet a patient's communication needs.

2. **Competence**
   Adults over 18 years of age in most states are legally competent and capable of giving valid consent for medical treatment. The patient must be of sound mind and free from any legal or mental impediments for making a binding decision regarding health care. Therefore, a patient who has a legal guardian or is a minor may not be legally competent to give consent. Each state has different rules about age of competence; it is therefore necessary to be mindful of the states' legalities.

3. **Voluntariness**
   For a patients consent to be voluntary, the patient must freely elect to undergo the treatment without any sort of physical or psychological coercion. If

the person is intimidated, threatened, or coerced by health care personnel, there could be a lack of valid consent.

Regarding the physician's responsibility in the communications process, the physician providing or performing the treatment and/or procedure (not a delegated representative) should disclose and discuss with the patient:

- The patient's diagnosis, if known
- The nature and purpose of a proposed treatment or procedure
- The risks and benefits of a proposed treatment or procedure
- Alternatives (regardless of their cost or the extent to which the treatment options are covered by health insurance)
- The risks and benefits of the alternative treatment or procedure
- The risks and benefits of not receiving or undergoing a treatment or procedure

In turn, the patient should have an opportunity to ask questions to elicit a better understanding of the treatment or procedure, so that he or she can make an informed decision to proceed or to refuse a particular course of medical intervention (American Medical Association, 2008).

The consent for treatment is given by a patient after three requirements are met—the individual has the capacity to consent, consent is voluntary, and the individual receives information regarding treatment in a manner that is understandable to him or her (Sullivan, 2005, p. 75).

Individual capacity to consent is determined by age and competence. The legal age is determined by state laws. Competency is determined when an individual has the ability to make choices and understands the consequences of their choices. When individuals make choices without force, fraud, deceit, or duress, they are acting voluntarily. And the information must contain all of the following (Sullivan, 2005, p. 74):

1. An explanation of the treatment to be performed and the expected results
2. A description of the anticipated risks and discomforts
3. A list of potential benefits
4. A disclosure of possible alternatives
5. An offer to answer the patient's questions
6. A statement that the patient may withdraw his or her consent at any time

Nurses are often asked to witness a patient's informed consent. In signing the document, the nurse is witnessing the patient's signature, not validating the patient's complete understanding. A nurse has a right to refuse to sign if he or she thinks that any of the above information is not met.

PATIENT RESTRAINTS

Basic human rights are not forfeited on entry into a health care facility. A competent patient has the right to refuse restraints unless he or she is at risk for harming others. Improper use of restraints may constitute assault or false imprisonment. If a patient has to be restrained, the patient has a right to the least restrictive restraint use at all times. As stated earlier, injuries resulting from improper use of restraints often are a cause of legal complaints.

The Omnibus Budget Reconciliation Act (OBRA) of 1987 provides patients the right to be free from any physical or chemical restraint imposed for the purpose of discipline or convenience and not required to treat medical symptoms.

Restraint use must meet the following requirements:
1. Physician's order for specific duration and circumstances for use
2. PRN orders not permitted
3. Continuous assessment and reassessment of patient as per hospital policy
4. Informed consent for use must be given (if patient unable, proxy consent necessary)

PATIENT SELF-DETERMINATION ACT

The Patient Self-Determination Act provides legislative support to the expression of a patient's consent to or refusal of medical treatment even when the patient is no longer able to verbalize them. Patients who can verbalize refusal of care are allowed to sign out "against medical advice" (AMA). Health care organizations have policies and procedures surrounding patients signing out "AMA." In this situation, the nurse documents in detail the events leading to the refusal of care and documents patient awareness of the consequences of refusal. Patients who are unable to verbalize consent or refusal can do so with the following documents:

1. Advance medical directive
2. Durable power of attorney
3. Health care proxy
4. Living will

ADVANCE MEDICAL DIRECTIVE

Advance medical directives are written instructions expressing an individual's health care wishes in the event of incapacitation (Fig. 18-1).

DURABLE POWER OF ATTORNEY

These are legal instructions enabling an individual to act on another's behalf. In health care, it is often part of an advance medical directive (Fig. 18-2).

HEALTH CARE PROXY

Documents delegate the authority to make health care decisions to another when the patient has become incapacitated.

LIVING WILL

This is a document in which an individual expresses in advance his or her wishes regarding the application of life-sustaining treatments if he or she becomes unable to do so.

As with all legal issues, it is important to know state statutes and laws that affect these documents. For further information, go to the websites www.partnershipforcaring.com and www.abanet.org/aging/toolkit/home.html.

It is important to note that an advance directive does not mean "do not resuscitate" (DNR). An advance directive spells out a patient's wishes in certain health care situations. A patient may desire to have full emergency care done in certain situations. A DNR order is placed on a patient's chart by the physician. If a patient does not have a DNR order, the standard of care requires that the nurse attempts resuscitation if necessary. Each health care organization has extensive policies surrounding the decision making for DNR orders.

NURSE'S RESPONSIBILITY IN ADVANCE DIRECTIVES

Most health care organizations have policies for the documentation of patient self-determination documents. Nurses are required to ask patients and families

Text continued on page 234

Combined Advance Directive for Health Care
(Combined Proxy and Instruction Directive)

I understand that as a competent adult, I have the right to make decisions about my health care. There may come a time when I am unable, due to physical or mental incapacity, to make my own health care decisions. In these circumstances, those caring for me will need direction concerning my care and will turn to someone who knows my values and health care wishes. I understand that those responsible for my care will seek to make health care decisions in my best interests, based upon what they know of my wishes. In order to provide the guidance and authority needed to make decisions on my behalf:

I, _____, hereby declare and make known my instructions and wishes for my future health care. This advance directive for health care shall take effect in the event I become unable to make my own health care decisions, as determined by the physician who has primary responsibility for my care, and any necessary confirming determinations. I direct that this document become part of my permanent medical records.

In completing Part One of this directive, you will designate an individual you trust to act as your legally recognized health care representative to make health care decisions for you in the event you are unable to make decisions for yourself.

In completing Part Two of this directive, you will provide instructions concerning your health care preferences and wishes to your health care representative and others who will be entrusted with responsibility for your care, such as your physician, family members and friends.

Part One: Designation of a Health Care Representative

A) Choosing a Health Care Representative:

I hereby designate:

name _____

address _____

city _____ state _____

telephone _____

as my health care representative to make any and all health care decisions for me, including decisions to accept or to refuse any treatment, service or procedure used to diagnose or treat my physical or mental condition, and decisions to provide, withhold or withdraw life-sustaining measures. I direct my representative to make decisions on my behalf in accordance with my wishes as stated in this document, or as otherwise known to him or her. In the event my wishes are not clear, or a situation arises I did not anticipate, my health care representative is authorized to make decisions in my best interests, based upon what is known of my wishes.

Figure 18-1 • Combined advance directive for health care. From New Jersey Commission on Legal and Ethical Problems in the Delivery of Health Care (The New Jersey Bioethics Commission), March 1991.

I have discussed the terms of this designation with my health care representative and he or she has willingly agreed to accept the responsibility for acting on my behalf.

_____

B) Alternate Representatives: If the person I have designated above is unable, unwilling or unavailable to act as my health care representative, I hereby designate the following person(s) to act as my health care representative, in order of priority stated:

1. name_____   2. name_____
address_____   address_____
city_____ state_____   city_____ state_____
telephone _____   telephone _____

Part Two: Instruction Directive

In Part Two, you are asked to provide instructions concerning your future health care. This will require making important and perhaps difficult choices. Before completing your directive, you should discuss these matters with your health care representative, doctor and family members or others who may become responsible for your care.

In **Sections C and D,** you may state the circumstances in which various forms of medical treatment, including life-sustaining measures, should be provided, withheld or discontinued. If the options and choices below do not fully express your wishes, you should use **Section E,** and/or attach a statement to this document which would provide those responsible for your care with additional information you think would help them in making decisions about your medical treatment. **Please familiarize yourself with all sections of Part Two before completing your directive.**

C) General Instructions. To inform those responsible for my care of my specific wishes, I make the following statement of personal views regarding my health care.

Initial ONE of the following two statements with which you agree:

1. _____ I direct that all medically appropriate measures be provided to sustain my life regardless of my physical or mental condition.

2. _____ There are circumstances in which I would not want my life to be prolonged by further medical treatment. In these circumstances, life-sustaining measures should not be initiated and if they have been, they should be discontinued. I recognize that is likely to hasten my death. In the following, I specify the circumstances in which I would choose to forego life-sustaining measures.

If you have initialed statement 2, on the following page please initial each of the statements (a, b, c) with which you agree:

Figure 18-1 • cont'd.

a. _____ I realize that there may come a time when I am diagnosed as having an incurable and irreversible illness, disease, or condition. If this occurs, and my attending physician and at least one additional physician who has personally examined me determine that my condition is **terminal,** I direct that life-sustaining measures which would serve only to artificially prolong my dying be withheld or discontinued. I also direct that I be given all medially appropriate care necessary to make me comfortable and relieve pain.

In the space provided, write in the bracketed phrase with which you agree:

To me, terminal condition means that my physicians have determined that:

_____

[I will die within a few days] [I will die within a few weeks]
[I have a life expectancy of approximately _____ or less (enter 6 months or 1 year)]
b. _____ If there should come a time when I become **permanently unconscious,** and it is determined by my attending physician and at least one additional physician with appropriate expertise who has personally examined me, that I have totally and irreversibly lost consciousness and my capacity for interaction with other people and my surroundings, I direct that life-sustaining measures be withheld or discontinued. I understand that I will not experience pain or discomfort in this condition, and I direct that I be given all medically appropriate care necessary to provide for my personal hygiene and dignity.

c. _____ I realize that there may come a time when I am diagnosed as having an **incurable and irreversible** illness, disease, or condition which may not be terminal. My condition may cause me to experience severe and progressive physical or mental deterioration and/or a permanent loss of capacities and faculties I value highly. If, in the course of my medical care, the burdens of continued life with treatment become greater that the benefits I experience, I direct that life-sustaining measures be withheld or discontinued. I also direct that I be given all medically appropriate care necessary to make me comfortable and to relieve pain.

(Paragraph **c.** covers a wide range of possible situations in which you may have experienced partial or complete loss of certain mental or physical capacities you value highly. If you wish, in the space provided below you may specify in more detail the conditions in which you would choose to forego life-sustaining measures. You might include a description of the faculties or capacities, which, if irretrievably lost would lead you to accept death rather than continue living. You may want to express any special concerns you have about particular medical conditions or treatments, or any other considerations, which would provide further guidance to those who may become responsible for your care. If necessary, you may attach a separate statement to this document or use **Section E** to provide additional instructions.)

Examples of conditions which I find unacceptable are:

_____
_____
_____
_____

Figure 18-1 • cont'd.

D) Specific Instructions: Artificially Provided Fluids and Nutrition; Cardiopulmonary Resuscitation (CPR). On page 3 you provided general instructions regarding life-sustaining measures. Here you are asked to give specific instructions regarding two types of life-sustaining measures-artificially provided fluids and nutrition and cardiopulmonary resuscitation.

In the space provided, write in the bracketed phrase with which you agree:

1. In the circumstances I initialed on page 3, I also direct that artificially provided fluids and nutrition, such as feeding tube or intravenous infusion,

_____

[be withheld or withdrawn and that I be allowed to die]
[be provided to the extent medically appropriate]

2. In the circumstances I initialed on page 3, if I should suffer a cardiac arrest, I also direct that cardiopulmonary resuscitation (CPR)

_____

[not be provided and that I be allowed to die]
[be provided to preserve my life, unless medically inappropriate or futile]

3. If neither of the above statements adequately expresses your wishes concerning artificially provided fluids and nutrition or CPR, please explain your wishes below.

_____

_____

_____

E) Additional Instructions: (You should provide any additional information about your health care preferences which is important to you and which may help those concerned with your care to implement your wishes. You may wish to direct your health care representative, family members, or your health care providers to consult with others, or you may wish to direct that your care be provided by a particular physician, hospital, nursing home, or at home. If you are or believe you may become pregnant, you may wish to state specific instructions. If you need more space than is provided here you may attach an additional statement to this directive.)

_____

_____

_____

F) Brain Death: (The state of New Jersey recognizes the irreversible cessation of all functions of the entire brain, including the brain stem (also known as whole brain death), as a legal standard for the declaration of death. However, individuals who cannot accept this standard because of their personal religious beliefs may request that it not be applied in determining their death.)

Figure 18-1 • cont'd.

Initial the following statement only if it applies to you:

_____To declare my death on the basis of the whole brain death standard would violate my personal religious beliefs. I therefore wish my death to be declared solely on the basis of the traditional criteria of irreversible cessation of cardiopulmonary (heartbeat and breathing) function.

G) After Death-Anatomical Gifts: (It is now possible to transplant human organs and tissue in order to save and improve the lives of others. Organs, tissues, and other body parts are also used for therapy, medical research and education. This section allows you to indicate your desire to make an anatomical gift and if so, to provide instructions for any limitations or special uses.)

Initial the statements which express your wishes:

1. _____ **I wish** to make the following anatomical gift to take effect upon my death:

A. _____ any needed organs or body parts.
B. _____ only the following organs or parts

_____

for the purposes of transplantation, therapy, medical research or education, or

C. _____ my body for anatomical study, if needed.
D. _____ special limitations, if any;

_____

If you wish to provide additional instructions, such as indicating your preference that your organs be given to a specific person or institution, or be used for a specific purpose, please do so in the space provided below.

_____
_____
_____

2. _____ **I do not wish** to make an anatomical gift upon my death.

Part Three: Signature and Witnesses

H) Copies: The original or a copy of this document has been given to the following people (Note: If you have chosen to designate a health care representative, it is important that you provide him or her with a copy of your directive):

1. name _____   2. name_____

address _____   address _____

city _____ state _____   city_____ state _____

telephone_____   telephone _____

Figure 18-1 • cont'd.

I) Signature: By writing this advance directive, I inform those who may become entrusted with my health care of my wishes and intend to ease the burdens of decision-making which this responsibility may impose. I have discussed the terms of this designation with my health care representative and he or she has willingly agreed to accept the responsibility for acting on my behalf in accordance with this directive. I understand the purpose and effect of this document and sign it knowingly, voluntarily and after careful deliberation.

Signed this _____ day of _____, 20 _____ .

signature _____

address _____

city_____ state _____

J) Witnesses: I declare that the person who signed this document, or asked another to sign this document on his or her behalf, did so in my presence, that he or she is personally known to me, and that he or she appears to be of sound mind and free of duress or undue influence. I am 18 years of age or older, and am not designated by this or any other document as the person's health care representative.

1. witness_____

address _____

city_____ state _____

signature _____

date _____

2. witness_____

address _____

city_____ state _____

signature _____

date _____

**New Jersey Commission on Legal and Ethical
Problems in the Delivery of Health Care
(The New Jersey Bioethics Commission)
March 1991**

Figure 18-1 ● cont'd.

Durable Power of Attorney for Health Care Decisions
■ *Take a copy of this with you whenever you go to the hospital or on a trip* ■

It is important to choose someone to make healthcare decisions for you when you cannot make or communicate decisions for yourself.   Tell the person you choose what healthcare treatments you want. The person you choose will be your agent. He or she will have the right to make decisions for your healthcare. If you DO NOT choose someone to make decisions for you, write NONE on the line for the agent's name.

I, _____ , SS# _____ (optional), appoint the person named in this document to be my agent to make my healthcare decisions.

This document is a Durable Power of Attorney for Healthcare Decisions, My agent's power shall not end if I become incapacitated or if there is uncertainty that I am dead. This document revokes any prior Durable Power of Attorney for Healthcare Decisions. My agent may not appoint anyone else to make decisions for me. My agent and my care-givers are protected from any claims based on following this Durable Power of Attorney for Healthcare. My agent shall not be responsible for any costs associated with my care. I give my agent full power to make all decisions for me about my healthcare, including the power to direct the withholding or withdrawal of life-prolonging treatment, including artificially supplied nutrition and hydration/tube feeding. My agent is authorized to:

• Consent, refuse or withdraw consent to any care, procedure, treatment, or service to diagnose, treat or maintain a physical or mental condition, including artificial nutrition and hydration;
• Permit, refuse, or withdraw permission to participate in federally regulated research related to my condition or disorder
• Make all necessary arrangements for any hospital, psychiatric treatment facility, hospice, nursing home, or other health-care organization; and, employ or discharge healthcare personnel (any person who is authorized or permitted by the laws of the state to provide health care services) as he or she shall deem necessary for my physical, mental, or emotional well-being;
• Request, receive, review and authorize sending any information regarding my physical or mental health, or my personal affairs, including medical and hospital records; and execute any releases that may be required to obtain such information;
• Move me into or out of any state or institution;
• Take legal action, if needed;
• Make decisions about autopsy, tissue and organ donation, and the disposition of my body in conformity with state law; and
• Become my guardian if one is needed.

In exercising this power, I expect my agent to be guided by my directions as we discussed them prior to this appointment and/or to be guided by my Healthcare Directive (*see reverse side*).

If you DO NOT want the person (agent) you name to be able to do one or other of the above things, draw a line through the statement and put your initials at the end of the line.

Agent's name _____ Phone _____ Email _____

Address _____

*If you do **not** want to name an alternate, write "none."*

Alternate Agent's name _____ Phone _____ Email _____

Address _____

Execution and Effective Date of Appointment
My agent's authority is effective immediately for the limited purpose of having full access to my medical records and to confer with my healthcare providers and me about my condition. My agent's authority to make all healthcare and related decisions for me is effective when and only when I cannot make my own healthcare decisions.

SIGN HERE for the *Durable Power of Attorney* and /or *Healthcare Directive* forms. Many states require notarization. It is recommended for the residents of all states. Please ask two person to witness your signature who are not related to you of financially connected to your estate.

Signature _____ Date _____

Witness _____ Date _____ Witness _____ Date _____

Notarization:

On this_____ day of _____ , in the year of _____ , personally appeared before me the person signing, known by me to be the person who completes this document and acknowledged it as his/ her free act and deed.

IN WITNESS WHEROF, I have set my hand and affixed my official seal in the Count of_____ ,

State of _____ , on the date written above.

Notary Public_____

Commission expires_____

Figure 18-2 • Sample durable power of attorney. Reprinted with permission from the Center for Practical Bioethics.

Healthcare Treatment Directive

■ *If you only want to name a Durable Power of Attorney for Healthcare Decisions, draw a large X through this page.*■

I, _____ , SS# _____ , want everyone who cares for me to know what
healthcare I want.   (optional)

I always expect to be given care and treatment for pain or discomfort even if such care may affect how I sleep, eat, or
breathe.

I would consent to, and want my agent to consider my participation in federally regulated research related to my disorder or
condition.

I want my doctor to try treatments/interventions on a time-limited basis when the goal is to restore my health or help me
experience a life in a way consistent with my values and wishes. I want such treatments/interventions withdrawn when they
cannot achieve this goal or become too burdensome to me.

I want my dying to be as natural as possible. Therefore, I direct that no treatment (including food or water by tube) be given
just to keep my body functioning when I have

- a condition that will cause me to die soon, or

- a condition so bad (including substantial brain damage or brain disease) that I have no reasonable hope of achieving
  a quality of life that is acceptable to me.

An acceptable quality of life to me is one that includes the following capacities and values. (Describe here the things that
are most important to you when you are making decisions to choose or refuse life-sustaining treatments.)

_____

_____

_____

_____

Examples:	• recognize family or friends	• make decisions	• communicate
	• feed myself	• take care of myself	• be responsive to my environment

*If you do not agree with one or other of the above statements, draw a line through the statement and put your initials at the end of
the end of the line.*

In facing the end of my life, I expect my agent (if I have one) and my caregivers to honor my wishes, values, and directives.

For further clarification, please refer to my *Caring Conversations* Workbook, which is located at _____ .

**Be sure to sign the reverse side of this page even if you do not wish
to appoint a Durable Power of Attorney for Healthcare Decisions**

**Talk about this form and your ideas about your healthcare with the person you have chosen to make decisions for you,
your doctors, family, friends, and clergy. Give each of them a completed copy.**

You may cancel or change this form at any time. You should review it often. Each time you review it, put your initials and the date
here. _____

This document is provided as a service by the Center for Practical Bioethics.
For more information, call the Center for Practical Bioethics at 816-221-1100
Email – *bioethic@practicalbioethics.org* • Website – *www.practicalbioethics.org*

Figure 18-2 • cont'd.

if there are advance directives on initial assessment. These documents are then placed in the chart for future reference if necessary. State statutes regarding advance directives vary from state to state, so it is important to know state practice.

GOOD SAMARITAN LAWS

While nurses are legally covered for professional actions within the workplace, there are often concerns about professional actions in times of emergency outside of the health care institution. Good Samaritan laws have been enacted to encourage professional to render help in an emergency or accident situation. The Hawaii Good Samaritan Act reads: "Any person who in good faith renders emergency care, without renumeration or

expectation of renumeration, at the scene of an accident or emergency to the victim of the accident or emergency shall not be liable for any civil damages resulting from the persons acts or omission, except for such damages as may result from the persons gross negligence or wanton acts or omissions" (US Legal Definitions, 2008).

SUMMARY

The practice of nursing occurs within situations guided by practice acts, law, and organizational policy and procedures. Awareness of the legalities of the professional workplace is a vital component of safe practice for all nurses. If there are any questions regarding legal issues surrounding practice, the state board in which the nurse practices is a valuable resource.

CLINICAL CORNER

How We Educate Staff in the Health Insurance Portability and Accountability Act
Denise Occhiuzzo, Denyse Addison

The overall education plan for the Health Insurance Portability and Accountability Act (HIPAA) of 1996 includes initial education and annual updates for all Hackensack University Medical Center (HUMC) employees across the organization in order to maintain competency and promote compliance with the established requirements.

The orientation plan for all new employees requires participation in the General Orientation Program. The curriculum includes regulatory education on HIPAA. The content outline consists of the definitions of HIPAA and protected health information, state requirements, use and disclosure of protected health information, and HUMC's related policies. The method for this educational segment is twofold. The first method is lecture by an instructor from the Compliance Department with an opportunity for questions and answers. Then, each employee completes an e-learning module on HIPAA , which is an electronic module that the learner accesses through our Learning Management System via HUMC's intranet.

Upon completion of general orientation, the new employee then embarks on department-specific orientation. HIPAA education is included in this phase of the orientation period to ensure that employees understand the implications specific to his/her assigned area, role, and responsibilities. For example, nursing has a required specialty orientation. HIPAA education is further addressed during this phase to ensure understanding and compliance with HUMC's philosophy and security of electronic documentation for protected health information.

Annual mandatory education for all employees requires completion of the HIPAA e-learning module. This module provides a general review followed by a 10-question final examination that the employee must pass with a score of at least 80%.

The overall education plan includes reinforcement of HIPAA regulations to be threaded throughout the curriculum as necessary and where applicable. For example, this content would be found in lectures on ethics, documentation, and patient's rights.

EVIDENCE-BASED PRACTICE

The Impact of Managed Care on Nursing Regulations in Nine Western States

Robinson, J. E. (2000). The impact of managed care on nursing regulations in nine western states. Journal of Health and Social Policy, 11, 17–31.

In a time of globalization and technology, the push toward a national standardized nursing practice is strong and supported by the Pew Commissions recommendations in 1995 as well as the National Council of Nursing. At first glance, it would appear that nursing in the United States is moving toward national standardization; however, the results of this qualitative study confirm that state-controlled nursing regulations remain the norm. In this study, funded by the Idaho Commission on Nursing and Nursing Education, a series of open-ended questions were addressed to officials from nine Western states' board of nursing in hopes of identifying major nursing issues in the respective states as well as common approaches to issues.

With the exception of North Dakota, the remaining eight Western states have various entry-to-nursing points including various combinations of diploma, associate's, and bachelor's prepared nurses. In addition, unlicensed personnel are playing a larger role in patient care as the need for providers increases without an equal increase in the availability of registered professional nurses. A common theme across all states was that nursing is in a constant state of flux and that there is not a single dominant approach for addressing nursing regulation and education in the Western states. The substitution of unlicensed personnel or "deskilling" of nursing is a potential risk to patients as economics demands that less-trained staff carry out more formerly nursing skills. This is a larger issue as no one group has evolved to balance the issues of quality and safety with cost. The research points to the existing vibrancy of state governments and autonomous state control of nursing care and licensing.

NCLEX® EXAM QUESTIONS

1. The purpose of risk management programs are to:
   1. identify and correct system problems and protect the institution from financial liability
   2. provide hospital quality improvement programs and staff support
   3. identify system problems and perform process improvement
   4. inspect hospital policies and offer advice on improvement
2. Good Samaritan laws do NOT:
   1. protect from blame those who aid injured persons
   2. reduce bystanders' hesitation to assist
   3. prevent bystander from being prosecuted for wrongful death
   4. provide legal protection to nurses working in the emergency department
3. Which of the following sets educational standards, examination requirements, licensing requirements and regulates the nursing profession in each particular state?
   1. the National League for Nursing (NLN)
   2. nurse practice acts
   3. state board of nursing
   4. the National Council of State Boards of Nursing
4. FLAT charting includes the following four items:
   1. factual, legible, accurate, timely
   2. factual, legal, accurate, timely
   3. factual, legible, active, timely
   4. factual, legible, accurate, thorough
5. To establish legal liability on the ground of malpractice (professional negligence), the injured client (plaintiff) does not have to prove:
   1. a duty of care was owed to the injured party
   2. there was a breach of that duty.
   3. the breach of the duty did not caused the injury.
   4. actual harm or damages were suffered by the plaintiff.
6. Which of the following states is NOT part of the nursing licensure compact states?
   1. Maryland
   2. Delaware
   3. New Jersey
   4. New Hampshire

Continued

NCLEX® EXAM QUESTIONS—cont'd

7. The direct application of physical force to a patient, with or without the patient's permission, to restrict his or her freedom of movement is:
   1. illegal
   2. arrest
   3. restraint
   4. nonrestraint
8. Both employee and patient health information are confidential and must not be released outside the organization without written consent. The employee or patient can sign a written consent for release of health information. This form is called:
   1. release of information
   2. chart reconciliation
   3. advance directive
   4. consent to treat

9. The responsibility of an organization for its own wrongful conduct is:
   1. corporate liability
   2. personal liability
   3. due cause
   4. protocol
10. Which of the following is TRUE regarding patient restraints?
    1. They are restricted in the acute care facility.
    2. They can be applied without a physician's order.
    3. They cannot be applied without a physician's order.
    4. A written physician's order is valid for length of stay.

Answers: 1. 1   2. 4   3. 2   4. 1   5. 3   6. 3   7. 3   8. 1   9. 1   10. 3

REFERENCES

Aiken, T. (2004). *Legal ethical and political issues in nursing*, 2nd ed. Philadelphia: F.A. Davis.

American Medical Association. (2008). Informed consent. Retrieved November 9, 2008, from http://www.ama-assn.org/ama/pub/category/4608.html.

Carroll, P. (2006). *Nursing leadership and management, a practical guide*. Clifton Park, NY: Thompson Delmar Learning.

Fiesta, J. (1999). Do no harm: when caregivers violate the golden rule. *Nursing Management, 30*, 10-11.

Kelly-Heidenthal, P., & Marthaler, M. T. (2005). *Delegation of nursing care*. Clifton Park, NY: Thomson Delmar Learning.

Martin, J. W., & Cain, K. (2003). Legal aspects of patient care. In P. Kelly-Heidenthal (Ed.), *Nursing leadership and management* (pp. 446-463). Clifton Park, NY: Thompson Delmar Learning.

Nathanson, M. (1996). *Home Health Care Law Manual*. Gaithersberg, MD: Aspen Publishers.

National Council of State Boards of Nursing (2008). Nurse licensure compact. Retrieved March 21, 2008, from https://www.ncsbn.org/nlc.htm.

Nurse Licensure Compact Administrators. (2008). Participating states in the NLC. Retrieved March 21, 2008, from https://www.ncsbn.org/158.htm.

Rowland, H., & Rowland, B. (1997). *Nursing administration handbook*, 4th ed. Gaithersburg, MD: An Aspen Publication, Aspen Publishers, Inc.

Sullivan, E. J., & Decker, P. J. (2001). *Effective leadership and management in nursing*, 5th ed. Upper Saddle River, NJ: Prentice Hall.

Sullivan, E., & Decker, P. (2005). *Effective leadership and management in nursing*. Upper Saddle River, NJ: Pearson, Prentice Hall.

The Joint Commission. (2007). *Hospital accreditation standards*. Oakbrook Terrace, IL: Author.

US Legal Definitions. (2008). Good Samaritan laws & legal definition. Retrieved November 9, 2008, from http://definitions.uslegal.com/g/good-samaritans/.

CHAPTER 19

Staffing and Scheduling

Chapter Objectives

1. Discuss the determination of staffing needs.
2. Review the different types of assignment systems.
3. Identify the difference between centralized and decentralized staffing.
4. Differentiate between the various types of staffing patterns.
5. Discuss activities used by the nurse manager to support fluctuating staffing needs.

Definitions

Staffing pattern Plan that articulates how many and what kind of staff are needed by shift and day to staff a unit or department

Staffing schedules Work schedules for personnel

Staffing formulas Calculations used to determine staffing needs

FTE Equal to the equivalent of a full-time employee (a full-time equivalent)

Patient acuity Measure of nursing workload that is generated for each patient

Centralized scheduling Scheduling done in one location

Decentralized scheduling Scheduling done in local areas

Self-scheduling Staff coordinating their own work schedules

Rotating work shifts Alternating work hours among days, evening, and nights

Permanent shifts Personnel working the same hours repeatedly

Block scheduling Using the same schedule repeatedly

Variable staffing Determining the number and mix of staff based on patient needs

Patient classification systems Systems developed to objectively determine workload requirements and staffing needs

STAFFING

One of the most time-consuming concerns of most nurse managers is the staffing of the unit. Staffing requires having enough staff to deliver care but also requires that the staff that are present are qualified to deliver the care. Staffing schedules are also a major concern of nurses as they enter a health care environment, and issues with schedules are often cited as a major job dissatisfier by nurses leaving the workplace (Halm, Peterson, & Kandelis, 2005).

There have been multiple studies in the recent literature supporting the importance of safe staffing and its relation to patient safety (Hugonnet, Chevrolet, & Pittet, 2007; Stone, Mooney-Kane, & Larsen, 2007; Weissman, Rothschild, & Bendavid, 2007). Higher numbers of hours of nursing care provided by registered nurses and a greater number of hours of care by registered nurses per day are associated with better care for hospitalized patients (Needleman, Buerhaus, Mattke, Stewart, & Zelevinsky, 2002; Needleman, Buerhaus, Stewart, Zelevinsky, & Mattke, 2006).

Health care staffing is a complicated issue, requiring knowledge of patient acuity, nursing productivity, nursing competence, organization finance, and health care regulations.

THE JOINT COMMISSION

The Joint Commission (TJC) surveys hospitals on the quality of care provided. TJC does not mandate staffing levels but does assess an organization's ability to provide the right number of competent staff to meet the needs of patients served by the hospital (TJC, 2007).

THE AMERICAN NURSES ASSOCIATION PRINCIPLES FOR NURSE STAFFING

In 1999, the American Nurses Association (ANA) published *Principles for Nurse Staffing*, which empha-sized the nursing work environment to provide safe patient care (Box 19-1). The ANA's *Principles for Nurse Staffing* (1999) offers standards to incorporate and balance the needs of patients, nurses, and organizations committed to positive patient outcomes. The principles recognize that providing nursing care services can be multivariate and complex.

Subsequently, the ANA advocated a work environment that supports nurses in providing the best possible patient care by budgeting enough positions, administrative support, good nurse-physician relations, career advancement options, work flexibility, and personal choice in scheduling (ANA, 1999).

State departments of health have staffing regulations for health care institutions; these regulations are often broad. Additionally, California has mandatory staffing guidelines. These guidelines have provoked court challenges and much discussion and review in other states. On October 10, 1999, California became the first state in the nation to require mandatory safe licensed nurse/

Box 19-1 THE AMERICAN NURSES ASSOCIATION PRINCIPLES FOR NURSE STAFFING

Policy Statements

- Nurse staffing patterns and the level of care provided should not depend on the type of payor.
- Evaluation of any staffing system should include quality of worklife outcomes, as well as patient outcomes.
- Staffing should be based on achieving quality of patient care indices, meeting organizational outcomes and ensuring that the quality of the nurse's worklife is appropriate.

Principles

The nine principles identified by the expert panel for nurse staffing and adopted by the ANA Board of Directors on November 24, 1998, are listed below. Discussion of each of the three categories follows the list.

  I. Patient Care Unit Related
   a. Appropriate staffing levels for a patient care unit reflect analysis of individual and aggregate patient needs.
   b. There is a critical need to either retire or seriously question the usefulness of the concept of nursing hours per patient day (HPPD).
   c. Unit functions necessary to support delivery of quality patient care must also be considered in determining staffing levels.

 II. Staff Related
   a. The specific needs of various patient populations should determine the appropriate clinical competencies required of the nurse practicing in that area.
   b. Registered nurses must have nursing management support and representation at both the operational level and the executive level.
   c. Clinical support from experienced RNs should be readily available to those RNs with less proficiency.

III. Institution/Organization Related
   a. Organizational policy should reflect an organizational climate that values registered nurses and other employees as strategic assets and exhibit a true commitment to filling budgeted positions in a timely manner.
   b. All institutions should have documented competencies for nursing staff, including agency or supplemental and traveling RNs, for those activities that they have been authorized to perform.
   c. Organizational policies should recognize the myriad needs of both patients and nursing staff.

patient ratios in all units in acute care facilities. The legislation (AB 394) requires that additional nurses be added to a minimum ratio in accordance with a patient classification system based on the severity of the patient's condition. Ten states have enacted legislation and/or regulations regarding nurse staffing plans and ratios: California, Washington, DC, Florida, Illinois, Maine, New Jersey, Oregon, Rhode Island, Texas, and Vermont (Robert Wood Johnson Foundation, 2007). Seventeen other states have introduced but have not enacted any legislation or regulations.

PROCESS OF STAFFING

A staffing plan addresses the requirements of the unit or organization over a defined period of time. Daily staffing plans outline what is necessary to meet the needs of the patients over a 24-hour period. An annual staffing plan is created to determine the budgetary needs of an organization. *Daily staffing* refers to filling in open shifts on the current work schedule.

Scheduling refers to making work assignments for the next work period. It is done from 4 to 8 weeks in advance depending on the institution (see Figure 19-1).

PROCESS OF DAILY STAFFING

The process of daily staffing begins with an assessment of the current staffing situation. The assessment includes

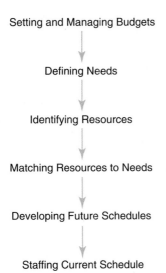

Setting and Managing Budgets

↓

Defining Needs

↓

Identifying Resources

↓

Matching Resources to Needs

↓

Developing Future Schedules

↓

Staffing Current Schedule

Figure 19-1 • Nurse scheduling and staffing. (From California Health Care Foundation [2005]. Adopting online nurse scheduling and staffing systems. Oakland, CA. Used with permission.)

the qualifications and competence of the staff needed and available (ANA, 2004). The next step is to formulate a plan to meet future needs. The staffing process culminates with a schedule (organized plan) of personnel to provide patient care services. Scheduling variables are defined as (Jones, 2007, p. 280):

1. The number of patients, complexity of patients' condition, and nursing care required
2. The physical environment in which nursing care is to be provided
3. The nursing staff members' competency levels, qualifications, skill range, knowledge or ability, and experience level
4. The level of supervision required
5. Availability of nursing staff members for the assignment of responsibilities

THE STAFFING PLAN

The staffing plan consists of four different elements that must be addressed—the health care setting, care delivery model, patient acuity, and nursing staff. They are then incorporated into the next step in the process—the scheduling and staffing system. A staffing plan can also be referred to as the staffing matrix.

STAFFING AND SCHEDULING SYSTEMS

There are various types of staffing systems in place in health care. The four major types are:

1. Centralized scheduling—Decision making occurs in a "centralized" location for the entire institution.
2. Decentralized scheduling—Decision making occurs with the nurse manager on the unit.
3. Mixed scheduling—Blends aspects of items 1 and 2. Individual units may manage staffing, but if they cannot fill open shifts, they might forward their needs to a centralized office.
4. Self-scheduling—Individual staff members schedule themselves. The nurse manager then works with staff members to fill empty slots.

Many organizations are moving toward computer-assisted staffing.

Centralized Scheduling

Two major advantages of centralized scheduling are fairness to employees through consistent, objective, and impartial application of policies and opportunities for cost containment through better use of resources (Tomey, 2004, p. 387).

Decentralized Scheduling

When managers are given authority and assume responsibility, they can staff their own units through decentralized scheduling (Tomey, 2004, p. 388).

Scheduling staff, which is very time consuming, takes managers away from other duties or forces them to do the scheduling while off duty. Decentralized scheduling may use resources less effectively and consequently make cost containment more difficult (Tomey, 2004, p. 389).

Mixed Scheduling

An individual may manage staffing but with the option of consulting a centralized office to help fill open shifts.

Self-Scheduling

In this type of scheduling system, the scheduling is coordinated by staff nurses. It saves the manager considerable scheduling time. This system also increases staff members' ability to negotiate with each other.

Table 19-1 provides pros and cons of centralized and decentralized scheduling.

Health care organizations must have in place a system to track available personnel. To match personnel with staffing needs, it is important that the organization is able to determine an individual's skills, competencies, license, certifications, etc. Most scheduling is done in advance; therefore, future scheduling is used. Institutions use one or more of the following four types of future scheduling in their planning:

- *Pattern scheduling*—Staff commit to work a set number of shift types in a given time frame. At the end of the time period, the pattern repeats (such as 3 weeks of day shift followed by 1 week of night shift, repeated every 4 weeks). Pattern scheduling can also include permanent shifts, block shifts, and rotating shifts (Box 19-2).
- *Preference scheduling*—Staff define their preference for shift type, days of the week, and unit. Defined rules can override preferences.
- *Rules scheduling*—Based on an organization's scheduling policies. Because it does not take pattern or preference into account, it is rarely used alone.
- *Self-scheduling*—Scheduling needs are defined, and then staff sign up for available shifts on a rotating, first-come, first-served basis.

Table 19-2 provides pros and cons of scheduling types.

Table 19-3 lists advantages and disadvantages of types of pattern scheduling.

FULL-TIME EQUIVALENT

No matter what the shift, the needs of the patient and unit must be accommodated. There is no end to creative ways that staffing can be accomplished, but the basic number that is used in staffing is the full-time equivalent (FTE). An FTE is a measure of the work commitment of a full-time employee. A full-time employee works to qualify for full-time employment. In institutions with a 40-hour full-time work week, this works out to 2080 hours of work time (40 hours per week for 52 weeks a year equals 2,080 hours of work time). In organizations with a 37.5-hour work week, this would work out to (37.5×52 weeks) 1950 hours of work time per year. Most institutions use a 40-hour workweek for the definition of an FTE (Table 19-4).

Therefore, if the nurse manager needed to cover 40 hours of work per week, it could be covered by one full-time employee or two half-time employees, etc. For budget purposes, it would be important to know the state rules and regulations covering benefits. When does an employee receive benefits (health care, vacation time, etc.)? Staff benefits are a costly expense to health care institutions.

Table 19-1	PROS AND CONS OF CENTRALIZED AND DECENTRALIZED SCHEDULING	
Scheduling Method	**Pros**	**Cons**
Centralized	Fairness Cost containment	Lack of individualized treatment
Decentralized	Managers have authority Staff get personalized attention Staffing is easier Staffing is less complicated	Schedule used to punish and reward Time consuming for managers Cost containment is more difficult

Box 19-2 TYPES OF PATTERN SCHEDULING

Alternating or rotating work shifts—Work schedule based on a predefined pattern, such an alternate weekends off, or rotating from days to evenings every 3 weeks. Sometimes, however, the rotating of shifts may only occur as needed, such as when the night nurse is off.

Permanent shifts—Individuals are hired to work specific shifts, such as nights only.

* *Block, or cyclical, scheduling*

This type of scheduling system uses the same schedule repeatedly. It may be similar to alternating or rotating shifts but may also include a pattern of days on and days off (four on; two off). Is often part of another type of scheduling pattern; see later.

* *Eight-hour shift, 5-day workweek*

This method uses the traditional 5-day, 40-hour workweek. This does not mean that weekends are not covered; the nurse works 5 days a week with 2 days off, and the nurse may work alternating weekends.

* *Ten-hour day, 4-day workweek*

This method utilizes the 10-hour day, 4-day workweek. It requires careful block scheduling to cover all shifts.

* *Twelve-hour shifts*

Three days on and 4 days off. Some studies demonstrate that this method allows for better use of nursing personnel, increased continuity of care, and improved job satisfaction and morale (Garret, 2008).

* *Baylor plan—weekend alternative*

Baylor University Medical Center in Dallas, Texas, started a 2-day alternative plan. Nurses have the option to work two 12-hour days on the weekends and be paid for 36 hours for day shifts, or 40 hours for night shifts, or to work five 8-hour shifts Monday through Friday. This plan required a larger nursing staff, filled weekend positions, and reduced turnover. Some hospitals have implemented the Baylor plan, indicating that the extra pay on weekends compensated for vacations, holidays, and sick time (Tomey, 2004, p. 393)

* *Variable staffing*

This type of staffing is dependent on the patient acuity and needs of the unit. If acuity is higher than budgeted, extra staff may be called in on overtime, or additional staff such as agency or float staff may be used.

Table 19-2 PROS AND CONS OF SCHEDULING TYPES

Scheduling Type	Pros	Cons
Rules based	Incorporates regulatory issues (hours of work, time off overtime, staffing ratios	Does not take preferences into account Does not take staffing patterns into account Scheduling can be erratic
Pattern	Predictable schedules	Little flexibility Impairs recruitment
Preference	Considers staff needs	Preferences may not match rules
Self	Enables more creativity in covering shifts Increased staff satisfaction Saves time for nurse managers	Less organization and manager control of staffing

From California Health Care Foundation (2005). *Adopting online nurse scheduling and staffing systems* (p. 13). Oakland, CA: Author. Used with permission.

Another variable in the staffing decision will be the amount of productive versus nonproductive hours. Not all of the 2080 hours of the FTE are productive. Benefit time such as vacation, sick time, and education time are considered nonproductive time. To determine the amount of productive time of an employee, you would subtract the hours of benefit time from the FTE of 2080 hours. So if an employee had:

5 Sick days (5 days × 8 hours/day) = 40 hours
20 Vacation days (20 × 8 hours/day) = 160 hours
Holidays (5 days × 8 hours/day) = 40 hours
Education time (3 days × 8 hours/day) = 24 hours
This all adds up to 264 hours of nonproductive time, and 2080 hours per year − 264 hours = 1816 hours of productive time. When calculating the number of FTEs needed to staff the unit, you would

Table 19-3 ADVANTAGES AND DISADVANTAGES OF TYPES OF PATTERN SCHEDULING

Type	Advantages	Disadvantage
Rotating work shifts	Can rotate teams	Rotate among shifts Increase stress Affect health Affect quality of work Disrupt development of work groups High turnover
Permanent shifts	Can participate in social activities Job satisfaction Commitment to the organization Few health problems Less tardiness Less absenteeism Less turnover	Most people want day shift New graduates predominantly staff evenings and nights Difficulty evaluation evening and night staff Nurses may not appreciate the workload or problems of other shifts Rigidity
Block, or cyclical, scheduling	Same schedule repeatedly Nurses not so exhausted Sick time reduced Personnel know schedule in advance Personnel can schedule social events Decreased time spent on scheduling Staff treated fairly Helps establish stable work groups Decreases floating Promotes team spirit Promotes continuity of care	
Variable staffing	Use census to determine number and mix of staff Little need to call in unscheduled staff Efficient	

From Tomey, A. M., (2004). *Guide to nursing management and leadership* (p. 390), 7th ed. St. Louis: Mosby.

Table 19-4 FTE CALCULATION FOR VARYING LEVELS OF WORK COMMITMENT

1.0 FTE = 40 hours per week or five 8-hour shifts per week

0.8 FTE = 32 hour per week or four 8-hour shifts per week

0.6 FTE = 24 hours per week or three 8-hour shifts per week

0.4 FTE = 16 hours per week or two 8-hour shifts per week

0.2 FTE = 8 hours per week or one 8-hour shift per week

From Kelly-Heidenthal, P. (2003). *Nursing leadership and management* (p. 240). Clifton Park, NY: Thomson Delmar Learning.

count only the number of productive hours available.

To determine staffing needs, the nurse manager needs to know the number of FTE employees and the amount of nursing hours per patient day. Nursing care hours per patient day are the number of hours worked by nursing staff that have direct patient care responsibilities. To calculate nursing care hours per patient day, use only productive hours.

Calculation of nursing care hours per patient day (Bernat, 2003):

20 Patients on the unit

5 Staff on each of three shifts = 15 staff

15 Staff each working 8 productive hours = 120 hours ÷ 24 hours

120 Nursing care hours ÷ 20 patients = 6.0 nursing care hours per patient

DEVELOPMENT OF A STAFFING PATTERN

One cannot assume that the number of nursing care hours is a permanent number. This number will change based on patient acuity. Patient acuity data are used to predict the amount of nursing care required by a group of patients. The higher the acuity level, the more nursing care is needed by the patient.

To develop a staffing pattern using nursing care hours per day (NCHPD), you would start with a goal nursing care hours. If your goal was 5 and you had 35 patients on your 40-bed unit, you would multiply 5 NCHPD × 35 patients to get 175 productive hours needed every day. Dividing 175 by 8-hour shifts worked by a FTE gives you 21.8 FTEs needed per day (adapted from Kelly-Heidenthal, 2003).

The staffing number calculated for the unit is 21.8, but that does not add for nonproductive hours. The manager must provide for the additional staff that will be needed for days off and benefit time. Each 8-hour shift for an FTE is equal to 0.2 FTE; therefore, to provide coverage for 2 days off a week, multiply the number of staff needed per day by 0.4 FTE. The 21.8 FTEs multiplied by 0.4 would be an additional 8.7 FTEs to cover 2 days off per week for a total of 30.5 FTEs (adapted from Kelly-Heidenthal, 2003).

The next step is to provide coverage for vacation time and other time away from work. If every employee receives 2 weeks of vacation and 2 educational days, this would equate to 1984 of productive time (2 weeks = 10 days × 8 hours + 2 days = 16 hours = 96 hours subtracted from the FTE 2080 hours = 1984 productive hours per FTE). Previously, it was decided that a total of 30.5 FTEs were needed to cover the unit. This was based on 2080 productive hours, but you have now found that there are only 1984 productive hours per FTE: 30.5 FTEs × 2080 equals 63,440 hours and 63,440 hours ÷1984 equals 31.9 FTEs needed to cover this unit (adapted from Kelly-Heidenthal, 2003).

The spread of staff across the 24-hour period depends on the type of patients. Typically, intensive care units have a relatively equal spread across the shifts. Typically, the spread of FTEs across the 24-hour period falls into the following pattern: days, 33% to 50%; evenings, 30% to 40%; nights, 20% to 33% (adapted from Kelly-Heidenthal, 2003).

PART-TIME STAFF

Part-time staff is used to decrease staffing shortages in an institution.

Nurses with part-time employment have the following benefits; they can:
- Broaden horizons beyond home
- Increase income
- Provide ego satisfaction
- Maintain nursing skills
- Continue education

Another option is for two nurses to share one full-time position. The disadvantages to an institution of position sharing are that educational and administrative expenses are higher proportionately for part-time than for full-time help because it costs as much to orient a part-time nurse as it does a full-time nurse, thereby costing more per hours worked. Also, maintaining continuity of care is complicated, because two or more part-time people may fill budgeted full-time positions. The disadvantages for the nurses are there are not full-time benefits such as vacation and sick time.

EXTERNAL TEMPORARY AGENCIES

Usually as a last resort, an institution may use temporary agency nurses. The staffing agency is a business that has a registry of nurses who have highly flexible schedules. Matching of nurses' credentials with the position is sometimes daunting. Replacement staff from agency pools are usually an expensive means of maintain the staffing. Most hospitals prefer to minimize the use of agency nurses due to the extra cost to the institution.

TRAVEL NURSES

"Travelers" are per diem nurses working for a business that places them in contracted hospitals. Unlike agency nurses, travelers usually sign longer-term contracts with hospitals (3 to 6 months or longer). There are many options used by health care institutions to deal with staffing and daily absences due to sick calls (Box 19-3).

OVERTIME

In a staffing emergency, institutions may ask nurses to work overtime. Overtime pay is usually on a par that is different than regular pay, and many nurses depend on the extra money provided by overtime. With overtime,

- Use a float, per diem, or agency nurse.
- Ask a nurse to work for the sick person and canceling a shift for that person later in the week.
- Ask a part-time person to work an extra shift, substituting one type of classification for another, such as an LPN for an RN.
- Ask one staff member to work a few hours of overtime and another to come in a few hours early.
- Do without a substitute.
- Manager covers the shift.

there are a number of issues with which the nurse and nurse manager need to be concerned.

- *Length of time* that the nurse will be working. In a 12-hour shift, the nurse has already worked 12 hours and an additional shift will have her working a full 24 hours! Sometimes 4 hours of overtime will be used in this situation.
- The nurse manager must be careful to evaluate the *exhaustion level* of the staff.

- There are documented instances of *increased errors* when the staff is exhausted (Garrett, 2008).
- On a budget end, overtime may increase the dollars spent on care provided. This *budget variance* will need to be documented.
- *State labor law* will need to be reviewed as well as *union guidelines*. They may define the number of hours required between shifts.

AUTOMATED STAFFING SYSTEMS

Many health care institutions are moving toward the use of computerized staffing and scheduling systems. These systems greatly enhance the manager's ability to properly schedule staff. They also free up much of the time that the manager spends on the creation of the schedule. Integrated online scheduling and staffing products are available for purchase under license.

SUMMARY

Staffing and scheduling represent one of the most challenging of the nurse managers responsibilities. It requires a keen sense of the day-to-day workings of the unit as well as a keen awareness of the staff's abilities and personalities. It also requires evaluation of the care delivered and the flexibility to create staffing levels that best meet the patient needs.

CLINICAL CORNER

Overview of the Recruitment and Retention Committee at St. Joseph's Regional Medical Center, Paterson, NJ
Cathy Hughes

The shortage of nurses makes staff retention a more pressing problem, and the shortage is expected to worsen (JCAHO, 2002; AACN, 2003). The first of the baby boomers will be reaching the age of retirement in a very short time, and the increasing elderly population will require that there are enough nurses to care for these patients. Some of these baby boomers are nurses who would love to be cared for by people with whom they worked for many years and who remember them. How do we keep nurses working for one hospital for their professional career, which could be 45 years of service?

Increasing salary and monetary perks are not the only things that are taken into consideration when new graduate nurses are getting their first jobs or when

experienced nurses are seeking employment because of hospital closings or downsizing. There have been two studies that show Magnet-recognized hospitals are more successful in the recruitment and retention of nurses (Buchan, 1999; Aiken, Havens, & Sloane, 2000).

Magnet-designated facilities have the following characteristics that assist in retaining nurses:

- Higher nurse-to-patient ratios
- Flexible schedules
- Decentralized administration
- Participatory management
- Autonomy in decision making
- Recognition
- Advancement opportunities

One committee of the professional Nurse Practice Council of St. Joseph's Regional Medical Center, in Paterson, NJ, is the Recruitment and Retention Committee. Since the development of the Recruitment and Retention Committee, the hard work of these commit-

CLINICAL CORNER—cont'd

tee members has made many changes in the organization. Examples include the implementation of peer review evaluations that are a part of the yearly review. Currently, the committee has been given the challenge to review and improve the peer review evaluation process, incorporating the language of Jean Watson, our nursing theorists, relationship-based care delivery model, and healthy work environment tenets. This committee was instrumental in human resource policy development such as a "no-float" policy for nurses with over 20 years of employment and the new merit raise policy, which is now housewide across all departments in the organization. We are also evaluating our clinical nurse ladder program, providing ideas for changes and improvements. With the collaboration of the nurse recruiter, there have been informal conversations with newly hired nurses to evaluate what the organization may need to change to retain them.

It is not just money that attracts people to a certain employer. For some, it is autonomy. For others, it is a safe work environment. Recruiting and retaining nurses throughout their careers, which could easily span 45 years, present a long-term challenge for employers. Nurses need to take the leadership role in shaping the policies and processes that govern not just their professional practice but their professional work environment as well. Magnet organizations embrace and support this type of nursing leadership.

References

American Association of Colleges of Nursing (AACN). (2003). *Nursing shortage fact sheet*. April 21, 2003:1-5.

Aiken, L. H., Havens, D. S., & Sloane, D. M. (2000). The Magnet Nursing Services Recognition Program. *American Journal of Nursing. 100*(3), 26-35.

Buchan, J. (1999). Still attractive after all these years? Magnet hospitals in a changing health care environment. *Journal of Advanced Nursing. 30*(1), 100-108.

Joint Commission on Accreditation of Healthcare Organizations (JCAHO). (2002). *Health care at the crossroads: strategies for addressing the evolving nursing crisis*. August, 2002:1-47.

EVIDENCE-BASED PRACTICE

Hospital Nurse Staffing and Patient Mortality, Nurse Burnout, and Job Dissatisfaction.

Aiken, L. H., Clarke, S. P., Sloane, D. M., Sochalski, J., & Silber, J. H. (2002). Hospital nurse staffing and patient mortality, nurse burnout, and job dissatisfaction. Journal of American Medical Association, 288*(16), 1987–1993.*

This work reports on findings from a comprehensive study of 168 hospitals and clarifies the impact of nurse staffing levels on patient outcomes and factors that influence nurse retention. Examination of whether serious surgical complications and mortality rates were lower in hospitals where nurses carry smaller patient loads was done. Also studied was the extent to which more favorable patient-to-nurse ratios were associated with lower burnout and lower job satisfaction among registered nurses.

Higher emotional exhaustion and greater job dissatisfaction in nurses were strongly and significantly associated with patient-to-nurse ratios. It was implied that nurses in hospitals with 8:1 patient to nurse ratios would be 2.29 times as likely as nurses with 4:1 patient to nurse ratios to show high emotional exhaustion and 1.75 times as likely to be dissatisfied with their jobs. The data further indicates that although 43% of nurses who reported high burnout and are dissatisfied with their jobs intend to leave their current job within the next 12 months, only 11% of the nurses who are not burned out and who remain satisfied with their jobs intend to leave.

Among the surgical patients studied there was a pronounced effect of nurse staffing on both mortality and deaths following complications. The results of the study showed that, all else being equal, substantial decreases in mortality rates could result from increasing registered nursing staffing, especially for patients who develop complications.

It is also suggested that the California hospital nurse staffing legislation represents a credible approach to reducing mortality and increasing nurse retention in hospital practice if it can be successfully implemented. These results further indicate that nurses in hospitals with the highest patient-to-nurse ratios are more likely to experience job related burnout and almost twice as likely to be dissatisfied with their jobs compared with nurse in hospitals with the lowest ratios. This effect of staffing on job satisfaction and burnout suggest that improvements in nurse staffing in California hospitals resulting from the new legislation could be accompanied by declines in nurse turnover. It was found that burnout and dissatisfaction predict nurses' intentions to leave their current jobs within a year.

These findings have important implications for two pressing issues: patient safety and the hospital nurse

Continued

EVIDENCE-BASED PRACTICE—cont'd

shortage. The association of nurse staffing levels with the rescue of patients with life-threatening conditions suggests that nurses contribute importantly to surveillance, early detection and timely interventions that save lives. Improving nurse staffing levels may reduce alarming turnover rates in hospitals by reducing burnout and job dissatisfaction which are major precursors of job resignation. The impact of staffing on patient and nurse outcomes suggest that by investing in registered nurse staffing, hospitals may avert both preventable mortality and low nurse retention in hospital practice.

NCLEX® EXAM QUESTIONS

1. Which of the following is NOT an acceptable option to be used for sick calls?
   1. using a float, per diem, or agency nurse
   2. doing without a substitute
   3. manager to cover the shift
   4. vice president of nursing to cover the shift
2. One advantage of centralized scheduling is:
   1. better use of resources
   2. lack of cost containment
   3. decreased use of resources
   4. increase in cost
3. One advantage of decentralized scheduling is:
   1. manager staffs own unit
   2. less time consuming for manager
   3. cost containment
   4. better use of resources
4. In self-scheduling, the personnel doing the scheduling is:
   1. the registered nurse
   2. the nursing assistant
   3. the licensed practical nurse
   4. the patient care technician
5. Which of the following is not an acceptable shifts?
   1. 8 hours
   2. 12 hours
   3. 17 hours
   4. 10 hours
6. The Baylor plan is:
   1. a weekend alternative plan
   2. a weekday alternative plan

   3. a plan developed for 12-hour shifts
   4. a plan developed for 10-hour shifts
7. Part-time staff are often utilized to decrease staffing shortages in an institution. Which of the following is an example of when part-time employment does NOT benefit the nurse.
   1. broaden horizons beyond home
   2. increase income
   3. continue education
   4. spending less time with family
8. Regarding overtime, the following is an issue that the nurse and nurse manager need to deal with:
   1. exhausted nurses
   2. decreased budget
   3. non-union labor laws
   4. increased incident reports
9. Which of the following is NOT an option that the nurse manager can utilize when replacing sick calls?
   1. using a float, per diem, or agency nurse
   2. asking a nurse to work for the sick person and canceling a shift for that person later in the week
   3. doing without a substitute
   4. allow the staffing level to fall below the need for acuity
10. External temporary agencies are:
    1. used as first line to replace sick calls
    2. used usually as a last resort
    3. not very expensive
    4. no longer used due to expense

Answers: 1. 4   2. 1   3. 1   4. 1   5. 3   6. 1   7. 4   8. 1   9. 3   10. 2

REFERENCES

Aiken, L., Clarke, S., Slaoan, D., Sochalski, J., & Silber, J. (2002). Hospital nurse Staffing and patient mortality, nurse burnout, and job dissatisfaction. *Journal of the American Medial Association, 288,* 1987-1993.

American Nurses Association. (1999). *Principles for nurse staffing.* Washington, DC: Author. Retrieved November 11, 2008, from http://www.nursing-world.orgn/readroom/stffprnchtm.

American Nurses Association. (2004). *Scope and standards for nurse administrators* (2nd ed.). Silver Spring, MD: author.

Bernat, A. (2003). Effective staffing. In P. Kelly-Heidenthal (Ed), *Nursing leadership and management* (pp. 238-265). Clifton Park, NY: Thomson Delmar Learning.

California Health Care Foundation. (2005). *Adopting online nurse scheduling and staffing systems.* Oakland, CA: Author.

Garrett, C. (2008). The effect of nurse staffing patterns on medical errors and nurse burnout. *AORN Journal, 87,* 1191-1192, 1194, 1196-1200, 1202-1204.

Halm, M., Peterson, M., & Kandelis, M. (2005). Hospital nurse staffing and patient mortality, emotional exhaustion, and job dissatisfaction. *Clinical Nurse Specialist, 19,* 241-251.

Hugonnet, S., Chevrolet, J., & Pittet, D. (2007). The effect of workload in infection risk in critically ill patient. *Critical Care Medicine, 35,* 76-81.

Kelly-Heidenthal, P. (2003). *Nursing leadership and management.* Clifton Park, NY: Thomson Delmar Learning.

Needleman, J., Buerhaus, P., Stewart, M., Zelevinsky, K., & Mattke, S. (2006). Nurse staffing in hospitals: is there a business case for quality? *Health Affairs, 25,* 204-211.

Needleman, J., Buerhaus, P., Mattke, S., Stewart, M., & Zelevinsky, K. (2002). Nurse staffing levels and the quality of care in hospitals. *New England Journal of Medicine, 346,* 1715-1722.

Stone, P., Mooney-Kane, C., & Larson, E. (2007). Nurse working conditions and patient safety outcomes. *Medical Care, 45,* 571-578.

The Joint Commission. (2007). *Comprehensive accreditation manual for hospitals.* Oakbrook Terrace, IL: Author.

Tomey, A. M., (2004). *Guide to nursing management and leadership* (7th ed.). St. Louis: Mosby.

Weissman, J., Rothschild, J., & Bendavid, E. (2007). Hospital workload and adverse events. *Meical Care, 45,* 448-455.

CHAPTER 20

Supervising and Evaluating the Work of Others

Chapter Objectives

1. Discuss nurse leader responsibility regarding group management.
2. Review techniques for working with groups.
3. Review techniques for leading groups and meetings.
4. Differentiate between functional and dysfunctional groups.
5. Review the different methods used to evaluate staff performance.
6. Identify the difference between supervising and evaluating the work of others.
7. Review the importance of supervising and leading groups, task forces, and patient care conferences.

Definitions

Group Aggregate of individuals who interact and mutually influence each other; several individuals assembled together or who have some unifying relationship

Formal groups Clusters of individuals designated by an organization to perform specified organizational tasks

Informal groups Groups that evolve from social interactions that are not defined by an organizational structure

Real (command) groups Groups that accomplish tasks in an organization and are recognized as legitimate organizational entities

Task group Several individuals who work together to accomplish specific time-limited assignments

Committees or task forces Groups that deal with specific issues involving several service areas

Teams Real groups in which people work cooperatively with each other to achieve a goal

Competing groups Groups in which members compete for resources or recognition

Team building Group development technique that focuses on task and relationship aspects of a group's functioning to build team cohesiveness

Norms Informal rules of behavior shared and enforced by group members

Role Set of expectations about behavior ascribed to a specific position in society

Productivity Measure of how well the work group or team uses the resources available to achieve its goals and produce its services

Cohesiveness Degree to which the members are attracted to the group and wish to retain membership in it

Formal committees Committees in an organization with authority and a specific role

Informal committees Committees with no delegated authority that are organized for discussion

Task forces Ad hoc committees appointed for a specific purpose and a limited time

GROUPS AND TEAMS

Nurses work as part of a team on the unit where they are employed. This does not necessarily mean that they are all practicing team nursing, but they are part of a larger group that is responsible for the overall delivery of care on the unit. As a team member, it is important to know how to work within a team. It is also important to know how to manage teams and to evaluate the performance of others.

A group consists of individuals who interact and influence each other. Groups exist in organizations. Group members include (Sullivan & Decker, 2005, p. 157):

- Individuals from a single work group or individuals at similar job levels from more than one work group
- Individuals from different job levels
- Individuals from different work groups and different job levels in the organization

As can be seen from this definition of group, there are a number of groups that function within a nursing unit. Some of these groups will be:

- Interdisciplinary teams—Sometimes called collaboratives, which are composed of the different functions caring for a patient. An example would be an ambulatory chemotherapy collaborative, in which the team composition includes the nurse, the pharmacist, the dietician, the admission clerk, and the intravenous therapist.
- Patient care team—This may be similar to the group of individuals actually providing actual care to the patient. It may be composed of all individuals responsible for care per shift or over 24 hours.
- Performance improvement team—May include individuals from various disciplines and from various levels of the organization (e.g., department head, staff nurse, environmental services member, etc.)

The nurse and nurse manager are also part of a much larger group—the patient care (or nursing) department. As a member of this larger group, it is important to support the overall goals of the patient care department and be a functional valued member of this team. The characteristics of your team will depend on the characteristics of the group (Box 20-1). Teams are real groups in which individuals must work cooperatively with each other to achieve some overarching goal (Sullivan & Decker, 2005, p. 157).

Box 20-1 CHARACTERISTICS OF GROUPS
Norms

Group Size and Characteristics
Roles
Group size and composition
Team building
Status
Group tasks
Team building
Evaluating team performance
Leading committees and task forces

ACTIVE LISTENING

The first rule for dealing with individuals as well as with teams is to be a good listener. As a good listener, you must listen actively. When a person listens actively, the person is completely focused and tuned in to the individual who is speaking. The active listener is nonjudgmental and comprehends the full conversation. See Box 20-2 for guidelines for active listening.

CONDUCTING MEETINGS

Nurse managers are often asked to lead group or team meetings. Many of these meetings may be staff meetings for review of issues of importance to the unit, performance improvement teams, or patient care teams. Some guidelines for leading group meetings follow (Sullivan & Decker, 2005, p. 168):

- Begin and end on time.
- Create a warm, accepting, and nonthreatening climate.
- Arrange seating to minimize differences in power, maximize involvement, and allow visualization of all meeting activities. (A U-shape is optimal.)
- Use interesting and varied visuals and other aids.
- Facilitate thoughtful problem solving.
- Allocate time for all problem-solving steps.
- Promote involvement.
- Facilitate integration of material and ideas.
- Encourage exploration of implications of ideas.

Box 20-2   GUIDELINES FOR ACTIVE LISTENING

1. Slow down your internal processes and seek data. Do not interrupt the speaker.
2. The more information you acquire through listening, the less interpretation you do (making up the missing pieces or motivations). The less information you have, the more interpretation you do.
3. Realize that the first words from the other person are not necessarily representative of inner thoughts and feelings. Be patient.
4. When listening, suspend your own beliefs and views and judgments, at least temporarily. Attempt to understand the perspective of the other person, particularly if it is different from yours.
5. Realize that any judgments or "labels" strongly influence the manner in which you listen to the other person.
6. Appreciate the difference between understanding other people's perspective and agreeing with them. First strive to understand. Then you may agree or disagree.
7. Effective listening is based on an inner desire to learn about another's unique experience of the world.

Modified from Olen, D. (1992). *Communicating speaking and listening to end misunderstanding and promote friendship*. Germantown, WI: JODA Communications.

- Clarify all terms and concepts. Avoid jargon.
- Foster cooperation in the group.
- Establish goals and key objectives.
- Keep the group focused.
- Focus the discussion on one topic at a time.
- Facilitate evaluation of the quality of the discussion.
- Elicit the expression of dissenting opinions.
- Summarize discussion.
- Finalize the plan of action for implementing decisions.
- Arrange for follow-up.

These guidelines can be further adapted to delineate guidelines for leading teams, such as patient care teams:

- Do not waste staff time.
- Create a warm, accepting, and nonthreatening climate.
- Be knowledgeable of all team members' abilities and values.
- Communicate in clear terms that are understood by all members of team.
- Clarify all terms and concepts. Avoid jargon.
- Foster cooperation in the group.
- Establish goals and key objectives for the day.
- Routinely check on performance of group and patient outcomes to determine if changes in plan are needed.
- Facilitate thoughtful problem solving as appropriate.
- Allocate time for all changes in delivery of care.
- Promote involvement of all members.
- Facilitate integration of work and ideas of all team members.
- Assist other team members if needed.
- Evaluate work at end of shift.
- Thank all team members for the work done.
- Assist any members who need improvement.

EFFECTIVE AND INEFFECTIVE TEAMS

Parker (1990) states that a team is a group of people with a high degree of interdependence geared toward the achievement of a goal or a task. Not all teams function well, and there are times when even the most qualified team has a dysfunctional day. If a team has a "bad day," it is important for the team member or leader to evaluate the reasons for the poor performance. If the reasons can be understood, it will be important to alter the way the team works to increase functionality, efficiency, and patient outcomes.

When a team functions effectively, a significant difference is evident in the entire work atmosphere the way in which discussions progress, the level of understanding of the team-specific goals and tasks, the willingness of members to listen, the manner in which disagreements are handled, the use of consensus, and the way in which feedback is given and received (Yoder-Wise, 2003, p. 343).

Table 20-1 ATTRIBUTES OF EFFECTIVE AND INEFFECTIVE TEAMS

Attribute	Effective Team	Ineffective Team
Working environment	Informal, comfortable, relaxed	Indifferent, bored; tense, stiff
Discussion	Focused Shared by almost everyone	Frequently unfocused Dominated by a few
Objectives	Well understood and accepted	Unclear, or many personal agendas
Listening	Respectful—encourages participation	Judgmental—much interruption and "grandstanding"
Ability to handle conflict	Comfortable with disagreement Open discussion of conflicts	Uncomfortable with disagreement Disagreement usually suppressed, or one group aggressively dominates
Decision-making	Usually reached by consensus Formal voting kept to a minimum General agreement is necessary for action; dissenters are free to voice	Often occurs prematurely Formal voting occurs frequently Simple majority is sufficient for action; minority is expected to go along with opinion
Criticism	Frequent, frank, relatively comfortable, constructive Directed toward removing obstacle	Embarrassing and tension-producing; destructive Directed personally at others
Leadership	Shared; shifts from time to time	Autocratic; remains clearly with committee chairperson
Assignments	Clearly stated Accepted by all despite disagreements	Unclear Resented by dissenting members
Feelings	Freely expressed, open for discussion	Hidden, considered "explosive" and inappropriate for discussion
Self-regulation	Frequent and ongoing, focused on solutions	Infrequent, or occurs outside meetings

Modified from McGregor, D. (1960). *The human side of enterprise.* New York: McGraw-Hill.

The original work done by McGregor (1960) shows significant differences between effective and ineffective teams (Table 20-1).

TEAM ASSESSMENT QUESTIONNAIRE

Instructions: Use the scale below to indicate how each statement applies to your team. It is important to evaluate the statements honestly and without overthinking your answers.

3 = Usually
2 = Sometimes
1 = Rarely

_____ 1. Teams are passionate and unguarded in their discussion of issues.

_____ 2. Team members call out one another's deficiencies or unproductive behaviors.

_____ 3. Team members know what their peers are working on and how they contribute to the collective good of the team.

_____ 4. Team members quickly and genuinely apologize to one another when they say or do something inappropriate or possibly damaging to the team.

_____ 5. Team members willingly make sacrifices (such as budget, turf, head count) in their departments or areas of expertise for the good of the team.

_____ 6. Team members openly admit their weaknesses and mistakes.

_____ 7. Team meetings are compelling, not boring.

_____ 8. Team members leave meetings confident that their peers are completely committed to the decisions that were agreed on, even if they were in initial disagreement.

_____ 9. Morale is significantly affected by the failure to achieve team goals.

_____ 10. During team meetings, the most important—and

difficult—issues are put on the table to be resolved.

_____ 11. Team members are deeply concerned about the prospect of letting down their peers.

_____ 12. Team members know about one another's

personal lives and are comfortable discussing them.

_____ 13. Team members end discussions with clear and specific resolutions and action plans.

_____ 14. Team members challenge

one another about their plans and approaches.

_____ 15. Team members are slow to seek credit for their own contributions, but quick to point out those of others.

Scoring

Combine your scores for the preceding statements as indicated below:

Dysfunction 1: Absence of Trust	Dysfunction 2: Fear of Conflict	Dysfunction 3: Lack of Commitment	Dysfunction 4: Avoidance of Accountability	Dysfunction 5: Inattention to Results
Statement 4: ___	Statement 1 : ___	Statement 3: ___	Statement 2: ___	Statement 5: ___
Statement 6: ___	Statement 7: ___	Statement 8: ___	Statement 11: ___	Statement 9: ___
Statement 12: ___	Statement 10: ___	Statement 13: ___	Statement 14: ___	Statement 15: ___
Total: ___	Total: ___	Total: ___	Total: ___	Total: ___

A score of 8 or 9 is a probable indication that the dysfunction is not a problem for your team.
A score of 6 or 7 indicates that the dysfunction could be a problem.
A score of 3 to 5 is probably an indication that the dysfunction needs to be addressed.
Regardless of your scores, it is important to keep in mind that every team needs constant work, because without it, even the best ones deviate toward dysfunction.
(From Lencioni, P. [2002]. The five dysfunctions of a team: a leadership fable. San Francisco: Jossey-Bass. Use with permission.)

POWER AND CONTROL

Whenever there is a team effort, power and control usually come into play. When a person reacts to a situation at the feeling level, there are often blame and judgment calls. People normally would like to believe that their input and contributions are respected and used by the group. For a team to be effective, each member of the group must be able to effectively communicate, offer constructive criticism, and also acknowledge the positive at every chance. (See Guidelines for Acknowledgment in Box 20-3.)

RECOGNIZE AND REWARD SUCCESS

Rewards are listed as one important principle of high performing organizations. The Studer Group (2007) has defined nine principles of high performing organizations. The ninth principle is to:

RECOGNIZE AND REWARD SUCCESS

Everyone makes a difference! Start creating legends in your organization. A legend is an example of those who live the organizational values. By creating legends we establish real-life examples for others to follow. Create win-win-wins for your staff. Never let great work go unnoticed! The first step in creating legend in your organization is to reward team members for a job well done.

QUALITIES OF A TEAM PLAYER

As a student you have learned how to pick out the leader of the group when doing group class assignments. The same holds true in the working environment. The only difference is that the leader is usually called the manager or the team leader.

Maxwell (2002) has identified 17 characteristics that make a good team player:

Box 20-3   GUIDELINES FOR ACKNOWLEDGMENT

1. Acknowledgments must be specific. The specific behavior or action that is appreciated must be identified in the acknowledgment; for example, "Thank you for taking notes for me when I had to go to the dentist. You identified three key points that appeared on the test."
2. Acknowledgments must be "eye to eye."
3. Acknowledgments must be sincere, that is, from the heart. Each of us recognizes insincerity. If you do not truly appreciate a behavior or action, do not say anything. Insincerity often makes people angry or upset, thus defeating the goal.
4. Acknowledgments are more powerful when they are given in public. Most people receive pleasure from public acknowledgment and remember these occasions for a long time. For people who are shy and may prefer no public acknowledgment, this is an opportunity to work on a personal growth issue with them. Public acknowledgment is an opportunity to communicate what is valued.
5. Acknowledgments need to be timely. The less time that elapses between the event and the acknowledgment, the more powerful and effective it is and the more the acknowledgment is appreciated by the recipient.

From Yoder-Wise, P. (2003). *Leading and managing in nursing* (p. 353). St. Louis: Elsevier.

1. Adaptability—Inflexibility does not work in teams. Being rigid in thinking or behavior is destructive to both the individual and to the team.
2. Collaboration—Collaboration is more than cooperation. It means each person brings something to the project that adds value to the team and supports the creation of synergy.
3. Commitment—It is a passion in the face of adversity to take action and make things happen. It is the passion to do whatever it takes to accomplish the team objectives.
4. Communicate—Communication should happen early and often. Frequency of interaction with other team members, talking with them and sharing thoughts, ideas, and experiences—these are the activities that support team-work.
5. Competence—Competence translates as someone who is quite capable, highly qualified, and does the job well.
6. Dependable—Team members who are dependable follow through and do what they have agreed to do well, without prodding or delay.
7. Disciplined—Discipline is doing what you really do not want to do so you can accomplish the goals you really want and includes paying attention to the details in thinking, in emotions, and in the actions they take.
8. Adding value—Helping a teammate advance or grow into a better person or team player; helping teammates advance the team; believing in your

teammates before they believe in themselves are examples of adding value.
9. Enthusiastic—Enthusiasm focuses on becoming a highly energetic team member who has a positive attitude and believes that the team, together, can be better than anyone dreamed they could.
10. Intentional—The team and its members have a purpose for themselves and for the team. Every action counts and is meaningful. Focusing on doing the right things in each moment and following through with these actions to their logical conclusion.
11. Awareness of the mission—Each team member has a sense of purpose and mission that drives all thoughts, ideas, and actions to do what is best for their team and their cause.
12. Prepared—Being prepared translates as preparation for every meeting and event and begins with a thorough assessment of what is needed, aligning the appropriate work with the appropriate effort, addressing the mental aspects of the right attitude, and being ready to take action.
13. Relationship-oriented—The ability to be connected to other members of the team, to be in a relationship with them is the core of being relationship-oriented. These relationships and the mutual respect upon which they are built create cohesiveness on the team.
14. Improve yourself—As a team member, you strive to continually grow and reflect, both routinely

and periodically, on how well each venture of assignment went and what you could have done better. This is a process of self-reflection.

15. Selflessness—Put others on the team ahead of yourself by being generous to team members, avoid "playing politics," show loyalty toward team members, and value interdependence among team members over the American value of being independent are all examples of selflessness.

16. Solution-Focused—Do not be consumed with all of the problems associated with the endeavor; rather, focus on finding the solutions; think about what is possible.

17. Tenacious—Being tenacious means giving your all, with determination, and refusing to stop until the goal has been accomplished.

INTERDISCIPLINARY TEAMS

Highly functional interdisciplinary teams are essential in today's health care system. The following are some of the different team members who work with nurses: physicians, dieticians, case managers, social workers, teachers, respiratory therapists, physical therapists, occupational therapists, psychologists, and pharmacists. The composition from varied disciplines oft times creates a more challenging team function in that everyone is attempting to protect their own "turf" and assume power. In the early stages of these groups, there may be some turf wars until the team forms a single identity.

Durskat and Wolf (2001) believe that three major components of smoothly functioning teams must be created:

- Mutual trust among the members
- A strong sense of team identity (that the team is unique and worthwhile)
- A sense of team efficacy (that the team performs well and its members are synergistic in their manner of working together)

An example of a highly functional team is the pre-admission evaluation committee that is charged with the complete evaluation of a child who has been referred by his physician in an acute care facility. The team members consist of physicians, nurses, psychologists, nurse practitioners, and pharmacists. The first process that takes place is the referral from an acute care facility. In the next step, the admission nurse makes a site visit to the acute care facility, evaluates the chart,

and interviews the primary care nurse, the primary physician, and the social worker to obtain critical health information. Parents with children being admitted to Children's Specialized Hospital in Westfield, NJ, are encouraged to see firsthand what happens when a child enters the rehabilitation facility. Again, questions are answered and parents' questions and fears are addressed. The finance department has had close contact with the social worker of the facility to obtain permission to admit from the insurance company. An admission application (Fig. 20-1) is then completed and the evaluation committee interdisciplinary team meets weekly to discuss the patients who have been referred. Specific goals of admission are noted, as well as a review of systems, the event that caused the acute care hospital admission, the family status, Division of Youth and Family Services evaluation if necessary, the medication and diet, and any treatments that are being provided. The admission criteria have been clearly established, and the team evaluates whether the child is a rehabilitation candidate. Once the decision has been made by the team to accept the child and the parents are in agreement to transfer the child, the next process of evaluation is seeking an appropriate bed for the child.

SUPERVISING THE WORK OF OTHERS

Nurses continuously supervise the work of others. This may include the nursing assistant, licensed practical nurse/licensed vocational nurse (LPN/LVN), other registered nurses, patient care technicians, and the unit clerk. The facilities' organizational chart clearly delineates the positions and links. For a discussion of the delegation of care to members of the health care team, see Chapter 3.

As a supervisor of care, nurse managers are expected to:

- Actively provide suitable working conditions, including adequate staffing, equipment, and supplies
- Understand the needs of assigned clients and which agency resources are required to meet them
- Orient, teach, and guide coworkers according to their individual learning styles and needs, consistent with their backgrounds, experience, and assignments
- Stimulate desire for self-improvement in supervisees

PATIENT INTAKE INFORMATION
Name: Last_____ First_____
Patient's Address   Street_____City_____
State_____ Zip Code_____ Home Phone_____
Date of Birth_____
Father's Name_____ Occupation_____
Address_____ Home Phone_____
Employer_____ Business Phone_____
Employer's Address_____
Mother's Name_____ Occupation _____
Mother's Address_____ Home Phone_____
Mother's Employer_____ Business Phone_____
Employer's Address_____ Cell Phone_____
Siblings' Ages and Sex_____
Primary Language_____
Facility Patient Being Transferred From_____
Please List All Physicians_____
Please List All Agencies (e.g., The Division of Youth and Family Services)_____
_____
Please List All Insurances_____

PAST HISTORY
School Attending_____
Grade_____
List All Pre-illness Special Education Requirements_____
Allergies_____
Past History
Birth (C-section, Normal Delivery, Apgar's, Birth Weight)_____
List All:
Medical Diagnoses_____
Surgeries_____

PRESENT ILLNESS
Diagnosis_____
Date of Illness/Injury_____
Weight on Admission, Present Weight_____
Vital Signs and Pulse Oximetry_____
Cognitive Level_____
Developmental Level_____
Rancho Los Amigos Scale Level_____
List All Lab and Procedure Results Including:
CBC, SMA, Drug Levels, X-rays, MRIs, Hearing Screenings, Swallow Studies_____
_____
DIET: Exact Physician's Order (GT Feeds, etc.)_____

MEDICATIONS
Exact Physician's Medication Orders_____
Allergies to Medications_____
Latex Allergy_____
Other Allergies_____
Weight upon Admission_____
Weight Today_____
Patient Care Conference Notes_____
Patient/Family Expectations of Admission to Rehab Facility_____
Family Living Arrangements During This Hospitalization_____

Figure 20-1 • Sample application from Morristown Memorial Hospital.

FALL RISK ASSESSMENT:
PREVIOUS FACILITY_____
REHAB FACILITY_____

The following information must be received one day prior to admission:

1. Transfer summary/discharge summary
2. Copy of medical progress notes and consultation notes
3. Operative notes
4. Laboratory reports and all special tests such as EEG, EKG, Genetics, Endocrine, etc.
5. Copies of pertinent X-rays, CAT scans
6. All medications and treatments
7. Latest social service assessment
8. Immunization record.

A PARENT OR LEGAL GUARDIAN MUST BE PRESENT AT TIME OF ADMISSION

Behavior Assessment
Psychosocial:
1   Any history of behavior problems at home or school?
2   History of previous neuropsych/psych testing or treatment?
3   Prior TBI?
4   Family History?
5   DYFS/Legal History
6   Current behavior at acute care

ENTRY INTO CARE

A   MEDICAL CONDITIONS
1   Failure to thrive
2   Developmental delayed/assessment and interventions
3   Feeding disorders
4   Chronic illnesses poorly controlled
5   Catastrophic injuries that may cause changes in physical, developmental, and cognitive functioning
6   Acquired illnesses that may cause changes in physical, developmental, and cognitive functioning
7   Developmental disabilities suspected or newly diagnosed that have the potential to cause long-term deficits and problems in functioning
8   Chronic developmental disabilities that are causing long-term deficits and problems in functioning
9   Prematurity with residual impairments
10   Technology-dependent children
11   Surgeries requiring postoperative rehabilitative care
12   Medical problems requiring subacute medical care

B   REHABILITATIVE SERVICES NEEDED
1   Requires extended delivery of integrated interventions including nursing and intensive therapy program
2   Requires in-depth and/or longitudinal interdisciplinary developmental assessment
3   Requires continued nutritional assessment and/or intervention
4   Requires adaptive and/or augmentative equipment for positioning, ADL, or communication
5   Requires cognitive rehabilitation including computer-assisted therapy to facilitate recovery
6   Intensive inpatient rehabilitation services will expedite recovery and/or improvement of function

Figure 20-1 ● cont'd.

C   PSYCHOSOCIAL CONDITIONS/INTERVENTION
Children having any medical problem with attendant psychosocial
Conditions such that adequate care cannot be delivered in the home

PSYCHOSOCIAL INTERVENTION
1   Requires intensive teaching of diet, medications, or other self care
2   Requires intensive behavior modification program to cope appropriately with medical problem
3   Requires medical or therapeutic care in a protective environment
4   At risk at home due to family inability to provide necessary medical care
5   Requires longer-term interagency networking for provision of support services and other programs

FAMILY
1   Requires further family and environmental evaluation
2   Requires extended counseling and/or teaching
3   Requires extended counseling and/or teaching

D   READINESS FOR TRANSFER TO REHAB FACILITY
1   Initial diagnostic procedures completed
2   Necessary surgical procedures completed
3   Regimen of medication stabilized though may still need adjustments
4   Fluid and electrolyte balance stabilized though may still need monitoring
5   Life support services (such as respiratory, parenteral nutrition) stabilized
6   Required direct care by nurses several times daily
7   Requires daily, but not constant, monitoring by and accessibility of physician
8   May require immediate access to physician
9   Requires 3 hours rehab
10   Discharge disposition has been clearly identified

Figure 20-1 • cont'd.

- Encourage supervisees to use unique talents and develop special skills
- Model desired attitudes, skills, interests, and work habits

TYPES OF CONVERSATIONS

In the evaluation of team members, some organizations are defining team members as high-medium-low (H-M-L) performers. Basically, high performers are people who bring solutions. Middle performers can identify the problem but may lack the experience or self-confidence to bring solutions. Low performers tend to blame others for the problem. They act like renters instead of owners. Studer (2007) suggests that leaders rate themselves. The best leaders are always willing to perform an honest self-assessment. Are you a high, middle, or low performer? What actions will you take as a result?

Often, leaders using this exercise to rank their employees ask, "What if I have an employee who is technically excellent, but nobody wants to work with him or her?" To qualify as a high performer, an individual must be excellent both technically and as a team member. In fact, Studer (2007) even suggests to terminate employees who get results but do not role model the organization's standards of behavior, because they are so damaging to overall employee morale.

According to Studer (2007), after the ranking of an employee as an H-M-L performer, use an employee tracking log to track the name, rating (H-M-L), initial meeting date, and follow-up date/comments. Always begin by holding meetings with high performers first, middle performers next, and low performers last. Ordering the meetings in this way accomplishes a few things. High performers, for example, can dispel fear about the meetings when other employees ask why the boss wanted to meet with them. Perhaps most important, leaders report that they feel energized and fortified for those difficult low-performer conversations once they have enjoyed so many positive conversations with employees they value.

H-M-L conversations are not evaluations tied to pay, so they should not take place at evaluation time. However, by repeating these meetings twice a year, conversations can complement staff evaluations so employees get the more frequent feedback they seek from managers. Leaders can help employees—especially middle performers—understand that these 15-minute meetings are opportunities for recognition, coaching, and professional development.

The objectives and outcomes are distinct for each type of conversation.

High-performer conversations. Re-recruit the best performers by giving specific positive feedback about what they do well, their accomplishments, and examples of positive attitude. Share information about where the organization is going, and ask if there is anything you can do for them to make their job better.

Middle-performer conversations. Use a support coach technique. The overall tone of the meeting must be positive. Begin by reassuring these individuals that you value their contributions and that your goal is to retain them as valuable employees. Thank them for what they do well. Then identify and discuss one specific area for development—something you would like them to improve. Complete the conversation by reaffirming their good qualities and expressing your appreciation.

Low-performer conversations. Do not start the meeting out on a positive note. Use the DESK approach:

- **D**escribe what has been observed.
- **E**valuate how you feel.
- **S**how what needs to be done.
- **E**nsure that employees **K**now the consequences of the continued poor performance.

Because low performers are so skilled at excuses, guilt, and indignation, these conversations can be difficult for managers. The manager needs to remain calm, objective, and clear about consequences if performance does not improve by a specified date. If the behavior has not improved, the nurse manager needs to follow through and take action.

See Table 20-2 for a differentiating staff worksheet.

Table 20-2	DIFFERENTIATING STAFF WORKSHEET		
	High	**Medium**	**Low**
Definition	Comes to work on time Good attitude Problem solves You relax when you know they are scheduled Good influence Use for peer interviews Five pillar ownership Brings solutions	Good attendance Loyal most of the time Influenced by high and low performers Want to do a good job Could just need more experience Helps manager be aware of problems	Points out problems in a negative way Positions leadership poorly Master of we/they Passive aggressive Thinks they will outlast the leader Says manager is the problem
Professionalism	Adheres to unit policies concerning breaks, personal phone calls, leaving the work area, and other absences from work.	Usually adheres to unit policies concerning breaks, personal phone calls, leaving the work area, and other absences from work.	Does not communicate effectively about absences from work areas. Handles personal phone calls in a manner that interferes with work. Breaks last longer than allowed.

Continued

Table 20-2   DIFFERENTIATING STAFF WORKSHEET—cont'd

	High	Medium	Low
Teamwork	Demonstrates high commitment to making things better for the work unit and organization as a whole.	Committed to improving performance of the work unit and organization. May require coaching to fully execute.	Demonstrates little commitment to the work unit and the organization.
Knowledge and competence	Eager to change for the good of the organization. Strives for continuous professional development.	Invested in own professional development. May require some coaching to fully execute.	Shows little interest in improving own performance or the performance of the organization. Develops professional skills only when asked.
Communication	Comes to work with a positive attitude.	Usually comes to work with a positive attitude. Occasionally gets caught up in the negative attitude of others.	Comes to work with a negative attitude. Has a negative influence on the work environment.
Safety awareness	Demonstrates the behaviors of safety awareness in all aspects of work.	Demonstrates the behaviors of safety awareness in most aspects of work.	Performs work with little regard to the behaviors of safety awareness.

From The Studer Group. (2007). *The nine principles.* Retrieved November 9, 2007, from http://www.studergroup.com/dotCMS/knowledgeAssetDetail? inode=217849.

GUIDELINES FOR OVERALL PERFORMANCE RATING

Peer review is used in many health care institutions. In a peer review evaluation, clinical performance is measured and assessed by peers. It is central to the drive for excellence and is part of a process to improve care. Nurses in many hospitals use peer review to strengthen the profession of nursing and to guide professional development.

Formal performance evaluations occur on an annual basis for most employees. These are most often done at a predetermined time based on the human resource policies of the institution. The formal evaluation is part of the employee record and is usually a competency-based assessment of the performance of the employee during the past year. In many institutions, the competencies are related to the overall mission, vision, and goals of the organization. The evaluation forms the basis for the retention/promotion of the individual as well as the compensation adjustment. It also provides information that assists in the development of the employee's goals and objectives for the upcoming evaluation period.

Box 20-4 provides guidelines for overall performance rating.

A sample evaluation for a beginning nurse and a peer evaluation process is shown in Box 20-5.

SUMMARY

The culture of a hospital and a unit is clearly delineated once you work on a specific unit for a period of time. Positive attitudes foster positive attitudes; negative work habits foster negative work habits. The nurse manager is charged with creating an environment conducive to high-quality patient care and staff satisfaction. The interactions within the team environment set the tone. Supervision and evaluation are part of a process of continuous improvement and staff development.

Box 20-4   GUIDELINES FOR OVERALL PERFORMANCE RATING
University of Michigan Health System

Important Points

- There should be no surprises at evaluation time that influence an employee's overall rating.
  Overall principle is preponderance
  At applicable to level of nurse
- Developmental tool to initiate discussion in regard to level movement.
- **Any rating other than "meets behavioral expectations" requires rationale.**

Scale	Guidelines
Behavioral Expectations Not Met/NA	• This category is used when employees have consistently not met their job expectations over the course of the last year. • It would be expected that you would have already documented and counseled the employee on the issues that led to this overall rating.

Approaching Behavioral Expectations	• This category can be used for two purposes. One is to indicate performance issues that need attention, the other is to indicate performance for a new hire or someone at a new level who has not been in the position long enough to fully evaluate performance.
	• For staff that are new to UMHHC or their roles:
	    Employment or transfer of less than 4-6 months (or whatever timeframe is appropriate for you to evaluate performance)
	    Still mastering new skills and responsibilities
	    You expect the employee will be able to meet expectations next year
	• For staff whose performance is less than meeting expectations:
	    Inconsistent demonstration of framework behaviors for applicable level
	    Needs to demonstrate growth and improvement in order to meet behaviors
	    Specific action plan should be developed to improve performance that includes measurable goals and expected outcomes

Meets Behavioral Expectations	• This category is used when the employee is meeting behavioral expectations, is effective, and provides value for the organization.
	    Work is thorough and accurate; is accountable for own outcomes
	    Contributes to the goals of the organization and the unit
	    Exhibits professional demeanor
	    Demonstrates commitment to meeting level expectations

Exceeds Behavioral Expectations	• This category is used when the employee regularly meets expectations plus:
	    Demonstrates excellence and exceeds expectations consistently; goes above and beyond
	    Continuously increases the quality and/or quantity of contribution
	    Demonstrates self-awareness related to performance

Box 20-5   UNIVERSITY OF MICHIGAN HEALTH SYSTEM
Performance Evaluation Process—Self-evaluation With Peer Input

1. The nurse will select a minimum of three peers to perform peer review.
   - Those selected must be educated in the peer review process.
   - At least one peer must be an RN.
   - Each nurse will be asked to evaluate the person on one or two different Framework domains, so that all five Framework domains are reviewed by peers. Clinical Skills and Knowledge domain must be completed by an RN whenever possible.

2. The nurse will submit the names of their chosen peers to the manager that will be completing their performance evaluation. The nurse distributes one or two domains of the peer feedback tool to selected peers.

3. The reviewers will use the current Development Framework Peer Input tool for their appraisal. They will complete their peer tool, sign it and **return it to the nurse** within 7 days.
   - Peers should circle the appropriate behavioral level. Peer reviewers would be encouraged to

Continued

Box 20-5   UNIVERSITY OF MICHIGAN HEALTH SYSTEM—cont'd

support their views with concrete examples on the right hand side of the page.

- Each peer will comment on one or two different Framework domains.

4. The peer review forms are **returned to the nurse**, who shall review the content and summarizes the information on the performance review form.

   The nurse will complete the level appropriate self-evaluation portion of the staff.

5. Performance Planning and Evaluation form, with consideration of the input provided by the peer evaluation.

6. The nurse will submit their completed Staff Performance Planning and Evaluation form and their Peer Review forms to the manager. If materials are not submitted within 2 weeks of the established due date, then the managers may proceed with completing the evaluation process. The manager will review the peer review form, peer summary, and self-evaluation and then complete the manager section of the evaluation form.

- The manager will utilize peer and self-evaluations as well as own knowledge of employee performance in determining ratings on the Performance Planning and Evaluation form.

- **Rationale for rating other than "meets expectations," must be provided in the evaluation summary section after each domain.**

- The manager will arrange an appointment with the nurse for the performance review.

7. The Peer Review forms will be returned to the nurse following the performance evaluation process, and a copy of the completed Performance Plan/Evaluation will be given to the nurse.

8. Completed evaluations are given to the administrative assistant for processing.

   Final 4/16/04 Perry

   Revised 7/15/05, 9/15/06 Jordan-Sedgeman, Minerath

   Revised 3/13/07 Professional Development Framework Performance Evaluation Workgroup

(From University of Michigan Health System. Performance evaluation process—self-evaluation with peer input. Used with permission.)

CLINICAL CORNER

Magnet Award Recognition: It's All About Staff RNs: Site Survey Preparation—Evaluating Yourselves, Your Practice, and Your Magnetism!

Maryann Hozak

Magnet appraisers conduct an on-site survey to verify that the written application of approximately 3000 pages of narratives, meeting minutes, committee membership lists and policies is "alive and well" in the applying organization. This is accomplished by meeting with the nurses and the leadership teams with the goal of hearing from them directly the information they read about in the document. Particularly, the appraisers look to see that the communication between the staff nurses and the chief nursing officer is a "two-way street." Both need to hear what the other is saying, have opportunity to ask questions and, most importantly, have opportunity to voice opinions and suggestions. Shared decision-making or Shared Governance fosters this "two-way street" approach to problem solving for issues in professional practice, healthy work environments, and positive patient outcomes. Such shared decision making also requires continual self-evaluation by each staff nurse related to individual practice, and evaluation of the practice on the unit.

In preparing for our redesignation survey, we held six-hour staff fairs off site with each fair divided into 4 sessions. Sitting at tables as teams and armed with posters and markers, nurses from all departments were asked to take 30 minutes and write down everything they could think of to tell a Magnet appraiser about a particular subject with each table having a different topic.

At the end of the 30 minutes, a spokesperson from each table then taped the poster to the wall and shared with everyone their list of ideas and examples of how St. Joseph nurses not only meet but exceed Magnet standards. The whole group then had opportunity to add to the list or reminisce about personal encounters related to the topic. By the end of the day and four sessions later, the staff had discussed 20 topics related to the Magnet application and survey. They didn't learn anything new—they simply held up a mirror to see themselves as the Magnet nurses they have grown to be. These nurses were now excited to sit with the appraisers to demonstrate how they meet Magnet standards.

CLINICAL CORNER—cont'd

Magnet Topics: Global Organizational Subjects Within the 14 Forces of Magnetism

	Team # 1	Team # 2	Team # 3	Team # 4	Team # 5
Session # 1	Role of the CNO	Budgets	Shared Governance	Nursing Care Delivery System & Watson's Caring Theory	Staffing Patterns
Session # 2	Interdisciplinary Collaboration	Experts & Resources	Peer Review & Performance Appraisals	PI Process	Patient and RN Satisfaction Surveys & Scores
Session # 3	Ethics & Confidentiality	Staff Education	Standards of Nursing Practice	Information Systems	Patient & Family Education
Session # 4	Healthy Work Environment	Cultural Care	Evidenced-based Practice & Research	Recruitment & Retention	Communication

EVIDENCE-BASED PRACTICE

Stress as Related to Team Citizenship

Haslam, S. A., Jetten, J., & Waghorn, C. (2009). Social identification, stress and citizenship in teams: a five phase longitudinal study. Stress and Health 25, 21–30.

Social identity theory argues that when individuals identify themselves in terms of social identity (on the basis of relevant group membership), they see their goals and actions to be similar with those of other group members and they attempt to advance the outcomes of the group. A large body of research has demonstrated that organizational identification is a predictor of key organizational outcomes—and that organizational identification is a basis for organizational citizenship, in which a person performs at a level that is essential for the success of the organization.

In a longitudinal study of theatre production teams (from audition to post performance), the authors found:

- That identification with the team at the onset predicted positive perceptions and attitudes at the completion of the team's work.
- High identifiers were willing to demonstrate organizational citizenship, had greater work satisfaction, and more pride in their work than those scoring lower in social identification.
- Compared with low identifiers, high social identifiers were less likely to experience burnout during the most demanding phases of the performance.
- Social identification may not only motivate individuals to work toward unit success, but may protect them from the stressors that are present in the work environment.

These findings suggest that social identification with the group played a role in protecting individuals from burnout in demanding work periods.

While this study dealt with individuals in the theatre business, the implications for nursing are clear.

NCLEX® EXAM QUESTIONS

1. A group consists of individuals who interact and influence each other. Groups exist in organizations. Group members usually do not include:
   1. individuals from a single work group
   2. individuals from different job levels
   3. individuals from the same job levels
   4. individuals from a different facility
2. Which of the following guidelines for leading group meetings is NOT an issue?
   1. Beginning on time
   2. Keeping the group focused

Continued

3. Focusing on one topic at a time
4. Having no need to end on time

3. Which of the following is NOT an attribute of an effective team?
   1. Informal
   2. Focused
   3. Understood
   4. Unrelaxed

4. Which of the following is NOT an attribute of an ineffective team?
   1. Bored
   2. Unfocused
   3. Judgmental
   4. Productive

5. Which of the following is NOT a characteristics of a good team player?
   1. Commitment
   2. Collaboration
   3. Adaptability
   4. Affordability

6. Patients should expect _____ during their hospital stay.
   1. high-quality hospital care
   2. a private room
   3. to choose their roommate
   4. none of the above

7. In an effort to prepare the patient and his or her family for when he or she leaves the hospital, discharge planning should start:

1. upon admission to facility
2. when the physician writes the discharge order
3. the day before discharge
4. the day of discharge

8. Nursing's role in patient rights includes:
   1. ensuring that patients participate in decisions regarding their health care
   2. ensuring that only families participate in health care decisions
   3. obtaining surgical consent in the absence of the surgeon
   4. obtaining advance directives in the absence of family member

9. Which of the following is NOT a guideline for active listening?
   1. Slow down your internal processes and seek data.
   2. Do not interrupt the speaker.
   3. Realize that the first words from the other person do not necessarily represent inner thoughts and feelings. Be patient.
   4. Never suspend your own beliefs, views, and judgments.

10. _____ is NOT a characteristic of a good team player.
    1. Adaptability
    2. Collaboration
    3. Commitment
    4. Change

Answers: 1. 4   2. 4   3. 4   4. 4   5. 4   6. 1   7. 1   8. 1   9. 4   10. 4

REFERENCES

Durskat, V., & Wolf, S. (2001). Building the emotional intelligence of groups. *Harvard Business Review, 79*, 81-91.

Lencioni, P. (2002). *The Five Dysfunctions of a Team: A Leadership Fable.* San Francisco: Jossey-Bass.

Maxwell, J. (2002). *The 17 essential qualities of a team player.* Nashville, TN: Thomas Nelson Publishers.

McGregor, D. (1960). *The Human Side of Enterprise.* New York: McGraw-Hill.

Parker, G. M. (1990). *Team players and teamwork.* San Francisco: Jossey-Bass.

Sullivan, E. J. & Decker, P. J. (2005). *Effective leadership and management in nursing* (6th ed.). Upper Saddle River, NJ: Pearson Prentice Hall.

The Studer Group. (2007). *The nine principles.* Retrieved November 9, 2007, from http://www.studergroup.com/dotCMS/knowledgeAssetDetail?inode=217849.

University of Michigan Health System. (2008). Performance evaluation process. Retrieved November 18, 2008, from www.med.umich.edu/nursing/jit/docs/forms/Performance%20Evaluation%20Instructions.doc.

Yoder-Wise, P. (2003). *Leading and managing in nursing.* St. Louis: Elsevier.

Congratulations

To those readers who are students, this chapter is about progression after graduation. First ... Congratulations! It is not yet time to relax, however. There is much work to be done on entry to the new role of a professional nurse. This chapter will review the process for registering and taking the licensure exam, the means to continue professional growth and continuation of your nursing education.

CHAPTER 21

New Graduates: The Immediate Future

Chapter Objectives

1. Review the process for registering for the licensing exam.
2. Identify states participating in Nurse Compact licensure.
3. Elaborate on the decision making surrounding selection of the first job.
4. Identify specialty organizations in nursing.
5. Review the types of certification exams available to the nurse.
6. Discuss the importance of continued education in nursing.

Definitions

NCLEX National Council Licensing Exam
NCSBON National Council of State Boards of Nursing
ANCC American Nurses Credentialing Center
Pearson Vue Company under contract with NCSBON to administer NCLEX examination

Nursing Licensure Compact States recognizing the license regulation of other states
Specialty certification Exam credential specifying the candidate's knowledge level within a specialty

PREPARING FOR LICENSURE EXAM

Entry into the practice of nursing in the United States and its territories is regulated by the licensing authorities within each jurisdiction. To ensure public protection, each jurisdiction requires a candidate for licensure to pass an examination that measures the competencies needed to perform safely and effectively as a newly licensed, entry-level registered nurse. The National Council of State Boards of Nursing (NCSBN) develops two licensure examinations—the National Council Licensure Examination for Registered Nurses and the National Council Licensure Examination for Practical Nurses—that are used by state and territorial boards of nursing to assist in making licensure decisions.

The new nurse needs to decide where he or she wishes to be licensed. Most graduates take the exam in the state where they intend to work. They first contact the state board of nursing in the state where they intend to work; Table 21-1 lists the addresses of the various state boards of nursing.

While many states require practicing nurses to take the exam in that state or to apply through the state board for reciprocity, the Nurse Licensure Compact of the National Council of State Boards of Nursing (NCSBON) is moving toward mutual recognition of licensure by the states. Not all state boards have enacted

Table 21-1   STATE BOARDS OF NURSING

State Boards of Nursing

Alabama Board of Nursing 770 Washington Ave. RSA Plaza, Suite 250 Montgomery, AL 36130-3900 Phone: (334) 242-4060 Fax: (334) 242-4360 http://www.abn.state.al.us/	Illinois Department of Professional Regulation James R. Thompson Center 100 West Randolph, Suite 9-300 Chicago, IL 60601 Phone: (312) 814-2715 Fax: (312) 814-3145 http://www.idfpr.com/dpr/WHO/nurs.asp	Montana State Board of Nursing PO Box 200513 Helena, MT 59620-0513 Phone: (406) 841-2345 Fax: (406) 841-2305 http://mt.gov/dli/nur/	Rhode Island Board of Nursing Registration and Nursing Education 105 Cannon Building Three Capitol Hill Providence, RI 02908 Phone: (401) 222-5700 Fax: (401) 222-3352 http://www.health.state.ri.us/hsr/professions/nurses.php
Alaska Board of Nursing Dept. of Comm. & Econ. Development Division of Occupational Licensing 3601 C St., Suite 722 Anchorage, AK 99503 Phone: (907) 269-8161 Fax: (907) 269-8196 http://www.dced.state.ak.us/occ/pnur.htm	Indiana State Board of Nursing Health Professions Bureau 402 W. Washington St., Room W401 Indianapolis, IN 46204 Phone: (317) 232-2960 Fax: (317) 233-4236 http://www.in.gov/pla/express/index.html	Nebraska Health and Human Services System Dept. of Regulation & Licensure, Nursing Section 301 Centennial Mall South Lincoln, NE 68509-4986 Phone: (402) 471-4376 Fax: (402) 471-3577 http://www.hhs.state.ne.us/crl/nursing/Rn-Lpn/rn-lpn.htm	South Carolina State Board of Nursing 110 Centerview Dr. Suite 202 Columbia, SC 29210 Phone: (803) 896-4550 Fax: (803) 896-4525 http://www.llr.state.sc.us/POL/NURSING/
Arizona State Board of Nursing 4747 N. 7th St. Suite 200 Phoenix, AZ 85014 Phone: (602) 889-5150 Fax: (602) 889-5155 http://www.azbn.gov/	Iowa Board of Nursing River Point Business Park 400 S.W. 8th St. Suite B Des Moines, IA 50309-4685 Phone: (515) 281-3255 Fax: (515) 281-4825 http://www.iowa.gov/nursing/	Nevada State Board of Nursing License Certification and Education 4330 S. Valley View Blvd. Suite 106 Las Vegas, NV 89103 Phone: (702) 486-5800 Fax: (702) 486-5803 http://www.nursingboard.state.nv.us/	South Dakota Board of Nursing 4300 South Louise Ave., Suite C-1 Sioux Falls, SD 57106-3124 Phone: (605) 362-2760 Fax: (605) 362-2768 http://doh.sd.gov/boards/nursing/
Arkansas State Board of Nursing University Tower Building 1123 S. University, Suite 800 Little Rock, AR 72204-1619 Phone: (501) 686-2700 Fax: (501) 686-2714 http://www.state.ar.us/nurse/	Kansas State Board of Nursing Landon State Office Bldg. 900 SW Jackson, Suite 551 S. Topeka, KS 66612-1230 Phone: (785) 296-4929 Fax: (785) 296-3929 http://www.ksbn.org/	New Hampshire Board of Nursing PO Box 3898 78 Regional Dr., Bldg. B Concord, NH 03302 Phone: (603) 271-2323 Fax: (603) 271-6605 http://www.nh.gov/nursing/	Tennessee State Board of Nursing 426 Fifth Ave. North 1st Floor-Cordell Hull Bldg. Nashville, TN 37247 Phone: (615) 532-5166 Fax: (615) 741-7899 http://health.state.tn.us/Boards/Nursing/

Table 21-1   STATE BOARDS OF NURSING—cont'd

State Boards of Nursing

California Board of Registered Nursing 400 R St., Suite 4030 PO Box 944210 Sacramento, CA 95814 Phone: (916) 322-3350 Fax: (916) 327-4402 http://www.rn.ca.gov	Kentucky Board of Nursing 312 Whittington Pkwy., Suite 300 Louisville, KY 40222 Phone: (502) 329-7000 Fax: (502) 329-7011 http://kbn.ky.gov/	New Jersey Board of Nursing PO Box 45010 124 Halsey St., 6th Floor Newark, NJ 07101 Phone: (973) 504-6586 Fax: (973) 648-3481 http://www.state.nj.us/oag/ca/medical/nursing.htm	Texas Board of Nurse Examiners 333 Guadalupe, Suite 3-460 Austin, TX 78701 Phone: (512) 305-7400 Fax: (512) 305-7401 http://www.bon.state.tx.us/
Colorado Board of Nursing 1560 Broadway, Suite 880 Denver, CO 80202 Phone: (303) 894-2430 Fax: (303) 894-2821 http://www.dora.state.co.us/nursing	Louisiana State Board of Nursing 17373 Perkins Rd. Baton Rouge, LA 70810 Phone: (225) 755-7500 Fax: (225) 755-7584 http://www.lsbn.state.la.us/	New Mexico Board of Nursing 6301 Indian School Rd. NE Suite 710 Albuquerque, NM 87110 Phone: (505) 841-8340 Fax (505) 841-8347 http://www.bon.state.nm.us/	Utah State Board of Nursing Heber M. Wells Bldg., 4th Floor 160 East 300 South Salt Lake City, UT 84111 Phone: (801) 530-6628 Fax: (801) 530-6511 http://www.dopl.utah.gov/licensing/nursing.html
Connecticut Board of Examiners for Nursing Dept. of Public Health 410 Capitol Ave., MS# 13PHO PO Box 340308 Hartford, CT 06134-0328 Phone: (860) 509-7624 Fax: (860) 509-7553 http://www.ct.gov/dph/cwp/view.asp?a=3143&q=388910	Maine State Board of Nursing 158 State House Station Augusta, ME 04333 Phone: (207) 287-1133 Fax: (207) 287-1149 http://www.maine.gov/boardofnursing/	New York State Board of Nursing Education Bldg. 89 Washington Ave. 2nd Floor West Wing Albany, NY 12234 Phone: (518) 474-3817 Ext. 120 Fax: (518) 474-3706 http://www.ncbon.com/	Vermont State Board of Nursing 109 State St. Montpelier, VT 05609-1106 Phone: (802) 828-2484 Fax: (802) 828-2484 http://www.professionals.org/opr1/nurses/
Delaware Board of Nursing 861 Silver Lake Blvd. Cannon Building, Suite 203 Dover, DE 19904 Phone: (302) 739-4522 Fax: (302) 739-2711 http://dpr.delaware.gov/boards/nursing/reciprocity.shtml	Maryland Board of Nursing 4140 Patterson Ave. Baltimore, MD 21215 Phone: (410) 585-1900 Fax: (410) 358-3530 http://www.mbon.org/main.php	North Carolina Board of Nursing 3724 National Dr., Suite 201 Raleigh, NC 27612 Phone: (919) 782-3211 Fax: (919) 781-9461 http:/www.ncbon.com/	Virginia Board of Nursing Perimeter Center 9960 Maryland Dr., Suite 300 Richmond, VA 23233-1463 Phone: (804) 367-4515 Fax: (804) 527-4455 http://www.dhp.virginia.gov/nursing/

Continued

Table 21-1 STATE BOARDS OF NURSING—cont'd

State Boards of Nursing

District of Columbia
  Board of Nursing
Department of Health
717 14th St., NW
Suite 600
Washington, DC 20005
Phone: 1-877-672-2174
Fax: (202) 727-8471
E-mail: hpla.doh@dc.
  gov

Massachusetts Nursing State
  Board
Commonwealth of
  Massachusetts
239 Causeway St.
Boston, MA 02114
Phone: (617) 973-0800
Fax: (617) 727-1630
http://www.mass.gov/?pageID=
  eohhs2subtopic&L=5&L0=H
  ome&L1=Provider&L2=Certi
  fication%2c+Licensure%2c+
  and+Registration&L3=Occu
  pational+and+Professional
  &L4=Nursing&sid=Eeohhs2

North Dakota Board of
  Nursing
919 South 7th St., Suite
  504
Bismark, ND 58504
Phone: (701) 328-9777
Fax: (701) 328-9785
http://www.ndbon.org/

Washington State
  Nursing Care Quality
  Assurance
  Commission
Department of Health
1300 Quince St. SE
Olympia, WA
  98504-7864
Phone: (360) 236-4740
Fax: (360) 236-4738
http://www.doh.wa.gov/
  hsqa/Professions/
  Nursing/default.htm

Florida Board of Nursing
4052 Bald Cypress Way,
  Bin # A07
Tallahassee, FL
  32399-1708
Phone: (850)245-4244
http://www.doh.state.fl.
  us/mqa/nursing/
  nur_home.html

Michigan CIS/Office of Health
  Services
Ottawa Towers North
611 W. Ottawa, 4th Floor
Lansing, MI 48933
Phone: (517) 373-9102
Fax: (517) 373-2179
http://michigan.gov/
  mdch/0.1607,7-132-27417_
  27529_27542---,00.html

Ohio Board of Nursing
17 South High St., Suite
  400
Columbus, OH
  43215-3413
Phone: (614) 466-3947
Fax: (614) 466-0388
http://www.nursing.ohio.
  gov/

West Virginia Board of
  Examiners for
  Registered
  Professional Nurses
101 Dee Dr.
Charleston, WV 25311
Phone: (304) 558-3596
Fax: (304) 558-3666
http://www.wvrnboard.
  com/

Georgia Board of
  Nursing
237 Coliseum Dr.
Macon, GA 31217-3858
Phone: (478) 207-1640
Fax: (478) 207-1660
http://www.sos.state.ga.
  us/plb/rn//

Minnesota Board of Nursing
2829 University Ave. SE
Suite 500
Minneapolis, MN 55414
Phone: (612) 617-2270
Fax: (612) 617-2190
http://www.state.mn.us/portal/
  mn/jsp/home.
  do?agency=NursingBoard

Oklahoma Board of
  Nursing
2915 N. Classen Blvd.,
  Suite 524
Oklahoma City, OK 73106
Phone: (405) 962-1800
Fax: (405) 962-1821
http://www.ok.gov/
  nursing/

Wisconsin Department
  of Regulation and
  Licensing
1400 E. Washington
  Ave.
PO Box 8935
Madison, WI 53708
Phone: (608) 266-0145
Fax: (608) 261-7083
http://drl.wi.gov/boards/
  nur/

Hawaii Board of Nursing
Professional &
  Vocational Licensing
  Division
PO Box 3469
Honolulu, HI 96801
Phone: (808) 586-3000
Fax: (808) 586-2689
http://www.state.hi.us/
  dcca/pvl/areas_nurse.
  html

Mississippi Board of Nursing
1935 Lakeland Dr., Suite B
Jackson, MS 39216-5014
Phone: (601) 987-4188
Fax: (601) 364-2352
http://www.msbn.state.ms.us/

Oregon State Board of
  Nursing
17938 SW Upper Boones
  Ferry Rd.
Portland, OR 97224
Phone: (971) 673-0685
Fax: (971) 673-0684
http://www.osbn.state.
  or.us/

Wyoming State Board
  of Nursing
1810 Pioneer Ave.
Cheyenne, WY 82002
Phone: (307) 777-7601
Fax: (307) 777-3519
http://nursing.state.
  wy.us/

Table 21-1 STATE BOARDS OF NURSING—cont'd

State Boards of Nursing

Idaho Board of Nursing 280 N. 18th St., Suite 210 PO Box 83720 Boise, ID 83720 Phone: (208) 334-3110 Fax: (208) 334-3262 http://www2.idaho.gov/ibn/	Missouri State Board of Nursing 3605 Missouri Blvd. PO Box 656 Jefferson City, MO 65102-0656 Phone: (573) 751-0681 Fax: (573) 751-0075 http://www.pr.mo.gov/nursing.asp	Pennsylvania State Board of Nursing 124 Pine St. Harrisburg, PA 17101 Phone: (717) 783-7142 Fax: (717) 783-0822 http://www.dos.state.pa.us/bpoa/cwp/view.asp?a=1104&q=432883

such legislation, but a list of states participating in the Nurse Licensure Compact is given in Table 21-2.

After the graduate decides where to take the exam, he or she needs to begin the registration process. NCSBON maintains a website for all candidates for the NCLEX examination, which provides answers for most questions that applicants have.

This process needs to begin before graduation. The eight steps identified by NCSBOB are listed in Box 21-1. The exam is administered by Pearson VUE; this company is contracted by NCSBON to provide test administration services.

An overview of the registration process follows:

REGISTRATION PROCESS OVERVIEW

1. Submit an application for licensure to the board of nursing where you wish to be licensed.
2. Meet all of the board of nursing's eligibility requirements to take the NCLEX examination.
3. Register for the NCLEX examination with Pearson VUE.
4. Receive Confirmation of Registration from Pearson VUE.
5. The board of nursing makes the candidate eligible to take the NCLEX examination.
6. Receive Authorization to Test (ATT) from Pearson VUE.

If you choose to provide an e-mail address at the time you register for the NCLEX examination (whether by mail, telephone, or via the Internet), please note that all of your correspondence from Pearson VUE will arrive ONLY by e-mail. If you do not provide an e-mail address when you register, your correspondence from Pearson VUE will arrive ONLY through U.S. mail.

Table 21-2 NURSE LICENSURE COMPACT (NLC) STATES

Compact States	Implementation Date
Arizona	7/1/2002
Arkansas	7/1/2000
Colorado	10/1/2007
Delaware	7/1/2000
Idaho	7/1/2001
Iowa	7/1/2000
Kentucky	6/1/2007
Maine	7/1/2001
Maryland	7/1/1999
Mississippi	7/1/2001
Nebraska	1/1/2001
New Hampshire	1/1/2006
New Mexico	1/1/2004
North Carolina	7/1/2000
North Dakota	1/1/2004
Rhode Island	7/1/2008
South Carolina	2/1/2006
South Dakota	1/1/2001
Tennessee	7/1/2003
Texas	1/1/2000
Utah	1/1/2000
Virginia	1/1/2005
Wisconsin	1/1/2000

If you have questions regarding NLC licensure, please contact your state board of nursing in your primary state of residence for specific requirements.
This table indicates which states have enacted the *RN and LPN/VN Nurse Licensure Compact (NLC)*. Please note that Missouri is pending implementation in June 2010. From Nurse Licensure Compact Administrators. (2008). Participating states in the NLC. Retrieved September 25, 2009, from https://www.ncsbn.org/158.htm. Last updated October 2009.

Box 21-1   THE EIGHT STEPS OF THE NCLEX EXAMINATION PROCESS

1. **Apply** for licensure to the board of nursing in the state or territory where you wish to be licensed. Contact the state board for the requirements.
2. **Register** for the NCLEX examination with Pearson VUE by mail, telephone or via the Internet.
   A. The name with which you register must **match exactly** with the printed name on the identification you present at the test center
   B. **If you provide an e-mail address** when registering for the NCLEX examination, all subsequent correspondences from Pearson VUE will arrive **ONLY BY EMAIL.** If you do not provide an e-mail address, all correspondences will arrive only through the U.S. mail.
   C. All NCLEX examination registrations will remain open for a 365-day time period during which a board of nursing may determine your eligibility to take the NCLEX examination.
   D. **There is no refund of the $200 NCLEX registration fee for any reason.**
3. **Receive** confirmation of registration from Pearson VUE.
4. **Receive** eligibility from the state board of nursing you applied for licensure with.
5. **Receive** the Authorization to Test (ATT) from Pearson VUE.
If more than two weeks have passed after you have submitted a registration for the NCLEX examination **and** you received a confirmation from Pearson VUE, and have not received an ATT, please call Pearson VUE.
   A. You must test within the validity dates of your ATT. These validity dates cannot be extended for any reason.
   B. The printed name on your identification must **match exactly** with the printed name on your ATT. IF the name with which you have registered is different from the name on your identification, you must bring legal name change documentation with you to the test center on the day of your test. **The only acceptable forms of legal documentation are: marriage licenses, divorce decrees, and/or court**

action legal name change documents. **All documents must be in English and must be the original documents.**
6. **Schedule** an appointment to test by visiting **www.pearsonvue.com/nclex** or by calling Pearson VUE.
   A. To change your appointment date:
   • For exams scheduled on: **Tuesday, Wednesday, Thursday and Friday,** call Pearson VUE at least 24 hours in advance of the day of the appointment.
   • For exams scheduled on **Saturday, Sunday** and **Monday,** call Pearson VUE no later than the Friday at least **1 full business day** in advance of your appointment.
7. **Present** one form of acceptable identification and your ATT on the day of the examination.
   A. The only acceptable forms of identification in test centers in the U.S., American Samoa, Guam, Northern Mariana Islands and Virgin Islands are:
   • U.S. driver's license (not a temporary or learner's permit)
   • U.S. state identification
   • Passport
   B. For all other test centers (international), only a passport is acceptable. All identification must be written in English, have a signature in English, be valid (not expired) and include a photograph. Candidates with identification from a country on the U.S. embargoed countries list will not be admitted to the test.
   C. You will not be admitted to the examination without acceptable identification and your ATT. If you arrive without these materials, you forfeit your test session and must re-register; this includes re-payment of the $200 registration fee.
8. **Receive** your NCLEX examination results from the board of nursing you applied for licensure with within one month from your examination date.
For more detailed information on the NCLEX examination and registration process consult the Candidate Bulletin by visiting www.ncsbn.org or www.pearsonvue.com/nclex.

From National Council of State Boards of Nursing (NCSBON). Used with permission.

If more than 2 weeks have passed after you have submitted a registration for an NCLEX examination and received confirmation from Pearson VUE and you have not received an ATT, please call Pearson VUE at the appropriate number listed on the inside front cover (NCSBON, 2008).

BEFORE THE EXAM

Some schools of nursing administer "readiness exams" as a requirement for graduation. These exams are also administered by companies that manage NCLEX review courses. Many students take such courses upon graduation as a preparation for the exam. Most of these courses are valuable preparation tools for exam candidates. They offer large test banks that allow the graduate to constantly practice and review NCLEX-type questions. While they are an additional expense for the student, many students believe that the continued exposure to testing situations is worth the expense. Most schools of nursing will assist the student in finding appropriate courses in the area.

YOUR FIRST JOB AS A NURSE

This is a very exciting time, and the decision about the first professional position is a challenging one. John (2006) has suggested a few tips to help the new graduate get through this decision and survive the first year as a nurse:

- Go on several interviews. Try to find a job that feels "right." That is important in making the decision. The culture of the institution; its mission, vision, and values; and the work environment are all important variables in determining if the institution is a "good fit." Evaluate your own strengths and challenges, and determine what type of work environment is important for your success.
- Get to know the new job. Gather all of the materials that you were given during the interview process. Read them and look at your job description … do they match what you want to do?
- Find out how long your orientation will be. Will you have a mentor? The first year of work is a period of tremendous learning and it is important that you be supported through this process. You need to realize that you are a novice nurse, with lots to learn and experience. Be realistic about your abilities and choose a workplace based on these abilities and expectations.
- Take some time off before you begin work. You have just finished an arduous journey through your nursing education. Take some time for yourself to recover and to prepare for the next challenge in your nursing life.
- Take care of yourself. One of the major challenges in the first work year has been found to revolve around balancing work and life. Watch your diet, sleep, and exercise! Try to maintain a balance. Also, find someone you can speak to about work outside of the workplace. Have you ever noticed

that when nurses get together, they all talk "shop"? You will need to talk about your experiences with someone who will understand. Keep in touch with the support group that you formed at school.
- Stay positive and motivated. Be positive every day, and avoid negative energy and negative people who will drain you.

YOUR FIRST JOB INTERVIEW

In the Leadership Course in the final semester, the graduate will, it is hoped, be exposed to the interview process. It is the graduate's responsibility to be fully prepared before the first job interview. At this time in the career path, it is the new nurse's responsibility to make a concerted effort in the job search. This decision should be made diligently with several factors taken into consideration. Preparation for the interview is key. Begin by listing your strengths and weaknesses. Take into consideration your student clinical evaluations from your professors. Was one of your weaknesses tardiness? If yes, you can list or discuss it as one of your weaknesses, but you can add ways in which you have made corrections to this issue. If one of your strengths was clinical group leadership, play this up during the interview process. Be prepared with a list in hand on the day of the interview. You will be asked for references, both personal and professional. Request a letter of recommendation from one of your clinical professors in a course where you did exceptionally well that will clearly point out your assets and strengths. Be prepared to answer the question, Why do you want to work at this facility? You may know the culture and the mission and vision of an association if you have worked there, but if you have not, do some investigation. Evaluate the web site for information about the organization, including the facility's mission and vision. Note this in answering a question that addresses why you have chosen to interview at this particular facility. If the health care organization holds Magnet status, you may say you would very much like to begin your nursing career at a facility with Magnet status. You may be asked about your short-term goals and long-term goals. For example, you may be interviewed for a 7 P.M.-to-7 A.M. nursing position on the Pediatric Unit. A short-term goal might be that you may want to be working the 7 A.M.-to-7 P.M. shift in 1 year's time. A long-term goal would be that you plan on taking the ANCC (American Nurses Credentialing Center) Pediatric

Nursing Certification when you are eligible. Some institutions will ask you to analyze clinical situations and to present potential solutions. For further information about interviews, see Chapter 15.

WHERE TO LOOK

Where do you look for a nursing position? There are endless ways to search for positions—the Sunday newspaper classified section, nursing journals, online at a facility's web site, by word of mouth, and on in-hospital human resources job postings, for example. Job fairs are also an excellent place to job search. The National Student Nurses Association website is one place to evaluate (http://www.nsna.org/).

HOW TO APPLY

Three items are baseline requirements to apply for a position: cover letter, resume, and facility application. The cover letter is one-page document that includes the specific job you are applying for, statement of attachment of resume and/or application, and specifics as to how to contact you, including home telephone number, cell phone number, home address, and e-mail address. Chapter 15 provides a sample résumé.

KNOWLEDGE BEFORE THE INTERVIEW

- Position shift
  - 7 A.M. to 7 P.M.?
  - 7 P.M. to 7 A.M.?
  - 7 A.M. to 3 P.M.? etc.
- Specific area of hospital
- Specific job requirements

Most hospitals have numerous components to the interviewing process. The first contact will be through the interview by human resources personnel or the nurse recruiter. This interview is usually used to determine the potential "fit" between the institution and candidate. After this, the candidate is usually interviewed by the nurse manager and perhaps staff.

KNOWLEDGE ABOUT THE FACILITY

Human Resources Representative
- When does health care coverage begin?
- Parking restrictions and designations
- When does holiday time begin?

Nurse Manager
- Length of unit-specific nursing orientation
- Culture of unit
- Type of nursing care delivery systems
- Nursing decision making

- Is the facility one of the "best places to work"?
- Do you have to use all vacation time and sick time in same year?
- What is carry-over of vacation time and sick time policy?
- Is there "cash-in" option at end of year?
- Childcare? On-site? Off-site? Fees?
- In-house amenities?
  Spa
  Nail, hair salons
  On-site banking

- Type of leadership style
- Patient mix of unit
- Mentor
- Preceptor program
- Baylor program
- Pull-policy to another unit
- Probationary period
- First evaluation
- Second evaluation
- Annual evaluation

EITHER OR BOTH

- Does facility hold Magnet status?
- Research facility?
- Teaching hospital?
- Service area

LEVEL OF COMFORT WITH TYPE OF FACILITY

Depending on the experience as a student as well as personality, new graduates may choose to begin employment at a large medical center or in a small community facility. Either way, they need to be equally prepared for the interview.

AFTER THE INTERVIEW

Once the interview is complete, it is very professional to send a brief message thanking the interviewer for his or her time and consideration for the position. The message should be handwritten, not a quick e-mail. If it is the candidate's first choice for a position, he or she should state interest in further discussion about the position at the interviewer's convenience. This is a perfect way to begin a professional future.

PROFESSIONAL GROWTH

As nurses mature in the profession, it is expected that they take a leadership role. How a nurse chooses to do this depends on their practice area. The most important thing is to maintain currency in the profession. Many states require nurses to obtain continuing education credits to renew the nursing license. While this is a way to maintain currency, much more work is required to keep up with the rapid changes that are occurring on a day-to-day basis in the profession. A good way to keep up to date is to belong to a professional organization that represents the area of practice and interest. There are numerous organizations representing the various specialties within the profession.

Professional nursing organizations, at both the national and local chapter level, provide opportunities to connect with peers in your specialty, share best practices, and learn about new trends, education, and technical advances. Many of these organizations also provide information about professional certification (Box 21-2).

Once the nurse has decided on a specialty, it is highly recommended that, when eligible, he or she sit for the certification examination in the chosen specialty field. Specialties have differing requirements for eligibility for the exam. There are advanced level exams for nurse practitioners and clinical nurse specialists.

Box 21-2 NURSING ORGANIZATIONS

Academy of Medical-Surgical Nurses
Alpha Tau Delta (National Fraternity for Professional Nurses)
American Academy of Ambulatory Care Nurses
American Academy of Nurse Practitioners (AANP)
American Association for the History of Nursing
American Association of Critical-Care Nurses (AACN)
American Association of Heart Failure Nurses
American Association of Legal Nurse Consultants
American Association of Nurse Assessment Coordinators
American Association of Nurse Attorneys
American Association of Occupational Health
American Association of Office Nurses
American Association of Spinal Cord Injury Nurses
American Assembly of Neuroscience Nurses (AANN)
American Association of Nurse-Anesthetists (AANA)
American College of Nurse-Midwives (ACNM)
American College of Nurse Practitioners (ACNP)
American Forensic Nurses
American Holistic Nurses Association
American Nephrology Nurses Association
American Nurses Association (ANA)
American Nurses Association-California
American Nursing Informatics Association
American Organization of Nurse Executives (AONE)
American Psychiatric Nurses Association (APNA)
American Society of PeriAnesthesia Nurses (ASPAN)
Association for Professionals in Infection Control and Epidemiology, Inc. (APIC)
Association of Camp Nurses
Association of Child Neurology Nurses
Association of Medical Esthetic Nurses
Association of periOperative Registered Nurses, Inc. (AORN)
Association of Rehabilitation Nurses (ARN)
Association of Women's Health, Obstetric, and Neonatal Nurses (AWHONN)
Baromedical Nurses Association
Council of Practical Nurse Programs NYS
Emergency Nurses Association (ENA)

Florida Nurse Practitioner Network
Infusion Nurses Society (INS)
National Alaska Native American Indian Nurses Association (NANAINA)
National Association of Catholic Nurses-USA
National Association of Directors of Nursing Administration (NADONA)
National Association of Hispanic Nurses (NAHN)
National Association of Neonatal Nurses
National Association of Orthopaedic Nurses, Inc. (NAON)
National Association of Pediatric Nurse Associates & Practitioners
National Association of School Nurses
National Black Nurses Association (NBNA)
National Federation of Licensed Practical Nurses, Inc. (NFLPN)
National League for Nursing (NLN)
National Maternal and Child Oral Health Resource Center
National Nurses in Business Association
National Nursing Staff Development Organization
National Organization for Associate Degree Nursing
National Organization of Nurse Practitioner Faculties
National Student Nurses Association
Nurses Christian Fellowship
Oncology Nursing Society (ONS)
Pediatric Endocrinology Nursing Society
Philippine Nurses Association of America
Rural Nurse Organization
Sigma Theta Tau International
Society for Gastroenterology Nurses and Associates, Inc.
Society of Otorhinolaryngology and Head-Neck Nurses
Society of Pediatric Nurses (SPN)
Society of Urologic Nurses and Associates
The National Association of Nurse Massage Therapists
Transcultural Nursing Society
Visiting Nurses Associations of America

From Orlovsky, C. (2008). How to avoid new nurse burnout. Retrieved June 4, 2008, from http://www.nursezone.com/Advancing-My-Career/professional-organizations.aspx.

Box 21-3 SOME SPECIALTY EXAMS FOR SPECIFIC PRACTICE AREAS

Nurse Practitioners
- Acute care
- Adult
- Adult psychiatric and mental health
- Diabetes management, advanced
- Family
- Family psychiatric and mental health
- Gerontological
- Pediatric

Clinical Nurse Specialists
- Diabetes management, advanced
- Adult health (formerly known as medical-surgical)
- Adult psychiatric and mental health
- Child/adolescent psychiatric and mental health
- Gerontological
- Pediatric
- Public/community health

Other Advanced-Level Exams
- Nurse executive, advanced (formerly nursing administration, advanced)

Specialty Certification
- Ambulatory care nurse
- Cardiac vascular nurse
- Case management nurse
- Gerontological nurse
- Informatics nurse
- Medical-surgical nurse
- Nurse executive (formerly nursing administration)
- Nursing professional development
- Pain management
- Pediatric nurse
- Psychiatric and mental health nurse

From American Nurses Credentialing Center. Data from http://www.nursecredentialing.org/cert/eligibility.html. June 18, 2008.

There are also specialty exams for specific practice areas; Box 21-3 lists some of the exams available.

Other certification exams are given by specialty organizations, such as the Certified Emergency Nurse (CEN) exam, which is administered by the Emergency Nurses Association, and the CCRN (Adult, Neonatal and Pediatric Acute/Critical Care Nursing Certification), as well as several other certification exams, which is administered by The Association of Critical Care Nurses Certification Corporation.

Some institutions recognize these accomplishments through monetary awards. It is also an accreditation that would provides the nurse with "an edge" if he or she were to seek an advanced position in nursing.

CONTACT HOURS

Many states have passed legislation that requires, to renew a nursing license, a nurse to have obtained a certain number of contact hours of continuing education. On hire, an important question to ask is the hospital policy on funding for continuing education, both within the facility and out of the facility. Ask whether the facility will pay a travel allowance for the nurse to attend a conference out of state. There are also contact hours offered in nursing magazines and online continuing education contact hours. It is up to the nurse to be aware of the state's licensure requirements for renewal.

RETURNING TO SCHOOL

As a nurse begins to assume a leadership role within the profession, it is time to think about advancing his or her education. Most hospitals have tuition reimbursement for nurses who return to school for an advanced degree. There has been movement in some states (New York and New Jersey) to require nurses to receive the bachelor's of science in nursing degree within 10 years of becoming a registered nurse. Some hospitals, especially Magnet certified hospitals, expect their nurses to continue their education and receive an advanced degree. There are numerous studies that document better patient outcomes in facilities with nurses with advanced education (Aiken et al., 2003; Aiken, 2004). What is important to realize is that while the new nurse has just finished his or her initial education, it is only the first step. Nursing is a profession that demands continued education and growth.

SUMMARY

You've finally done it! You've graduated; but this is only the first step. You will need to prepare for the NCLEX licensing exam, decide on your first job, and settle into the profession. The profession will demand that you keep up to date with changes in patient care, evidence, practice, and professional issues. You will need to join a professional organization, consider taking the certification exam, and return to school for an advanced degree.

CLINICAL CORNER

Lifelong Learning as a Nurse
Patricia D. Fonder

In a research study by Linda Aiken and her colleagues, improved surgical patient outcomes were seen in hospitals that had a higher proportion of nurses with baccalaureate or higher degrees in nursing. The National Institutes of Health funded this project, and the results were published in the *Journal of the American Medical Association*. The study reported, "Each 10% increase in the proportion of nurses with higher degrees decrease the risk of mortality and failure to rescue by a factor of 0.95, or by 5% after controlling for patient and hospital characteristics" (Aiken, Clarke, Cheung, Sloane, and Silber, 2003, p. 1620).

Promoting lifelong learning and the pursuit of advanced degrees is an acquired attribute, not one that is taught in the academic arena. As a graduate nurse from a diploma school, I was excited to begin my career. With high expectations and the knowledge and skills recently learned, I was ready to care for my patients. I soon realized that the expert guidance offered from the experienced nurses was essential. Each week brought new challenges, and I discovered how limited my global knowledge of nursing was and my confidence wavered.

As the months passed, the guidance of the seasoned nurses continued, but many times it was now me seeking them out for advice. I was now confident enough to ask questions without fear of reprisal. Realizing the burden of caring for patients, I soon recognized my limited scope of knowledge. Desiring the best for my patients and seeking self-satisfaction in rendering state-of-the-art compassionate care, I began attending nursing conferences. The first conference was happenstance; I was a last-minute substitute and this conference opened new avenues for me.

I cannot remember the topic of the conference, but I do remember that it was sponsored by the local region of the American Nurses Association (ANA). I listened in awe and enhanced my knowledge and discovered this was a means to state-of-the-art care for my patients. I joined the ANA that day and read each journal that I received cover to cover. Soon I was a regular at conferences and began networking with other nurses.

At work, I became involved in committees and realized my limited scope of practice away from the bedside.

Most members had their certification in nursing specialties, and many had advanced education and degrees. Desiring the best for my patients, I focused on my certification as a critical care nurse. At first, I attended conferences, and as my knowledge and practice standards advanced, I set my sight on the certifying exam. The day of the exam arrived. As I waited in anticipation of the results, I knew that regardless of the outcome, the continued learning benefited me as a professional and my patients. The results arrived; I was now a CCRN, and this achievement fostered my desire to return to school for my baccalaureate in nursing.

The return to the collegiate setting was daunting but exciting. I savored every moment and enjoyed using my new-found knowledge on a daily basis. When I attended committee meetings, I knew I was an integral part, and my contributions were scholarly and well received by my peers. I soon realized that my career as a nurse was now my profession. I had expanded my knowledge base but also realized that nursing is a dynamic profession that is always changing in the care we administer to patients. As a professional nurse, one must be a lifelong learner.

My professional goals have come full circle; I returned to school for my master's in nursing education. This degree has enhanced my ability as a preceptor, which benefits my orientees. I appreciate their varied learning styles and adapt their program accordingly. If change is needed, I recognize the problem and offer solutions to enhance the new graduate's learning needs. I always share with my protégé the excitement I have discovered in nursing, that it is ever evolving and dynamic; so for me, continued education is essential to success.

In addition, I have had the opportunity to work with student nurses, and I always promote nursing organizations as the backbone of their profession. I understand the stresses of the first year as a nurse, but I also know that the networking and educational offerings of these groups will enhance the graduate's career and confidence. With continued involvement, the new nurse will become a professional who understands and appreciates the value of lifelong learning.

Reference
Aiken, L. H., Clarke, S. P., Cheung, R. B., Sloane, D. M., Silber, J. H. (2003). Educational levels of hospital nurses and surgical patient mortality. *Journal of the American Medical Association, 290*, 1617-1623.

EVIDENCE-BASED PRACTICE

Graduate Nurse Perceptions of the Work Experience

Halfer, D., & Graf, E. (2006). Graduate nurse perceptions of the work experience. Nursing Economics 24*(3), 150–155.*

The nursing literature reports that the inability to handle the intense working environment, advanced medical technology, and high patient acuity result in new graduate nurse turnover rates of 35% to 60% within the first year of employment. This high turnover rate has substantial financial and emotional costs. Turnover affects new graduates personally and professionally and disrupts healing relationships. As job satisfaction increases, turnover decreases. Studies have shown the major predictor of job satisfaction was psychological empowerment. It has been found that graduates who intend to remain in their positions are more satisfied with certain aspects of their jobs that they thought were important. Those aspects that were cited included their schedule, coworker interaction, professional opportunities, recognition, control, and responsibility.

Many factors influence the satisfaction of new graduates. One study describes "reality shock." This occurs with the transition from the educational to the service setting, where there are different priorities and pressures. The new graduate must learn to balance the needs of the patient and the needs of the setting. Stresses cited by new graduates in rank order were lack of experience, interactions with physicians, lack of organizational skills, and new situations. Other stresses included administering medications, managing a large number of patients, receiving interruptions, having to rely on others, and perceiving a lack of support from other registered nurses. A positive correlation was found between social support and the development of confidence in new graduates.

It is important for nurse leaders and educators to understand the new graduate nurse experience, so they can offer effective strategies to ease transition and thereby enhance satisfaction and retention of these new professionals. Studies suggest that the role adjustment period for new graduates in an acute care setting may range from 6 to 12 months after hire. They also showed that for new nurses under the age of 32, life–work balance was ranked as the number one source of job dissatisfaction. It appears that novice nurse adjustment extends beyond mastering clinical skills and includes an adjustment to a profession that requires a 24-hour, 7-day-a-week commitment to patients and their families.

In conclusion, findings from recent studies have several implications for nursing practice and education:

- Work schedules are integrally linked to job satisfaction.
- There appears to be a grieving process that a new nurse goes through with loss of the academic schedule.
- Professional development or mentoring may also be a way to positively modify attitudes toward work schedules.

Mentoring by leaders, educators, preceptors, colleagues, and peer support groups may help new graduates adjust to the demands of the nursing profession during the critical 18 months of a first job. Internship programs designed to provide additional mentoring strategies to promote critical thinking and foster peer networking and discussion that support professional role transition throughout the first year of employment have been successful in increasing retention rates of new nurses.

REFERENCES

Aiken, L. H. (2004). RN education: a matter of degrees. *Nursing, 34,* 50-51.

Aiken, L. H., Clarke, S. P., Cheung, R. B., Sloane, D. M., & Silber, J. H. (2003). Education levels of hospital nurses and patient mortality. *Journal of the American Medical Association, 290,* 1617-1623.

American Nurses Credentialing Center. Retrieved June 18, 2008, from http://www.nursecredentialing.org/cert/eligibility.html.

Halfer, D., & Graf, E. (2006). Graduate nurse perceptions of the work experience. *Nursing Economics, 24,* 150-155.

John, T. (2006). Your first year as a nurse. *NSNA Imprint,* January.

National Council of State Boards of Nursing (NCSBON). Candidate bulletin. Retrieved June 4, 2008, from https://www.ncsbn.org/2008_NCLEX_Candidate_Bulletin.pdf.

Orlovsky, C. (2008). How to avoid new nurse burnout. Retrieved June 4, 2008, from http://www.nursezone.com/Advancing-My-Career/professional-organizations.aspx.

Index